The Psychedelic Landscape

Navigating Evidence, Regulation, and Therapeutic Potential

New York

Pharmacology - Research, Safety Testing and Regulation Series

Dietary Polyphenols for Infectious Diseases
Md. Faiyazuddin and Sumel Ashique
ISBN: 979-8-89530-750-2
eBook ISBN: 979-8-89530-841-7

Drug Shortages: Health, Security, and Policy Perspectives
Duncan Sawyer (Editor)
ISBN: 979-8-89530-660-4
eBook ISBN: 979-8-89530-683-3

Therapeutic Targets for Drug Repurposing in Osteoarthritis
Anca Zanfirescu, PhD and Corina Andrei, PhD
eBook ISBN: 979-8-89530-416-7

Drug Repurposing: Novel Therapeutic Avenues and Innovations in Healthcare
Shah Alam Khan, PhD and Md. Jawaid Akhtar, PhD
ISBN: 979-8-89530-422-8
eBook ISBN: 979-8-89530-478-5

Phyto-Nanomedicine: Advancements and Development in Drug Discovery and Delivery Systems
Hitesh Chopra, PhD, Vinod Kumar Gauttam, PhD, Ajmer Singh Grewal, PhD and Kavita Munjal, PhD
ISBN: 979-8-89530-317-7
eBook ISBN: 979-8-89530-356-6

More information about this series can be found at
https://novapublishers.com/product-category/series/pharmacology-research-safety-testing-and-regulation/

James P. Macintosh
Editor

The Psychedelic Landscape

Navigating Evidence, Regulation, and Therapeutic Potential

snova
New York

NOTICE TO THE READER

The Publisher has taken reasonable care in the preparation of this book, but makes no expressed or implied warranty of any kind and assumes no responsibility for any errors or omissions. No liability is assumed for incidental or consequential damages in connection with or arising out of information contained in this book. The Publisher shall not be liable for any special, consequential, or exemplary damages resulting, in whole or in part, from the readers' use of, or reliance upon, this material. Any parts of this book based on government reports are so indicated and copyright is claimed for those parts to the extent applicable to compilations of such works.

Independent verification should be sought for any data, advice or recommendations contained in this book. In addition, no responsibility is assumed by the Publisher for any injury and/or damage to persons or property arising from any methods, products, instructions, ideas or otherwise contained in this publication.

The Publisher assumes no responsibility for any statements of fact or opinion expressed in the published contents.

This publication is designed to provide accurate and authoritative information with regard to the subject matter covered herein. It is sold with the clear understanding that the Publisher is not engaged in rendering legal or any other professional services. If legal or any other expert assistance is required, the services of a competent person should be sought. FROM A DECLARATION OF PARTICIPANTS JOINTLY ADOPTED BY A COMMITTEE OF THE AMERICAN BAR ASSOCIATION AND A COMMITTEE OF PUBLISHERS.

Additional color graphics may be available in the e-book version of this book.

Library of Congress Cataloging-in-Publication Data

ISBN: 979-8-89530-991-9 (Hardcover)
ISBN: 979-8-90134-032-5 (eBook)

Published by Nova Science Publishers, Inc. † New York

Contents

Preface

Psychedelic and dissociative drugs have the capacity to temporarily alter mood, cognition, and perception of reality. Their effects vary widely, with users reporting intense emotional experiences—ranging from euphoria and profound connectedness to anxiety, confusion, and fear. While concerns remain about their safety and potential risks, scientific interest in these substances has surged in recent years, particularly in their potential to treat medical conditions such as mental health disorders.

Beyond clinical research, increasing numbers of individuals use these drugs recreationally, in pursuit of enhanced well-being, spiritual insight, or self-exploration. This book examines the health impacts of psychedelic and dissociative substances, exploring their therapeutic possibilities—especially in the context of substance use disorder treatment within medical settings.

Chapter 1

Psychedelic and Dissociative Drugs*

National Institute on Drug Abuse

Highlights

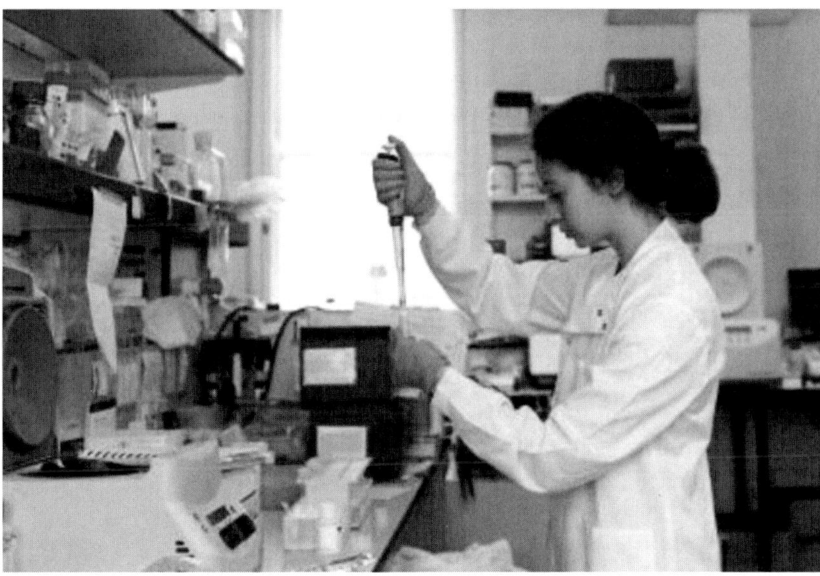

@Getty Images/Nick David.

- Psychedelic and dissociative drugs can temporarily alter a person's mood, thoughts, and perceptions. Among other health effects and

* This is an edited, reformatted and augmented version of National Institute on Drug Abuse Publication.

In: The Psychedelic Landscape
Editor: James P. Macintosh
ISBN: 979-8-89530-991-9

safety concerns, people who use these substances report feeling strong emotions ranging from bliss to fear and experiencing vast changes in how they perceive reality.

- In recent years, there has been growing research interest in the potential of psychedelic and dissociative drugs to treat medical conditions, including mental health disorders. An increasing number of people also report taking these drugs outside of medical settings for recreation, to improve well-being, or for spiritual or self-exploration.
- NIDA supports and conducts research to better understand the health effects of psychedelic and dissociative drugs and to learn whether some of these drugs may help treat substance use disorders in medical settings.

What Are Psychedelic and Dissociative Drugs?

Psychedelic and dissociative drugs can temporarily alter a person's mood, thoughts, and perceptions of reality [1]. Among other health effects and safety concerns, people who use psychedelic and dissociative drugs report feeling strong emotions, ranging from intense happiness and a feeling of connectedness to fear, anxiety, and confusion [2, 3]. People who use these drugs also report experiencing intense or distorted visions or sensations.1

Many psychedelic drugs derive from plants and fungi, and some have been used for thousands of years in traditional or religious rituals. Some psychedelic and dissociative drugs are also synthetic (lab-made).2 People report using psychedelic and dissociative drugs for a variety of reasons, including seeking new, fun, healing, or spiritual experiences [1, 3].

NIDA conducts and supports research on psychedelic and dissociative drugs to help inform policies and health decisions around their use. Researchers are also studying whether some of these substances may be effective treatments for mental health disorders, including addiction, when administered in a clinical setting [4, 5].

While researchers debate how to describe and classify psychedelic and dissociative drugs and other drugs with similar properties, they generally group these drugs according to how they work in the brain.3 Some people use the term "hallucinogens" to refer to all or some psychedelic and dissociative drugs.

Psychedelic drugs	Dissociative drugs	Other
Drugs that primarily influence the way the brain processes the chemical serotonin. They can bring on vivid visions and affect a person's sense of self [2]. *Includes:* psilocybin, LSD, DMT, mescaline, NBOMes	Drugs that primarily affect how the brain processes the chemical glutamate. These drugs can make people feel disconnected from their body and environment [6]. *Includes:* ketamine, PCP	Drugs such as MDMA, [7] ibogaine, [8] and salvia [9] affect a variety of brain functions to cause psychedelic and/or dissociative effects.
All of these substances have mind-altering properties with the potential to cause changes in thought processes, mood, and perception of reality [3, 7, 8, 9].		

Psychedelic drugs (also called "classic psychedelics" or "psychedelics"), including psilocybin and LSD, mainly interact with specific receptors, which are molecular structures in the brain. Known as 5-hydroxy-tryptamine (5-HT)$_{2A}$ receptors, these are targets for the neurotransmitter (chemical messenger) serotonin. At certain doses, psychedelics may bring on vivid visions or sensations, alter a person's sense of self, and promote feelings of insightfulness or connection [10].

Dissociative drugs, including ketamine and PCP, block the action of N-methyl-D-aspartate (NMDA) receptors. These are part of the brain's system for transporting glutamate, another neurotransmitter. While dissociative drugs can alter perception, they also typically make people feel disconnected from their body and environment [6].

Other drugs such as MDMA, ibogaine, and salvia work on a variety of brain functions to cause psychedelic or dissociative effects. For more information, see "How do psychedelic and dissociative drugs work in the brain?"

How Do Psychedelic and Dissociative Drugs Affect the Mind and Body?"

NIDA supports and conducts research on the short- and long-term health effects of psychedelic and dissociative drugs to better inform health decisions and policies related to their use. While research is ongoing, scientific studies have revealed important information about how these drugs work:

- Effects vary widely. Effects of psychedelic and dissociative drugs may be difficult to predict and depend on many factors. These include the amount taken and potency (concentration and strength), as well as a person's unique biology, age, sex, personality, mood, expectations, mindset—commonly called "set"—and environment, or "setting" [3, 11]. Using psychedelic and dissociative drugs that contain contaminants or using them in combination with other substances may also produce effects not associated with using these drugs alone [12].
- Psychedelic and dissociative drugs temporarily alter thought patterns, mood, and perceptions of reality. People who use these substances report feeling strong emotions, ranging from intense happiness and a feeling of connectedness to fear, anxiety, and confusion [1, 3] Many people who use psychedelic drugs, such as psilocybin and LSD, report seeing vibrant shapes, colors, and scenes and reliving vivid memories [10]. People who use dissociative drugs, such as ketamine and PCP, describe experiencing distorted vision and hearing [6].
- Dissociative drugs can make people feel "detached." Many people who use dissociative drugs report feeling as though they are floating or are disconnected from their body [13].
- People may experience adverse health effects. Physical side-effects of these substances, such as headache, nausea, or changes in heart rate, are generally not life-threatening [14]. However, illicitly manufactured or processed drugs may be contaminated with colorless and odorless fentanyl or other dangerous substances that can cause serious adverse events, including overdose and death [15]. Psychedelic or dissociative drugs may also produce adverse or debilitating psychological effects such as fear or anxiety. [3, 16].Research is ongoing to better understand short- and long-term health effects of psychedelic and dissociative drugs. For more information, see "Are psychedelic and dissociative drugs safe?"
- Using psychedelic and dissociative drugs has been linked to dangerous behavior and injuries. People using these drugs may have impaired thought processes and perception that cause them to behave in unusual and sometimes dangerous ways. This may lead to injuries

and other safety issues, particularly if there is not another individual present who can help prevent or respond to an emergency [14]. For more information, see "Are psychedelic and dissociative drugs safe?"

How Do Psychedelic and Dissociative Drugs Work in the Brain?

More studies are needed to better understand how psychedelic and dissociative drugs work. While researchers debate how to describe these drugs and how specific drugs should be classified, they generally group them according to what is known about how they work in the brain. Better understanding these mechanisms is an active area of NIDA-funded research. This basic research plays an important role in identifying their health effects and potential therapeutic uses.

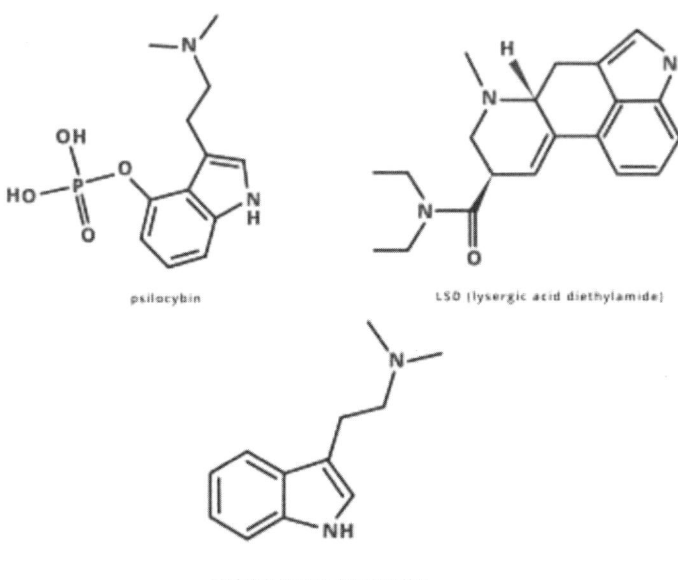

Top left: 2D chemical structure depiction of psilocybin Top right: 2D chemical structure depiction of LSD (lysergic acid diethylamide) Bottom: 2D chemical structure depiction of DMT (N,N-dimethyltryptamine)

Although research is ongoing, studies suggest psychedelic drugs—such as psilocybin, LSD, and DMT—primarily affect 5-HT2A receptors in the brain, which ordinarily are activated by the neurotransmitter (chemical messenger) serotonin [10].

Research suggests that the most prominent psychedelic effects stem from activity in the brain's prefrontal cortex, an area involved in mood, cognition, and perception [17, 18]. Psychedelic drugs also temporarily disrupt communication between different brain regions, including the regions collectively known as the default mode network (DMN). The DMN is most active during brain activity that's related to self-awareness—such as reflecting on past events or making plans [19]. This may account for why psychedelic drugs can make a person's thoughts less self-centered and more expansive, promoting a sense of connectedness with others and the world [10].

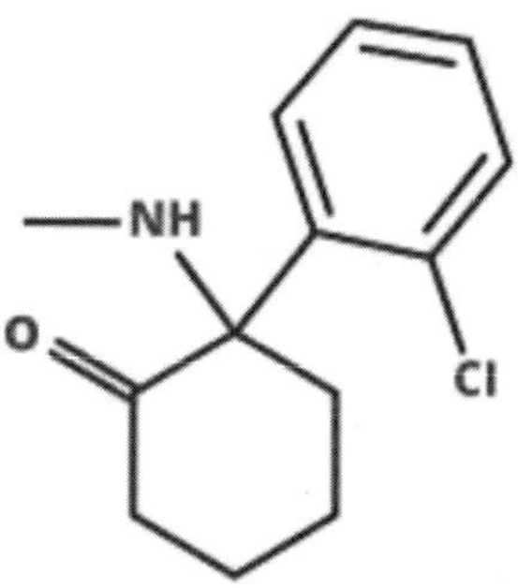

ketamine

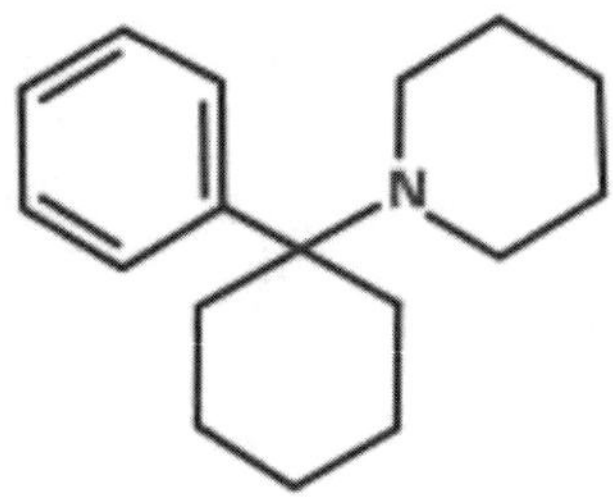

PCP (phencyclidine)

Left: 2D chemical structure depiction of ketamine

Right: 2D chemical structure depiction of PCP (phencyclidine)

Dissociative drugs, such as ketamine and PCP, also affect the balance of certain chemicals in the brain [6]. Some of these changes lead to altered perception, as well as feelings of being disconnected from the body or environment [20]. Ketamine and PCP disrupt the actions of the brain chemical glutamate at a type of receptor called the N-methyl-D-aspartate (NMDA) receptor [6]. Glutamate plays a major role in learning and memory, emotion, and the perception of pain [7].

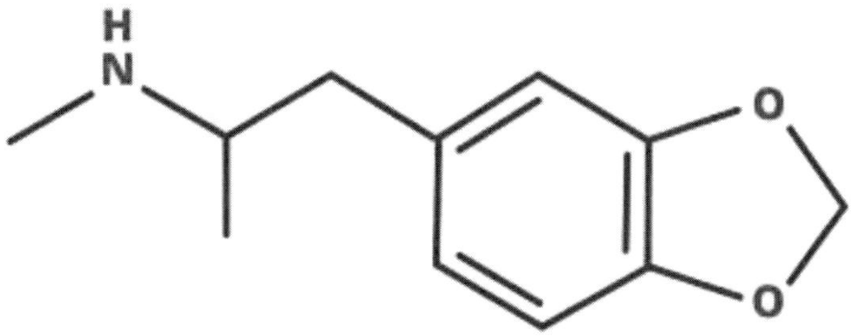

MDMA (3,4-methylenedioxymethamphetamine)

IMAGE: 2D chemical structure depiction of MDMA (3,4-methylenedioxymethamphetamine)

Researchers are also investigating *other drugs* sometimes classified as psychedelic and dissociative drugs, such as MDMA, and the way they work in the brain.

MDMA stimulates the brain to release serotonin and weakly activates serotonin receptors in the brain, producing some mind-altering effects associated with psychedelic drugs. MDMA also increases activity of other neurotransmitters, such as dopamine and norepinephrine, which are involved in mood and attention [7].

Other drugs that produce effects associated with psychedelic and dissociative drugs work differently. For example, salvia activates kappa opioid receptors in the brain [21] while ibogaine affects a variety of brain receptors [8].

How is NIDA Advancing Research on Psychedelic and Dissociative Drugs?

NIDA conducts and supports research on psychedelic and dissociative drugs to help inform health decisions and policies related to their use. This research includes efforts to better understand the health effects of psychedelic and dissociative drugs, how chemicals in—or similar to—these drugs work in the brain, and whether they may be able to treat substance use disorders and other conditions. NIDA also funds research on how and why people use these substances.

In June 2022, NIDA's Office of Translational Initiatives and Program Innovations also announced a new program to support small businesses to develop psychedelic-based therapies for substance use disorders.

Along with other agencies, NIDA also supports major coordination efforts in this evolving field, such as the 2022 Psychedelics as Therapeutics workshop co-sponsored by the National Institute on Mental Health and the National Institute on Alcohol Abuse and Addiction.

See NIDA-funded projects related to psychedelic and dissociative drugs, and learn more about related clinical trials.

Why Do People Use Psychedelic and Dissociative Drugs?

People report using psychedelic and dissociative drugs for a variety of reasons. People may use them for their mind- and mood-altering effects, for recreation, or to have an emotional or spiritual experience. Individuals also report using these drugs in the hopes of improving their mental health or well-being or easing pain or stress, but more research is needed to determine their effectiveness for these purposes [1, 3, 22].

Some psychedelic drugs are derived from plants and fungi that have a long history of use in many different cultures around the world [23]. Aztec shamans used psilocybin in healing rituals, and some Native American tribes used peyote as long ago as 5,700 B.C. in religious ceremonies [24]. References to psychedelic drug use have been found in ancient texts from India and Greece [2].

More recently, researchers are exploring the use of psychedelic and dissociative drugs in medical settings as treatments for substance use disorders and for other mental health disorders such as depression, anxiety, and post-traumatic stress disorder (PTSD) [4, 25].

Are Psychedelic and Dissociative Drugs Safe?

While more research is needed, the reported incidence of serious adverse events from professionally supervised use of specific psychedelic and dissociative drugs, such as in clinical trials, is relatively low [2, 10, 11, 26].

However, many past clinical studies on these drugs have not adequately assessed or reported on adverse events [27].

Most people who report using psychedelic and dissociative drugs do so outside of medical or research settings [1, 28]. While further research is also needed to better understand the health and safety impacts of typical use of these drugs, some serious adverse effects and safety issues have been identified [14, 27].

- *Effects vary widely.* Effects of psychedelic and dissociative drugs may be difficult to predict and depend on many factors. These include the amount taken and potency (concentration and strength), as well as a person's age, unique biology, sex, personality, history of drug use, mood, expectations, mindset, and surroundings (sometimes called "set and setting") [3, 10, 11]. Using psychedelic and dissociative drugs that contain contaminants or using them in combination with other substances may also produce effects not associated with using these drugs alone [12, 13, 15].
- *Short-term physical side effects are typically mild or moderate but may require professional care.* People who take psychedelic or dissociative drugs may experience short-term side effects such as a headache, abdominal pain, nausea or vomiting, high blood pressure, rapid heartbeat, trembling, and diarrhea [4, 29]. These are typically mild or moderate but may require medical care [30]. Importantly, reported cases of side-effects likely represent only a very small number of people who use psychedelic or dissociative drugs, and most people who use these drugs do not seek emergency services.

However, related data can provide insights on the side effects that may lead people to seek help. For example, according to U.S. poison control hotline data from 2000-2016, the most common negative short-term effects experienced by people who called in about using LSD and psilocybin were agitation, rapid heartbeat, pupil dilation, confusion, and vomiting. An analysis of these data found about 17% of these callers (600 people) who had used LSD and 6% of callers (363 people) who had used psilocybin mushrooms were admitted to critical care [31].

- *Adverse reactions include fear and anxiety.* People may also feel extreme emotions such as fear, confusion, or panic. These challenging experiences are also known as having a "bad trip"[32]. Research on the extent to which such experiences occur and their impact on health is limited, in part because definitions and reporting of these experiences vary.

- *Using psychedelic and dissociative drugs has been linked to dangerous behavior and injuries.* People using these drugs may have impaired thought processes and perception that causes them to behave in unusual or dangerous ways. This may lead to injuries and other safety issues, particularly if there is no one else present who can help prevent or respond to an emergency [14]. In a survey of almost 2,000 people who took psilocybin outside of a medical setting and had a challenging experience, 11% said they had put themselves or others at risk of harm [33]. More research is needed to better understand the impact of psychedelic and dissociative drugs on driving, operating heavy machinery, or performing other tasks that could be dangerous if impaired.
- *Emerging evidence suggests certain psychedelic and dissociative drugs may contain dangerous adulterants.* For more information, see "Can psychedelic and dissociative drugs be adulterated with fentanyl and other dangerous contaminants?"
- *Fatal overdoses and serious adverse effects are rarely associated with typical use of commonly used psychedelic and dissociative drugs* [14, 34, 35]. A 2004 analysis of multiple studies estimated that psilocybin and LSD both have a safety ratio of 1000, meaning that the lethal dose of either drug is about 1000 times larger than a person would typically take for non-medical use [36]. However, some psychedelic and dissociative drugs—including NBOMes, [37, 38] ibogaine, [39] and PCP [40] —have been associated with a small number of reported deaths and serious adverse health effects. Though more research is needed, evidence to date shows that fatal overdoses involving these substances are typically associated with taking very high doses or using combinations of drugs, particularly combining these substances with alcohol, or being placed in excessive physical restraints while displaying unsafe behavior [16]. More research is needed to understand to what extent certain psychedelic and dissociative drugs may be mixed with contaminants (such as fentanyl) that may cause an overdose. For more information, see "Can

psychedelic and dissociative drugs be adulterated with fentanyl and other dangerous contaminants?"

- *Drug interactions may influence effects.* Though more study in this area is needed and reported cases are exceedingly rare, some researchers suspect psychedelic drugs may interact with other drugs or medications a person has taken, including prescription medicines that also increase levels of the hormone serotonin in the brain. Too much serotonin in the brain is called serotonin toxicity or serotonin syndrome. Symptoms are typically mild but can be life-threatening in rare cases [41, 42].
- *Use of some psychedelic and dissociative drugs rarely cause a condition called hallucinogen persisting perception disorder (HPPD).* Some people report recurrently perceiving the same images or scenes and having the same mood changes they experienced when they were under the influence of a psychedelic or dissociative drug sometime in the past. These perceptions, or "flashbacks," are typically mild and brief, lasting for seconds or minutes and occurring within a week of taking a substance [43]. However, people with HPPD report that these episodes last longer and can reoccur even years after an experience with a substance, causing distress and other problems that impact their lives [44, 45]. Research on HPPD so far is limited and has relied mainly on self-reports on types and doses of the drugs believed to have caused these symptoms. More research is needed to assess how and why HPPD occurs and to find ways to help prevent and treat it.
- *Some psychedelic and dissociative drugs have been associated with specific long-term health problems. Research* shows that long-term use of ketamine may cause ketamine-induced uropathy, a treatable but potentially serious condition that causes symptoms similar to those of a urinary tract infection [46].Limited research also suggests using MDMA (considered by some to have psychedelic properties) may be associated with mild or moderate heart valve disease, in which one or more of the four valves controlling blood flow from the heart do not function normally [47]. In an analysis of studies conducted from 2015 through 2020, ibogaine use was associated with long QT syndrome, in which the electric impulses that control heartbeats function irregularly [48].

- *Research on long-term mental health effects of psychedelic and dissociative drugs is ongoing.* More research is needed to better understand the long-term impacts of psychedelic and dissociative drugs on mental health. Mental health complications from psychedelic and dissociative drugs are currently extremely rare in clinical research settings, in part because these studies are highly controlled and participants are screened for existing mental illnesses [32] For more information, see "*What is the relationship between psychedelic and dissociative drugs and mental illness?*"

Can Psychedelic and Dissociative Drugs Be Used as Medicine?

The U.S. Food and Drug Administration (FDA) has approved the ketamine derivative esketamine (under the brand name Spravato®) as a treatment for severe depression in patients who do not respond to other treatments [49]. The FDA has also granted Breakthrough Therapy designation for two formulations of psilocybin being studied as potential medical treatments for depression.

NIDA supports and conducts research to learn whether some of these drugs may help treat substance use disorders in medical settings.

What Is the Relationship Between Psychedelic and Dissociative Drugs and Mental Illness

While scientists are still studying their effects, research suggests that some psychedelic and dissociative drugs may promote positive changes in thinking and mood [3]. Researchers have suggested that these effects, including changes in brain functions that promote openness to new thoughts and experiences, may be valuable for supplementing mental health treatment [50]. The U.S. Food and Drug Administration (FDA) has approved the ketamine derivative esketamine (under the brand name Spravato®) as a treatment for severe depression in patients who do not respond to other treatments. The FDA has also granted Breakthrough Therapy designation for two formulations of psilocybin being studied as potential medical treatments for depression.

While short-term positive and negative mood changes are common with psychedelic and dissociative drugs, more research is needed to better understand the long-term effects these substances may have on mental health.

There is some evidence that psychedelic drugs might bring about or trigger schizophrenia-like illness in people with predisposing factors, but little evidence that they cause long-term psychiatric problems for most people. In a 1996 study where people with pre-existing psychoses were given LSD, three of 65 participants experienced persistent worsening of their psychiatric symptoms lasting 3-8 months [51].

In modern psychedelic research, as a precaution, participants with previously diagnosed psychosis or bipolar disorder, and sometimes other mental illnesses, are excluded from participation. Under these conditions, the risk of psychosis or suicide among people who participate in research on psychedelic drugs, or who receive them as medication, is extremely low [52]. An analysis of 34 clinical studies of LSD, psilocybin, or ayahuasca, published from 2006-2020 and involving 549 participants, found no evidence of longer-term adverse effects [26]. However, poor mental health outcomes may be more likely outside of clinical use [14].

Research suggests, though, that the dissociative drugs PCP [41] and ketamine [53] can make symptoms worse in people who have schizophrenia, and can cause short-term episodes of psychosis, in which a person experiences hallucinations and delusions, and has trouble experiencing what is real and what is not. PCP can also cause psychosis that persists for days to weeks [6, 54]. While it is not clear whether ketamine raises the risk of long-term psychosis, people who engage in regular recreational use of ketamine are more likely to experience delusions, even after weeks of abstinence [55]. Animal studies show that long-term use of PCP or ketamine can cause brain changes resembling those seen in people with schizophrenia [56].

One analysis found higher rates of suicidal ideation—thinking about, considering or planning suicide—but not attempted or completed suicide, in people who took esketamine, a ketamine derivative, compared to venlafaxine, an antidepressant medication [57]. In another analysis of 25 studies, medically unsupervised ketamine use was associated with related substance use disorder symptoms, memory loss, depression, and anxiety [58].

Can Psychedelic and Dissociative Drugs Be Adulterated with Fentanyl and Other Dangerous Contaminants?

Many illicitly manufactured or processed drugs are increasingly found to contain contaminants that produce effects—including overdose and death—

not associated with the substance or amount of substance a person intended to take [28, 59]. Adulteration of heroin, cocaine, and other drugs with highly potent fentanyl and related substances is a major contributor to rising drug overdose deaths [60]. Because fentanyl and related substances are colorless and odorless, they are difficult to detect without chemical testing. This means adulteration of psychedelic and dissociative drugs with fentanyl and similar compounds is possible, but more research is needed to understand to what extent this occurs. Some organizations are using harm reduction practices to help avoid drug overdose deaths related to possible adulteration of certain psychedelic and dissociative drugs, particularly those taken in pill, powder, or liquid form [15].

How Do Psychedelic and Dissociative Drugs Affect Pregnancy?

The effects of psychedelic and dissociative drugs during pregnancy are not well understood, as data are limited. PCP use during pregnancy has been linked to a range of congenital abnormalities in an infant's heart, lung, urinary, cardiovascular, respiratory, urinary, and musculoskeletal systems [61]. Some laboratory and epidemiological studies suggest MDMA (considered by some to have psychedelic properties) may cause motor delays and congenital abnormalities (particularly heart defects) in infants exposed to it during pregnancy [62, 63].

Are Psychedelic and Dissociative Drugs Addictive? Can People Experience Withdrawal?

To be diagnosed with a substance use disorder, a person must meet specific diagnostic criteria for continued substance use despite negative consequences. The *Diagnostic and Statistical Manual of Mental Disorders, Fifth Edition* (DSM-5)—a reference text professionals use to diagnose substance use disorders and other psychiatric disorders—includes diagnoses of phencyclidine (PCP) use disorder and "other hallucinogen use disorder" [64, 65] but does not include substance use disorder diagnoses related to other specific psychedelic and dissociative drugs.

Limited research suggests that use of psychedelic drugs, such as psilocybin and LSD, does not typically lead to addiction [1, 35]. Researchers think that one reason may be because people commonly experience unpleasant side effects when taking these substances, including headaches and nausea, which reduces their desire to take them again [66].

A small laboratory study published on psilocybin, DMT, and mescaline suggested that these psychedelic drugs are "weakly reinforcing," indicating their use is not likely to lead to a substance use disorder [67]. However, some evidence suggests people may quickly develop a tolerance to psychedelic drugs, meaning they must keep taking more of the drug to experience the same level of effects [24].

While more research is needed, laboratory research and a few human studies suggest that using the dissociative drug ketamine outside of a clinical setting can lead to cravings as well as symptoms of withdrawal [68].

NIDA conducts and supports research to better understand how often and to what extent people experience tolerance, withdrawal, and other substance use disorder symptoms related to the use of psychedelic and dissociative drugs.

What Is the Scope of Psychedelic and Dissociative Drug Use in the United States?

Information on the use of psychedelic and dissociative drugs is collected by several national surveys. These surveys use the terms "hallucinogen" and "hallucinogen use disorder" and data from those surveys are reported below.

How Many People Use Hallucinogens*?

Among people aged 12 or older in 2021, 2.6% (or about 7.4 million people) reported using hallucinogens in the past 12 months.

Source: 2021 National Survey on Drug Use and Health

How Many Young Students Use Hallucinogens**?

Among young people in 2022:

- An estimated 1.2% of 8th graders, 2.1% of 10th graders, and 4.4% of 12th graders reported using any hallucinogen
- *in the past 12 months.
- An estimated 0.6% of 8th graders, 1.3% of 10th graders, and 2.5% of 12th graders reported using LSD in the past 12 months.
- An estimated 1% of 8th graders, 1.6% of 10th graders, and 3.4% of 12th graders reported using hallucinogens other than LSD in the past 12 months.
- An estimated 0.6% of 8th graders, 0.7% of 10th graders, and 1.4% of 12th graders reported using MDMA
- An estimated 1.2% of 12th graders reported using ketamine in the past 12 months.
- An estimated 0.8% of 8th graders, 0.8% of 10th graders, and 0.8% of 12th graders reported using salvia in the past 12 months.

Source: 2022 Monitoring the Future Survey.

How Many Young Adults Use Hallucinogens?

Among young adults aged 19 to 30 in 2021:

- An estimated 8% reported using any hallucinogen*, representing an all-time high since the category was first surveyed in 1988.

Source: 2021 Monitoring the Future Panel Study Annual Report

How Many People Have a Hallucinogen Use Disorder?

Among people aged 12 or older in 2020, 0.2% (or about 493,000 people) had a hallucinogen use disorder in the past 12 months.

Source: 2021 National Survey on Drug Use and Health

* Types of hallucinogens reported by participants in the National Survey on Drug Use and Health include DMT/AMT/Foxy, ketamine, LSD, MDMA, PCP, peyote/mescaline, psilocybin mushrooms, and *Salvia divinorum*.

**Types of hallucinogens reported by participants in the Monitoring the Future surveys included LSD, MDMA, mescaline, peyote, "shrooms" or psilocybin, and PCP.

What Are Examples of Psychedelic and Dissociative Drugs?

While many emerging and established substances are classified as psychedelic and dissociative drugs, NIDA-supported research mainly focuses on the following substances, which are more commonly used and/or are being investigated as potential medical treatments. While some debate remains on how to describe these drugs and how specific drugs are classified, researchers generally classify them according to how they work in the brain.

Psychedelic Drugs

Among other health effects, psychedelic drugs alter a person's perception of their surroundings. They can change a person's sense of self, their mood, and their perception of reality [1, 3,10].

- *Psilocybin* is a chemical compound in certain types of mushrooms, also called "shrooms" or "magic mushrooms" [23].
- *LSD (lysergic acid diethylamide)*, or "acid," is a clear or white, odorless, lab-made (synthetic) substance derived from chemicals in fungi that grow on rye and other grains [69].
- *DMT (N,N-dimethyltryptamine)* is a chemical compound found in plants native to the Amazon rainforest. These plants are sometimes used to make a tea called *ayahuasca* [70]. Lab-made (synthetic) DMT is a white crystalline powder that is usually smoked [71].
- *Mescaline* is a chemical compound found in *peyote,* a small cactus native to America's southwest and northern Mexico. Mescaline can also be lab-made (synthetic) [72].
- *NBOMes* (*N*-Benzylphenethylamines) are lab-made (synthetic) chemical compounds originally developed for use in brain research [73]. They are sometimes sold as LSD but are more potent with higher risk of adverse effects.

Dissociative Drugs

Among other health effects, dissociative drugs can also alter people's perception of reality. They also typically make people feel as if they are disconnected from their body and environment [6].

- Ketamine is a chemical compound used in prescription medications for anesthesia in humans and animals. It is also illegally manufactured as a liquid or off-white powder [28]. A derivative called esketamine is FDA-approved for treatment-resistant depression.
- PCP (phencyclidine) is a synthetic chemical compound most commonly used as a liquid or white crystal powder [40].

Other

Researchers are also interested in the psychedelic and dissociative properties of other drugs. These include:

- MDMA (3,4-methylenedioxy-methamphetamine), also called "Molly" or "Ecstasy," is a lab-made (synthetic) drug that has effects similar to stimulants like methamphetamine. Some researchers and organizations consider MDMA to be a psychedelic drug because it can also mildly alter visual and time perception [7].
- Ibogaine is a chemical compound that comes from the bark of certain plants. These include the iboga shrub, which is used in religious rites in Western Africa. While ibogaine does have psychedelic properties, it affects a different spectrum of brain activity than psychedelic or dissociative drugs [8].
- Salvia (salvia divinorum) is a plant common to southern Mexico and Central and South America. Salvia leaves are typically chewed, extracted as juices, smoked, or vaporized. Unlike psychedelic or dissociative drugs, it primarily activates kappa opioid receptors in the brain [21].

What Is Microdosing?

Some people report "microdosing" psychedelic drugs, typically LSD or psilocybin. Microdosing refers to regularly taking these drugs in very small amounts, typically one tenth to one twentieth of a typical non-clinical dose. People report that they microdose to lessen mental health symptoms such as depression and stress, improve productivity, and ease pain. However, research to date has not established that microdosing is safe or effective [22, 74].

Are Psychedelic and Dissociative Drugs Legal?

While laws vary by specific substance, the U.S. Drug Enforcement Administration (DEA) lists most psychedelic and dissociative drugs on the U.S. schedule of controlled substances. However, the legal status of some of these drugs is evolving. Though most of these substances remain federally controlled, some states and the District of Columbia have decriminalized possession of psilocybin and some similar drugs (meaning there are no criminal penalties for possessing smaller amounts of the substance for personal use) or deprioritized enforcement of laws against the substances. Other jurisdictions are considering similar changes [75].

Learn more about psychedelic and dissociative drugs and their legal status in the United States from the DEA.

Find More Resources on Psychedelic and Dissociative Drugs

- Learn more about psychedelic and dissociative drugs and their legal status in the United States from the U.S. Drug Enforcement Administration (DEA).
- Browse consumer health information on psychedelic and dissociative drugs from MedlinePlus.

References

[1] Nichols D. E. Psychedelics. *Pharmacol. Rev* 2016;68:264–355.doi:10.1124/pr.115.011478.

[2] Johnson M. W., Hendricks PS, Barrett F. S., Griffiths R. R. Classic psychedelics: An integrative review of epidemiology, therapeutics, mystical experience, and brain network function. *Pharmacol Ther.* 2019;197:83-102. doi:10.1016/j.pharmthera. 2018.11.010.

[3] Garcia-Romeu A., Kersgaard B., Addy P. H. Clinical applications of hallucinogens: A review. *Exp Clin Psychopharmacol.* 2016;24 (4):229-268. doi:10.1037/pha0000084.

[4] Bender D., Hellerstein D. J. Assessing the risk-benefit profile of classical psychedelics: a clinical review of second-wave psychedelic research. *Psychopharmacology (Berl).* 2022;239(6):1907-1932. doi:10.1007/s00213-021-06049-6.

[5] Ivan Ezquerra-Romano I., Lawn W., Krupitsky E., Morgan C. J. A. Ketamine for the treatment of addiction: Evidence and potential mechanisms. *Neuropharmacology.* 2018;142:72-82. doi:10.1016/j.neuropharm. 2018.01.017.

[6] Lodge D., Mercier M. S. Ketamine and phencyclidine: the good, the bad and the unexpected. *Br. J. Pharmacol.* 2015;172(17):4254-4276. doi:10.1111/bph.1222.

[7] Dunlap L. E., Andrews A M., Olson DE. Dark Classics in Chemical Neuroscience: 3,4-Methylenedioxymethamphetamine. *ACS Chem. Neurosci.* 2018;9(10):2408-2427. doi:10.1021/acschemneuro.8b00155.

[8] Wasko M. J., Witt-Enderby P. A., Surratt C. K. DARK Classics in Chemical Neuroscience: Ibogaine. *ACS Chem. Neurosci.* 2018;9(10):2475-2483. doi:10.1021/acschemneuro.8b00294.

[9] Johnson M. W., MacLean K. A., Reissig C. J., Prisinzano T. E., Griffiths R. R. Human psychopharmacology and dose-effects of salvinorin A, a kappa opioid agonist hallucinogen present in the plant Salvia divinorum. *Drug Alcohol Depend.* 2011;115(1-2):150-155. doi:10.1016/j.drugalcdep.2010.11.005.

[10] Vollenweider FX, Smallridge JW. Classic Psychedelic Drugs: Update on Biological Mechanisms. *Pharmacopsychiatry.* 2022;55(3):121-138. doi:10.1055/a-1721-2914.

[11] Studerus E, Gamma A, Kometer M, Vollenweider FX. Prediction of psilocybin response in healthy volunteers. *PLoS One.* 2012;7(2):e30800. doi:10.1371/journal.pone.0030800.

[12] Oliver C. F., Palamar J. J., Salomone A., et al. Synthetic cathinone adulteration of illegal drugs. *Psychopharmacology (Berl).* 2019;236(3):869-879. doi:10.1007/s00213-018-5066-6.

[13] Jansen K. L. A review of the nonmedical use of ketamine: use, users and consequences. *J. Psychoactive Drugs.* 2000;32(4):419-433. doi:10.1080/02791072.2000.10400244.

[14] Breeksema J. J., Kuin B. W., Kamphuis J., van den Brink W., Vermetten E., Schoevers RA. Adverse events in clinical treatments with serotonergic psychedelics and MDMA: A mixed-methods systematic review. *J. Psychopharmacol.* 2022; 36(10):1100-1117. doi:10.1177/02698811221116926.

[15] Palamar J. J., Salomone A., Barratt M. J. Drug checking to detect fentanyl and new psychoactive substances. *Curr. Opin. Psychiatry.* 2020;33(4):301-305. doi:10.1097/YCO.0000000000000607.

[16] Schlag A. K., Aday J., Salam I., Neill J. C., Nutt D. J. Adverse effects of psychedelics: From anecdotes and misinformation to systematic science [published online ahead of print, 2022 Feb 2]. *J. Psychopharmacol.* 2022;2698811211069100. doi:10.1177/02698811211069100.

[17] Calvey T., Howells FM. An introduction to psychedelic neuroscience. *Prog. Brain Res.* 2018;242:1-23. doi:10.1016/bs.pbr.2018.09.013.

[18] Lee H. M., Roth B. L. Hallucinogen actions on human brain revealed. *Proc. Natl. Acad. Sci. U S A.* 2012;109(6):1820-1821. doi:10.1073/pnas.1121358109.

[19] Zhang R., Volkow N. D. Brain default-mode network dysfunction in addiction. *Neuroimage.* 2019;200:313-331. doi:10.1016/j.neuroimage.2019.06.036.

[20] Jansen K. L. A review of the nonmedical use of ketamine: use, users and consequences. *J. Psychoactive Drugs.* 2000;32(4):419-433. doi:10.1080/02791072.2000.10400244.

[21] Hernández-Alvarado R. B., Madariaga-Mazón A., Ortega A., Martinez-Mayorga K. DARK Classics in Chemical Neuroscience: Salvinorin A [published online ahead of print, 2020 Nov 9]. *ACS Chem. Neurosci.* 2020;10.1021/acschemneuro.0c00608. doi:10.1021/acschemneuro.0c00608.

[22] Kuypers K. P., Ng L., Erritzoe D., et al. Microdosing psychedelics: More questions than answers? An overview and suggestions for future research. *J. Psychopharmacol.* 2019;33(9):1039-1057. doi:10.1177/0269881119857204.

[23] Van Court R. C., Wiseman M. S., Meyer K. W., et al. Diversity, biology, and history of psilocybin-containing fungi: Suggestions for research and technological development. *Fungal Biol.* 2022;126(4):308-319. doi:10.1016/j.funbio.2022.01.003.

[24] Nichols D. E. Hallucinogens. *Pharmacol. Ther.* 2004;101(2):131-181. doi:10.1016/j.pharmthera.203.11.002.

[25] Castro Santos H., Gama Marques J. What is the clinical evidence on psilocybin for the treatment of psychiatric disorders? A systematic review. *Porto Biomed. J.* 2021;6(1):e128. Published 2021 Feb 11. doi:10.1097/j.pbj.0000000000000128.

[26] Goldberg S. B., Shechet B., Nicholas C. R., et al. Post-acute psychological effects of classical serotonergic psychedelics: a systematic review and meta-analysis. *Psychol. Med.* 2020;50(16):2655-2666. doi:10.1017/S003329172000 389X.

[27] Breeksema JJ, Kuin BW, Kamphuis J, van den Brink W, Vermetten E, Schoevers RA. Adverse events in clinical treatments with serotonergic psychedelics and MDMA: A mixed-methods systematic review. *J. Psychopharmacol.* 2022;36(10):1100-1117. doi:10.1177/02698811221116926.

[28] Morgan C. J., Curran HV; Independent Scientific Committee on Drugs. Ketamine use: a review. *Addiction.* 2012;107(1):27-38. doi:10.1111/j.1360-0443.2011.03576.x.

[29] van Amsterdam J, Opperhuizen A, van den Brink W. Harm potential of magic mushroom use: a review. *Regul. Toxicol. Pharmacol.* 2011;59(3):423-429. doi:10.1016/j.yrtph.2011.01.006.

[30] van Amsterdam J., Van Den Brink W. Harm related to recreational ketamine use and its relevance for the clinical use of ketamine. A systematic review and

comparison study. *Expert Opin. Drug Saf.* 2022;21(1):83-94. doi:10.1080/147 40338. 2021.1949454.

[31] Leonard J. B., Anderson B., Klein-Schwartz W. Does getting high hurt? Characterization of cases of LSD and psilocybin-containing mushroom exposures to national poison centers between 2000 and 2016. *J. Psychopharmacol.* 2018;32(12):1286-1294. doi:10.1177/0269881118793086.

[32] Johnson M., Richards W., Griffiths R. Human hallucinogen research: guidelines for safety. *J. Psychopharmacol.* 2008;22(6):603-620. doi:10.1177/0269881108093587.

[33] Carbonaro T. M., Bradstreet M. P., Barrett F. S., et al. Survey study of challenging experiences after ingesting psilocybin mushrooms: Acute and enduring positive and negative consequences. *J. Psychopharmacol.* 2016;30(12):1268-1278. doi:10.1177/ 0269881116662634.

[34] Johnson M. W., Griffiths R. R., Hendricks P. S., Henningfield J. E. The abuse potential of medical psilocybin according to the 8 factors of the Controlled Substances Act. *Neuropharmacology.* 2018;142:143-166. doi:10.1016/j.neuro pharm.2018.05. 012.

[35] Nichols D. E., Grob CS. Is LSD toxic? *Forensic Sci. Int.* 2018;284:141-145. doi:10.1016/j.forsciint.2018.01.006.

[36] Gable R. S. Comparison of acute lethal toxicity of commonly abused psychoactive substances. *Addiction.* 2004;99(6):686-696.doi:10.1111/j.1360-0443.2004. 00744. x.

[37] Gee P., Schep L. J., Jensen B. P., Moore G., Barrington S. Case series: toxicity from 25B-NBOMe--a cluster of N-bomb cases - PubMed (nih.gov). *Clin Toxicol (Phila).* 2016;54(2):141-146. doi:10.3109/15563650.2015.1115056.

[38] Wood D. M., Sedefov R., Cunningham A., Dargan P. I. Prevalence of use and acute toxicity associated with the use of NBOMe drugs. *Clin. Toxicol. (Phila).* 2015;53(2):85-92. doi:10.3109/15563650.2015.1004179.

[39] Köck P., Froelich K., Walter M., Lang U., Dürsteler K. M. A systematic literature review of clinical trials and therapeutic applications of ibogaine. *J. Subst. Abuse Treat.* 2022;138:108717. doi:10.1016/j.jsat.2021.108717.

[40] Bertron J. L., Seto M., Lindsley C. W. DARK Classics in Chemical Neuroscience: Phencyclidine (PCP). *ACS Chem Neurosci.* 2018;9(10):2459-2474. doi:10.1021 /acschemneuro.8b0026.

[41] Malcolm B., Thomas K. Serotonin toxicity of serotonergic psychedelics [published online ahead of print, 2021 Jul 12]. *Psychopharmacology (Berl).* 2021;10.1007/ s00213-021-05876-x. doi:10.1007/s00213-021-05876-x.

[42] Volpi-Abadie J., Kaye A. M., Kaye A. D. Serotonin syndrome. *Ochsner J.* 2013;13(4):533-540.

[43] Müller F., Kraus E., Holze F., et al. Flashback phenomena after administration of LSD and psilocybin in controlled studies with healthy participants [published online ahead of print, 2022 Jan 25]. *Psychopharmacology (Berl).* 2022;10.1007/s00213-022-06066-z. doi:10.1007/s00213-022-06066-z.

[44] Halpern J. H., Lerner A. G., Passie T. A Review of Hallucinogen Persisting Perception Disorder (HPPD) and an Exploratory Study of Subjects Claiming

Symptoms of HPPD. *Curr Top Behav. Neurosci.* 2018;36:333-360. doi:10.1007/ 7854_2016_457.

[45] Martinotti G., Santacroce R., Pettorruso M., et al. Hallucinogen Persisting Perception Disorder: Etiology, Clinical Features, and Therapeutic Perspectives. *Brain Sci.* 2018;8(3):47. Published 2018 Mar 16. doi:10.3390/ brainsci8030047.

[46] Castellani D., Pirola G. M., Gubbiotti M., et al. What urologists need to know about ketamine-induced uropathy: A systematic review. *Neurourol Urodyn.* 2020;39(4):1049-1062. doi:10.1002/nau.24341.

[47] Fonseca D. A., Ribeiro D. M., Tapadas M., Cotrim M. D. Ecstasy (3,4-methylenedioxymethamphetamine): Cardiovascular effects and mechanisms. *Eur. J. Pharmacol.* 2021;903:174156. doi:10.1016/j.ejphar.2021.174156.

[48] Ona G., Rocha J. M., Bouso J. C., Hallak J. E. C., Borràs T., Colomina M. T., Dos Santos R. G. The adverse events of ibogaine in humans: an updated systematic review of the literature (2015-2020). Psychopharmacology (Berl). 2021 Aug 18. doi: 10.1007/s00213-021-05964-y. *Epub ahead of print.* PMID: 34406452.

[49] Hashimoto K. Rapid-acting antidepressant ketamine, its metabolites and other candidates: A historical overview and future perspective. *Psychiatry Clin. Neurosci.* 2019;73(10):613-627. doi:10.1111/pcn.12902.

[50] Reiff C. M., Richman E. E., Nemeroff C. B., et al. Psychedelics and Psychedelic-Assisted Psychotherapy. *Focus (Am Psychiatr Publ).* 2021;19(1):95-115. doi:10. 1176/appi.focus.19104

[51] Fink M., Simeon J., Haque W., Itil T. Prolonged adverse reactions to LSD in psychotic subjects. Arch Gen Psychiatry-.1966;15(5):450-454. doi:10.1001/ archpsyc. 1966.01730170002002.

[52] Zeifman R. J., Singhal N., Breslow L., Weissman C. R. On the Relationship between Classic Psychedelics and Suicidality: A Systematic Review [published correction appears in ACS Pharmacol Transl Sci. 2022 Feb 22;5(3):176]. *ACS Pharmacol. Transl Sci.* 2021;4(2):436-451. Published 2021 Mar 11. doi:10.1021/ acsptsci.1c00024.

[53] Tyler M. W., Yourish H. B., Ionescu D. F., Haggarty S. J. Classics in Chemical Neuroscience: Ketamine. *ACS Chem Neurosci.* 2017;8(6):1122-1134. doi:10.1021/ acschemneuro.7b00074.

[54] Javitt D. C., Zukin S. R. Recent advances in the phencyclidine model of schizophrenia. *Am. J. Psychiatry.* 1991;148(10):1301-1308. doi:10.1176/ajp. 148.10. 1301

[55] Morgan C. J., Muetzelfeldt L, Curran HV. Consequences of chronic ketamine self-administration upon neurocognitive function and psychological wellbeing: a 1-year longitudinal study [published correction appears in Addiction. 2010 Apr;105(4):766].*Addiction.* 2010;105(1):121-133. doi:10.1111/j.1360-0443.2009. 02761.x.

[56] Kristiansen L. V., Huerta I., Beneyto M., Meador-Woodruff J. H. NMDA receptors and schizophrenia. Curr Opin Pharmacol. 2007 Feb;7(1):48-55. doi: 10.1016/j. coph.2006.08.013. Epub 2006 Nov 9. PMID: 17097347.

[57] Gastaldon C., Raschi E., Kane J. M., Barbui C., Schoretsanitis G. Post-Marketing Safety Concerns with Esketamine: A Disproportionality Analysis of Spontaneous

Reports Submitted to the FDA Adverse Event Reporting System. *Psychother. Psychosom.* 2021;90(1):41-48. doi:10.1159/000510703.

[58] van Amsterdam J., Van Den Brink W. Harm related to recreational ketamine use and its relevance for the clinical use of ketamine. A systematic review and comparison study. *Expert Opin. Drug Saf.* 2022;21(1):83-94.doi:10. 1080/ 14740338.2021. 1949454.

[59] Ivory S. T., Rotella J. A., Schumann J., Greene S. L. A cluster of 25B-NBOH poisonings following exposure to powder sold as lysergic acid diethylamide (LSD). *Clin. Toxicol. (Phila).* 2022;60(8):966-969. doi:10.1080/15563650.2022.2053150.

[60] D'Errico S. Commentary. Fentanyl-related death and the underreporting risk. *J. Forensic Leg. Med.* 2018;60:35-37. doi:10.1016/j.jflm.2018.09.007.

[61] Holbrook BD, Rayburn WF. Teratogenic risks from exposure to illicit drugs. *Obstet Gynecol Clin North Am.* 2014;41(2):229-239. doi:10.1016/j.ogc.2014.02.008.

[62] McElhatton P. R., Bateman D. N., Evans C., Pughe KR, Thomas SH. Congenital anomalies after prenatal ecstasy exposure. *Lancet.* 1999;354(9188):1441-1442. doi:10.1016/s0140-6736(99)02423-x.

[63] Singer L. T., Moore D. G., Min M. O., et al. Motor delays in MDMA (ecstasy) exposed infants persist to 2 years. *Neurotoxicol Teratol.* 2016;54:22-28. doi:10.1016/j.ntt.2016.01.003.

[64] Ryu I. S., Kim O. H., Lee Y. E., Kim J. S., Li Z. H., Kim T. W., Lim R. N., Lee Y. J., Cheong J. H., Kim H. J., Lee Y. S., Steffensen S. C., Lee B. H., Seo J. W., Jang E. Y. The Abuse Potential of Novel Synthetic Phencyclidine Derivative 1-(1-(4-Fluorophenyl)Cyclohexyl) Piperidine (4'-F-PCP) in Rodents. *Int. J. Mol. Sci.* 2020 Jun 29;21(13):4631. doi: 10.3390/ijms21134631.

[65] American Psychiatric Association, Substance-Related and Addictive Disorders, Diagnostic and Statistical Manual of Mental Disorders, 10.1176/appi.books. 9780890425787, (2022).

[66] Johnson M. W., Sewell R. A., Griffiths R. R. Psilocybin dose-dependently causes delayed, transient headaches in healthy volunteers. Drug Alcohol. Depend. 2012;123(1-3):132-140. doi:10.1016/j.drugalcdep.2011.10.029.

[67] Fantegrossi W. E., Woods J. H., Winger G. Transient reinforcing effects of phenylisopropylamine and indolealkylamine hallucinogens in rhesus monkeys. *Behav. Pharmacol.* 2004;15(2):149-157. doi:10.1097/00008877-200403000-00007.

[68] Kokane S. S., Armant R. J., Bolaños-Guzmán C. A., Perrotti LI. Overlap in the neural circuitry and molecular mechanisms underlying ketamine abuse and its use as an antidepressant. *Behav Brain Res.* 2020;384:112548. doi:10.1016/j.bbr. 2020.112548.

[69] Passie T., Halpern J. H., Stichtenoth D. O., Emrich H. M., Hintzen A. The pharmacology of lysergic acid diethylamide: a review. *CNS Neurosci Ther.* 2008;14(4):295-314. doi:10.1111/j.1755-5949.2008.00059.x.

[70] Domínguez-Clavé E., Soler J., Elices M., et al. Ayahuasca: Pharmacology, neuroscience and therapeutic potential. *Brain Res. Bull.* 2016;126(Pt 1):89-101. doi:10.1016/j.brainresbull.2016.03.002.

[71] Carbonaro T. M., Gatch MB. Neuropharmacology of N, N-dimethyltryptamine. *Brain Res. Bull.* 2016;126(Pt 1):74-88. doi:10.1016/j.brainresbull.2016.04.016.

[72] Dinis-Oliveira R. J., Pereira C. L., da Silva D. D. Pharmacokinetic and pharmacodynamic aspects of peyote and mescaline: clinical and forensic repercussions. *Curr. Mol. Pharmacol.* 2019;12(3):184-194. doi:10.2174/18744 67211 666181010154139.

[73] Poulie C. B. M., Jensen A. A., Halberstadt A. L., Kristensen J. L. DARK Classics in Chemical Neuroscience: NBOMes [published online ahead of print, 2019 Nov 12]. *ACS Chem. Neurosci.* 2019;10.1021/acschemneuro.9b00528. doi:10.1021/ acschemneuro.9b00528.

[74] de Wit H., Molla H. M., Bershad A., Bremmer M., Lee R. Repeated low doses of LSD in healthy adults: A placebo-controlled, dose-response study [published online ahead of print, 2022 Feb 1]. *Addict. Biol.* 2022;e13143. doi:10.1111/adb.13143.

[75] Siegel J. S., Daily J. E., Perry D. A., Nicol G. E. Psychedelic Drug Legislative Reform and Legalization in the US . *JAMA Psychiatry.* Published online December 07, 2022. doi:10.1001/jamapsychiatry.2022.4101.

Chapter 2

Medical Use of Psychedelics*

United States Government Accountability Office

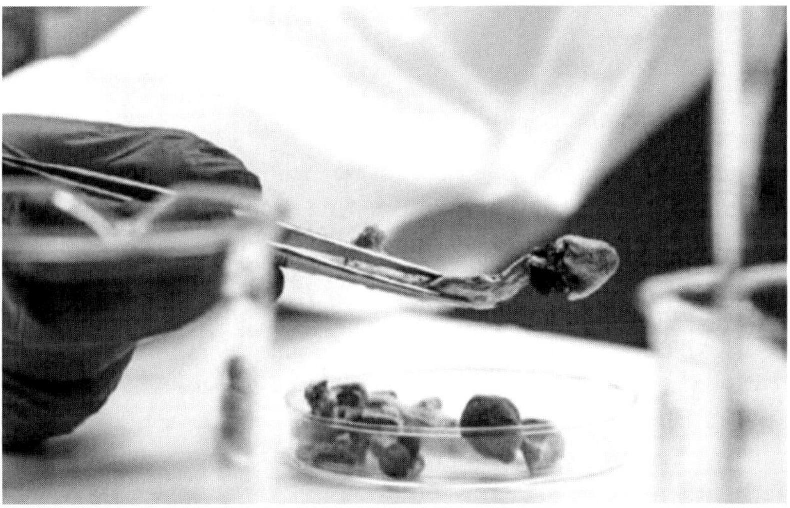

Why This Matters

Psychedelics can change a person's perceptions and sense of self, which has promising medical applications. While more research is needed, including on adverse effects, psychedelics may reduce depression and other conditions.

---

* This is an edited, reformatted and augmented version of the United States Government Accountability Office Publication No. GAO-25-108021, dated March 2025.

In: The Psychedelic Landscape
Editor: James P. Macintosh
ISBN: 979-8-89530-991-9

Key Takeaways

- Hundreds of clinical trials have examined psychedelics, including for treating PTSD and depression.
- Researchers struggle to distinguish genuine effects of psychedelics from the placebo effect.
- The medical use of psychedelics also raises questions for policymakers about how to balance potential benefits with research limitations and patient safety.

The Science

What are psychedelics? Psychedelics are hallucinogenic drugs that can temporarily alter a person's mood and perceptions. Like a class of drugs known as selective serotonin reuptake inhibitors (SSRI), which are often prescribed for mental health care, psychedelics affect serotonin levels (see fig. 1). At certain doses, psychedelics may be used for medical purposes. For example, MDMA (also called ecstasy), LSD, and psilocybin (a hallucinogen found in some mushrooms) have been examined as potential treatments for PTSD and depression.

What is known? Psychedelics work primarily by changing how a person's brain processes serotonin. This may cause vivid visions, or feelings of insightfulness or connection.

Between 2015 and early 2025, over 340 trials on psychedelics began or were completed, according to ClinicalTrials.gov. For example, one study found that psilocybin reduced depression symptoms more than escitalopram, an SSRI.

While most psychedelics have no federally approved medical uses, several U.S. government agencies have supported such research. For example, in December 2024, the Department of Veterans Affairs planned research to combine MDMA and psychotherapy to treat veterans with PTSD. Several states have also considered or passed legislation allowing medical use of psychedelics.

Psychedelics may have non-life-threatening side effects, such as headaches or vomiting. In some cases, the use of these drugs can lead to safety risks due to impairment, or illicit psychedelics may be contaminated with dangerous substances such as fentanyl. While some research suggests that the use of psychedelics does not typically lead to physical addiction, the adverse effects of these drugs have not been fully studied.

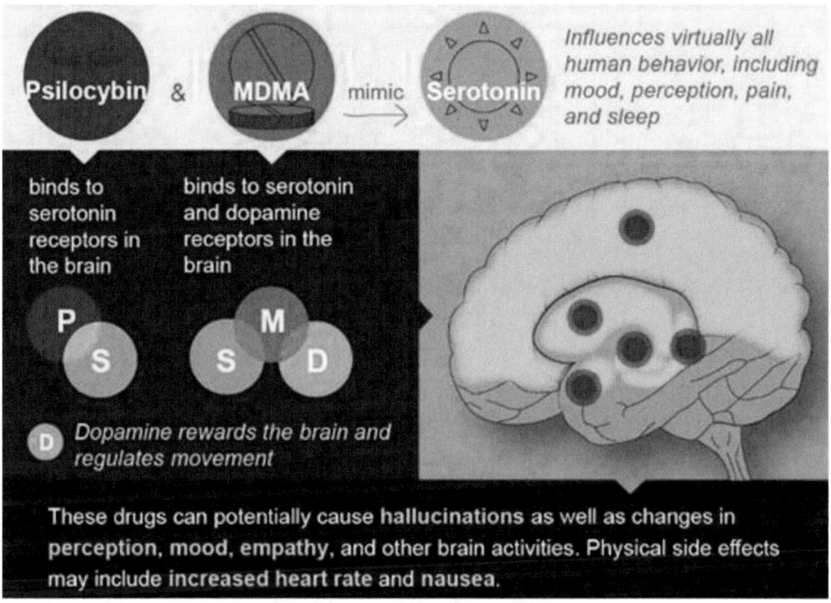

Source: GAO (analysis and illustration). | GAO-25-108021.

Figure 1. The Science Behind Psilocybin (Psychedelic Mushrooms) and MDMA.

What are the knowledge gaps? There is still much to learn about the potential benefits and adverse effects of psychedelics, including how they may be influenced by preexisting conditions or used in combination with psychotherapy. The effects of psychedelics can be difficult to predict and may depend on factors such as the dosage and unique biology of the person receiving the treatment. Moreover, data are limited since many of these clinical trials have been conducted on small groups of participants.

In blind clinical trials, participants are typically randomly selected to receive either a treatment or a placebo without being told which. This allows researchers to more easily differentiate between the effects of a given treatment and any placebo effect, in which participants who receive a placebo still report a benefit because they expect that the treatment will help.

Because of the distinct effects of psychedelics on recipients, it is difficult to prevent trial participants from knowing whether they received the treatment. This may complicate efforts to design such trials and interpret their findings. Clinical trials have tried to work around this by using an active placebo, such as a low dose of a psychedelic. Alternatively, researchers might compare the treatment with a more typical one, such as an SSRI.

Opportunities

- Mental health. Research has shown that psychedelics, such as psilocybin and MDMA, decrease fear and anxiety,
- with the potential to positively affect behavior in combination with therapy. For example, a clinical trial with patients with treatment-resistant PTSD demonstrated that combining MDMA and psychotherapy was effective, well- tolerated, and had no major adverse effects years later.
- Pain management. Psychedelics appear to show promise for patients with certain headache disorders and cancer pain. According to a few studies, drugs such as LSD and psilocybin appeared to alter pain perception by activating serotonin receptors and reducing inflammation.

Challenges

- Accessibility. LSD, MDMA, and psilocybin remain illegal at the federal level, categorized as Schedule I substances, which have no federally approved medical uses. To conduct research on these drugs, scientists need to follow several steps. These include obtaining permission from the U.S. Drug Enforcement Administration, finding clinical grade drugs to test, and identifying appropriate spaces in which to test and store these drugs.
- Federal approval. Difficulties associated with conducting large, blind trials of psychedelics have limited researchers' ability to determine the safety and effectiveness of these drugs, which is required for them to gain approval from the Food and Drug Administration (FDA). FDA approval is generally required before prescription drugs can be marketed for sale in the U.S.

Policy Context And Questions

- How could research be structured to help policymakers better understand any potential benefits and adverse effects of the medical use of psychedelics?
- How could research on medical use of psychedelics be conducted to better reflect requirements for FDA approval?
- What steps could policymakers take to weigh the potential benefits and risks of psychedelics, considering policy implications, resource demands, and patient needs?

Selected References

National Institute on Drug Abuse. "Psychedelic and Dissociative Drugs." Accessed January 21, 2025. https://nida.nih.gov/research-topics/psychedelic-dissociative-drugs.

A. Wem et al., "A Systematic Review of Study Design and Placebo Controls in Psychedelic Research," Psychedelic Medicine, vol. 2, no. 1 (March 2024).

Gao Support

The Government Accountability Office (GAO) meets congressional information needs in several ways, including by providing oversight, insight, and foresight on science and technology issues. GAO staff are available to brief on completed bodies of work or specific reports and answer follow- up questions. GAO also provides targeted assistance on specific science and technology topics to support congressional oversight activities and provide advice on legislative proposals.

For more information, contact: Karen L. Howard, PhD, at (202) 512-6888 or howardk@gao.gov Congressional Relations: A. Nicole Clowers, Managing Dir., (202) 512-4400, clowersa@gao.gov Public Affairs: Sarah Kaczmarek, Managing Dir., (202) 512-4800, kaczmareks@gao.gov.

This document is not an audit product and is subject to revision based on continued advances in science and technology. It contains information prepared by GAO to provide technical insight to legislative bodies or other external organizations. This document has been reviewed by Sterling Thomas, PhD, the Chief Scientist of the U.S. Government Accountability Office.

Staff Acknowledgments: Rich Hung (Assistant Director), Lauren Gomez (Analyst-in-Charge), Nicole Catanzarite, Cory Gerlach, Allison Henn, Rachael Johnson, Anika McMillon, and Jenique Meekins.

Source (cover photo): 24K-Production/stock.adobe.com. | GAO-25-108021.

Chapter 3

Evidence Brief: Psychedelic Medications for Mental Health and Substance Use Disorders*

U.S. Department of Veterans Affairs

Authors

Author roles, affiliations, and contributions to the present report (using the CRediT taxonomy) are summarized in the table below.

Author	Role and Affiliation	Report Contribution
Katherine M. Mackey, MD, MPP	Clinician Investigator, Evidence Synthesis Program (ESP) Coordinating Center, Portland VA Health Care System Portland, OR	Conceptualization, Methodology, Investigation, Formal analysis, Writing – original draft, Writing – review & editing, Supervision
Johanna K. Anderson, MPH	Senior Research Associate, ESP Coordinating Center, Portland VA Health Care System	Methodology, Investigation, Writing – original draft, Writing – review & editing, Project administration

* This is an edited, reformatted and augmented version of U.S. Department of Veterans Affairs, Evidence Synthesis Program Publication No. VA ESP Project #09-199; 2022, dated October 2022.

In: The Psychedelic Landscape
Editor: James P. Macintosh
ISBN: 979-8-89530-991-9

	Portland, OR	
Beth E. Williams, NP, MPH	Clinician Investigator, ESP Coordinating Center, Portland VA Health Care System Portland, OR	Investigation, Writing – original draft, Writing – review & editing
Rachel M. Ward, BA	Research Assistant, ESP Coordinating Center, Portland VA Health Care System Portland, OR	Project administration, Investigation
Nicholas J. Parr, PhD	Associate Director, ESP Coordinating Center, Portland VA Health Care System Portland, OR	Conceptualization, Methodology, Formal analysis, Writing – original draft, Writing – review & editing, Project administration

Preface

The VA Evidence Synthesis Program (ESP) was established in 2007 to provide timely and accurate syntheses of targeted health care topics of importance to clinicians, managers, and policymakers as they work to improve the health and health care of Veterans. These reports help:

- Develop clinical policies informed by evidence;
- Implement effective services to improve patient outcomes and to support VA clinical practice guidelines and performance measures; and
- Set the direction for future research to address gaps in clinical knowledge.

The program comprises four ESP Centers across the US and a Coordinating Center located in Portland, Oregon. Center Directors are VA clinicians and recognized leaders in the field of evidence synthesis with close ties to the AHRQ Evidence-based Practice Center Program. The Coordinating Center was created to manage program operations, ensure methodological consistency and quality of products, interface with stakeholders, and address urgent evidence needs. To ensure responsiveness to the needs of decision-makers, the program is governed by a Steering Committee composed of health system leadership and researchers. The program solicits nominations for review topics several times a year via the program website.

The present report was developed in response to a request from the VA Office of Research and Development (ORD) and VHA Office of Mental Health and Suicide Prevention (OMHSP). The scope was further developed with input from Operational Partners (below) and the ESP Coordinating Center review team.

Acknowledgments

The authors are grateful to Kathryn Vela, MLIS for literature searching, Sarah Young, MPH for study selection assistance, and the following individuals for their contributions to this project:

Operational Partners

Operational partners are system-level stakeholders who help ensure relevance of the review topic to the VA, contribute to the development of and approve final project scope and timeframe for completion, provide feedback on the draft report, and provide consultation on strategies for dissemination of the report to the field and relevant groups.

Ilse Wiechers, MD
Deputy Executive Director
Office of Mental Health and Suicide Prevention

Peer Reviewers

The Coordinating Center sought input from external peer reviewers to review the draft report and provide feedback on the objectives, scope, methods used, perception of bias, and omitted evidence (see Appendix D in Supplemental Materials for disposition of comments). Peer reviewers must disclose any relevant financial or non-financial conflicts of interest. Because of their unique clinical or content expertise, individuals with potential conflicts may be retained.

The Coordinating Center works to balance, manage, or mitigate any potential nonfinancial conflicts of interest identified.

Executive Summary

Key Findings

- In a clinical research setting, use of MDMA with intensive psychotherapy led by 2 mental health professionals may improve posttraumatic stress disorder (PTSD symptom severity and result in remission for some participants in the short term (1 month to 18 weeks) (low strength of evidence [SOE]). Findings are based on several small trials of adults with moderate to severe symptoms at baseline who did not improve with prior medication or therapy trials. Most studies did not include Veterans.
- Psilocybin-assisted psychotherapy may reduce depression severity and lead to sustained remission for some participants at 12 months compared to wait list controls, but these benefits were not observed when psilocybin-assisted psychotherapy was compared to intensive psychotherapy and daily escitalopram (low SOE).
- Psilocybin-assisted psychotherapy may reduce heavy drinking days and average daily alcohol consumption among adults with alcohol use disorder (low SOE).
- Ayahuasca use may be associated with a short-term reduction in depression symptoms and suicidality (low SOE). Whether ayahuasca is effective for substance use disorder treatment is unclear.
- Ibogaine may not reduce opioid withdrawal symptoms or short- term opioid use (low SOE) and has been associated with serious adverse events including prolonged QTc, cardiac arrhythmia, and death.
- Studies conducted in the US have predominantly included non-Veteran, young, non-Hispanic white populations with access to a clinical research center or treatment program. Whether benefits can be replicated in more diverse populations and treatment settings including within VHA is unclear.
- Critical gaps to address in future research include whether treatment effects vary according to patient characteristics and disease severity and whether benefits are durable over time. The feasibility of

implementing intensive psychotherapy protocols in real-world settings is another critical gap, as is determining how psychedelic treatments could fit into current standard of care and usual care pathways.

Background

The Evidence Synthesis Program Coordinating Center is responding to a request from the VA Office of Research and Development (ORD) and VHA Office of Mental Health and Suicide Prevention (OMHSP) for an Evidence Brief on the use of psychedelics for treating mental health and substance use disorders. Findings from this Evidence Brief will be used to inform VA research and clinical care.

Methods

To identify studies, we searched MEDLINE, Cochrane Database of Systematic Reviews, Cochrane Central Register of Controlled Trials, and other sources up to April 2022. We used prespecified criteria for study selection, data abstraction, and rating internal validity and strength of the evidence. See the Methods section and our PROSPERO protocol for full details of our methodology.

Clinical Bottom Line

MDMA-assisted psychotherapy for PTSD has been the most extensively studied therapeutic intervention involving psychedelics. Results from several small RCTs demonstrate that thistreatment may improve PTSD symptom severity to a clinically meaningful degree and lead to disease remission for some individuals in the short term. Similarly, psilocybin-assisted psychotherapy for depression shows some promise. However, study interventions included intensive psychotherapy protocols that may be challenging to implement in everyday practice. Moreover, US studies primarily enrolled young non-Hispanic white individuals and few studies included Veterans. Results may not be generalizable to more diverse populations and settings including within the Veterans Health Administration (VHA). Evidence on psychedelics for treatment of mental health and substance use disorders is therefore very preliminary. Several critical gaps need to be addressed by future research.

Overview

The term psychedelics refers to a group of substances that temporarily alter perception and mood and may impact numerous cognitive processes. The term is used to describe naturally derived substances with these properties, such as psilocybin, as well as synthetic substances like lysergic acid diethylamide (LSD) and 3,4-methylenedioxymethamphetamine (MDMA). Naturally derived psychedelics have been used for millennia, and starting in the 1940s through the 1960s, natural and synthetic psychedelics were used in clinical research as potential treatments for a range of medical conditions. However, study of psychedelics largely paused in the US in 1970 when most were codified as Schedule I drugs with no accepted medical use. In recent years, a growing number of researchers have been revisiting the potential therapeutic benefits of psychedelics and have sought out legal and regulatory pathways to study them.

Psychedelics and psychedelic-assisted psychotherapy have been proposed as novel treatments for adults with mental health and substance use disorders based on the supposition that intentional use of psychedelics over a limited period can disrupt problematic thought patterns, facilitate psychotherapy, and potentially lead to behavior change. New treatment options are needed given the limitations of existing therapies. The aim of this review is to inform VHA program planning by synthesizing available evidence on the benefits and harms of psychedelics as primary or adjunct treatment for mental health and substance use disorders.

From 2,532 potentially relevant articles, 15 RCTs and 23 observational studies (in 44 publications) met eligibility criteria. Studies enrolled adults with PTSD, depression, obsessive compulsive disorder (OCD), social anxiety, opioid use disorder (OUD), alcohol use disorder, tobacco use, or mixed substance use disorders and mood symptoms. Interventions involved treatment with MDMA, psilocybin, ayahuasca, 5-methoxy-N,N-dimethyltryptamine, and ibogaine with or without psychotherapy or other co-interventions.

The most extensively studied intervention involving psychedelics is MDMA-assisted psychotherapy for PTSD. We identified 9 small RCTs (including 1 study that pooled results from 6 smaller trials) and 3 observational studies of MDMA-assisted psychotherapy among adults with moderate or severe PTSD who had not improved with at least 1 past trial of medication or psychotherapy. All trials were conducted by researchers affiliated with the Multidisciplinary Association for Psychedelic Studies (MAPS) or were sponsored by this organization and thus had several features in common. Intervention group participants typically received MDMA 80– 125mg with or without a 40–62.5mg supplemental dose. Comparator group participants received an 0mg placebo or a low dose of MDMA (low-dose placebo) intended to maintain participant blinding by producing some sensations of having ingested a psychedelic. Intervention and control group participants underwent the same intensive psychotherapy protocol, typically consisting of several preparatory sessions and follow-up sessions in addition to day-long MDMA or placebo dosing sessions. Psychotherapy sessions were all co-led by 2 mental health professionals using a standardized therapy manual. If participants were receiving treatment for PTSD prior to the study start, they were required to stop it to avoid confounding and potential drug interactions with MDMA. Studies reported outcomes in terms of changes in mean total severity scores on the Clinician-Administered PTSD Scale (CAPS). Some studies reported whether participants experienced a clinically meaningful improvement in total CAPS score (defined as at least 30% improvement) and PTSD remission.

MDMA paired with intensive psychotherapy may reduce PTSD symptom severity and lead to clinically meaningful improvement and remission for some. In trials reporting these outcomes, 50% to 100% of participants experienced clinically meaningful improvements on CAPS total severity scores and remission rates ranged from 33% to 88% when assessed at 1 month to 18 weeks. Additionally, results of a meta-analysis of 7 trials indicate that participants receiving MDMA experienced significantly greater improvements in mean symptom severity compared with control group participants (pooled standardized mean difference in change scores = -0.91, 95% CI [-1.33, -0.50]). Symptoms among control group participants also improved in most studies regardless of the type of placebo used, although to a lesser degree than MDMA group participants. While the relative importance of different intervention components (MDMA, psychotherapy, and other factors such as participation effects) is unclear, a comparison of findings across trials using different forms of placebo suggests that benefits are at least partially attributable to the effects of MDMA. Although results are fairly consistent and direct, trial sample sizes are small and at risk of prognostic imbalance (a failure of randomization to balance groups on participants' responsiveness to treatment). Our confidence in these findings is low.

Other interventions involving psychedelics have been less extensively studied. Psilocybin- assisted psychotherapy for depression may reduce symptom severity and lead to sustained remission at 12 months for a proportion of recipients compared to wait list controls, but these same benefits were not observed (in a separate trial) when psilocybin-assisted psychotherapy was compared with the same psychotherapy protocol and daily escitalopram. We have low confidence in these findings, which are based on 1 small trial for each comparator. Ayahuasca use for depression may be associated with a reduction in short-term symptoms and suicidality.

However, our confidence in these findings is also low due to a smaller number of trials overall with small sample sizes and some inconsistency.

Among treatments evaluated for substance use disorders, we have low confidence that psilocybin-assisted psychotherapy for alcohol use disorder may reduce alcohol consumption (heavy drinking days and the number of drinks per day) based on results of 1 small trial.

Psilocybin has also been used as an adjunct to psychotherapy to reduce tobacco use, but results are limited to 1 small observational study and are insufficient to draw conclusions. Ibogaine, used most often to treat opioid withdrawal, did not improve withdrawal symptoms in 1 small trial despite observational data showing benefits. Unlike other psychedelics studied, ibogaine has been associated with serious adverse events, including death and cardiac events.

Psychedelic treatments for mental health and substance use disorders are still in an early phase of development and many gaps in the evidence exist, including whether treatment effects vary by patient characteristics or disease severity and whether observed benefits are maintained over time. Other critical gaps in the evidence include whether psychedelic treatment protocols are reproducible and scalable in real-world settings and whether the benefits of discontinuing mental health medications to undergo psychedelic treatments outweigh the risks. In addition to addressing these gaps, areas for future research include study of Veterans with combat-related trauma and study of more diverse populations, particularly with respect to race/ethnicity, socioeconomic status, and rurality.

ES Table. Summary of evidence

Outcome	Psychedelic	Evidence	Findings
Posttraumatic Stress Disorder			
Remission	MDMA	4 RCTs [1-4]	*Low SOE:* MDMA-assisted psychotherapy may result in PTSD remission
Clinically meaningful improvement	MDMA	4 RCTs [2-5]	*Low SOE:* MDMA-assisted psychotherapy may result in a clinically meaningful reduction in symptom burden (defined as a ≥30% improvement on CAPS total severity scores).
Difference in symptom change scores	MDMA	7 RCTs1-8 and 3 pre-post studies [9-11]	Low SOE: MDMA-assisted psychotherapy may reduce PTSD symptoms (in 7 trials, the pooled standardized mean difference in PTSD symptom change for intervention dose MDMA compared with 0mg or low-dose placebo is -0.91, 95% CI [-1.33, -0.50]).
Major Depressive Disorder			
	Psilocybin	1 RCT [12] and 3 pre-post studies [13-16][a]	Low SOE: Psilocybin-assisted psychotherapy may reduce depressive symptoms and lead to clinically meaningful improvement (defined as ≥ 50% improvement on GRID-HAMD) and/or remission in some individuals.
Depressive symptoms		1 RCT [17]	Low SOE: Psilocybin-assisted psychotherapy may not reduce depressive symptoms compared to psychotherapy and daily escitalopram.
	Ayahuasca	1 RCT18 and 2 pre-post studies [19, 20]	Low SOE: Ayahuasca may reduce depressive symptoms.
	Psilocybin	1 RCT [12]	Insufficient SOE: It is unclear whether psilocybin reduces suicidal ideation compared to no treatment.

ES Table. (Continued)

Outcome	Psychedelic	Evidence	Findings
		1 RCT [17]	*Insufficient SOE:* It is unclear whether psilocybin reduces suicidal ideation compared to escitalopram.
Suicidal ideation	Ayahuasca	1 RCT [18, 21] and 1 pre-post study [19, 22]	Insufficient SOE: It is unclear whether ayahuasca reduces suicidal ideation compared to placebo.
Opioid Use			
Opioid use	Ibogaine	1 RCT [23] and 3 pre-post studies [24-26]	*Low SOE:* Ibogaine may not reduce short-term opioid use compared to placebo.
Withdrawal	Ibogaine	1 RCT [23] and 5 pre-post Studies [24-28]	*Low SOE:* Ibogaine may not reduce short-term opioid withdrawal symptoms compared to placebo.
Alcohol Use Disorder			
	Psilocybin	1 RCT29 and 1 pre-post study [30]	*Low SOE:* Psilocybin may decrease drinking behavior.
Drinking behavior	MDMA	1 pre-post study [31]	*Insufficient SOE:* It is unclear whether MDMA decreases drinking behavior.
Tobacco Use			
Tobacco use	Psilocybin	1 pre-post study [32, 33]	Insufficient SOE: It is unclear whether psilocybin influences tobacco use.
Mixed Substance Use			
	Ayahuasca	1 pre-post study [34]	*Insufficient SOE:* It is unclear whether ayahuasca reduces substance use among participants of a substance use program.
Substance use	Ibogaine	1 pre-post study [35].	Insufficient SOE: It is unclear whether ibogaine reduces substance use in participants of a substance use program.

Outcome	Psychedelic	Evidence	Findings
Opiate or cocaine craving	Ibogaine	3 pre-post studies [36, 37]	Insufficient SOE: It is unclear whether ibogaine reduces opiate and cocaine craving.
Other Conditions			
Social anxiety symptoms	Ayahuasca	1 RCT [38]	*Insufficient SOE:* It is unclear whether ayahuasca improves symptoms in adults with social anxiety disorder.
Obsessive compulsive symptoms	Psilocybin	1 pre-post study [39]	*Insufficient SOE:* It is unclear whether psilocybin impacts symptoms in adults with obsessive compulsive disorder.
Mood and anxiety symptoms	Ibogaine and 5-MeO-DMT	1 pre-post study [40]	*Insufficient SOE:* It is unclear whether ibogaine reduces PTSD, depressive, or anxiety symptoms in Veterans of US special operations forces.

Notes. a Studies included overlapping populations, 2 studies included comparison to healthy, non-treated control groups.

Abbreviations. 5-MeO-DMT=5-methoxy-N,N-dimethyltryptamine; CAPS=Clinician-Administered PTSD Scale; CI=confidence interval; GRID-HAMD=GRID-Hamilton Depression Rating Scale; MDMA=3,4- methylenedioxymeth amphetamine; PTSD=posttraumatic stress disorder; RCT=randomized controlled trial; SOE=strength of evidence.

Evidence Brief Introduction Purpose

The ESP Coordinating Center (ESP CC) is responding to a request from the VA Office of Research and Development (ORD) and VHA Office of Mental Health and Suicide Prevention (OMHSP) for an Evidence Brief on the use of psychedelic substances for treating mental health and substance use disorders. Findings from this Evidence Brief will be used to inform VA research activities and clinical care in the areas of mental health and substance use disorder treatment.

Background

The term psychedelics refers to a group of substances that temporarily alter perception and mood and may impact numerous cognitive processes [41, 42]. The term is used to describe naturally derived substances with these properties, such as psilocybin, as well as synthetic substances like lysergic acid diethylamide (LSD) and 3,4-methylenedioxymethamphetamine (MDMA) [43]. Over time, various other terms have been used to describe and distinguish psychedelic substances including hallucinogens, psychotomimetics, psycholytics, and in the case of MDMA, entactogens [44, 45]. For brevity, the term psychedelics is used in this report. Table 1 presents the derivation and proposed mechanism of selected psychedelic substances.

Naturally derived psychedelics have been used for millennia, often in the context of religious or spiritual practices. From the 1940s through the 1960s, psychedelics were studied in clinical research as potential treatments for a range of medical conditions including mood and substance use disorders. Despite some promising early findings, [46]. research on psychedelic substances largely ceased in the US with passage of the 1970 Controlled Substances Act, [47] which codified psychedelics as drugs with no accepted medical use [48]. In recent years, a growing number of researchers have been revisiting the potential therapeutic benefits of psychedelics and have sought out legal and regulatory pathways to study them. Alongside renewed research interest, increasing media attention has raised public awareness of potential therapeutic uses of psychedelics. Although psychedelics are still categorized as Schedule I controlled substances, MDMA and psilocybin have received "breakthrough therapy" designation from the Food and Drug Administration (FDA) to be studied in adults with post-traumatic stress disorder (PTSD) and treatment-resistant depression, respectively [49, 50]. In 2020, Oregon was the first state to create a regulatory framework for therapeutic psilocybin use, [51] with plans to allow psilocybin service centers with licensed facilitators to begin operating in 2023.

Most psychedelics used in research act as agonists or partial agonists at serotonin 5- hydroxytryptamine 2A receptors in the brain. This group includes LSD, psilocybin, and ayahuasca and are often referred to as classical psychedelics. In clinical contexts, classical psychedelics have most often been used to treat depression and substance use disorders. For these indications, it is thought that psychedelic use can disrupt problematic thought patterns and potentially lead to behavior change [30]. So-called non-classical psychedelics include MDMA and ibogaine. MDMA has most often been used to treat

PSTD, as it is thought to reduce the anxiety and fear that can accompany memories of past trauma and thereby facilitate psychotherapy [52].

MDMA works by complex mechanisms to promote release of serotonin, (nor)epinephrine, and dopamine and may stimulate signaling of oxytocin and other hormones. Ibogaine, used predominantly to treat substance use disorders, has a poorly understood mechanism of action but may work through a mix of neurotransmitters [23]. In general, psychedelics are intended to be used for therapeutic purposes once or a limited number of times and are not meant to be used as long- term treatment of mental health or substance use disorders.

Table 1. Characteristics of selected psychedelic substances

Substance	Derivation	Proposed Mechanism of Action
Ayahuasca, a brewed drink containing N, N-dimethyltryptamine (N, N-DMT) and harmine, harmaline, and/or tetrahydroharmine	*Psychotria viridis* and *Banisteriopsis caapi*, plants indigenous to South America	Serotonin agonist (N, N-DMT) and monoamine oxidase inhibition (harmine, harmaline, and tetrahydroharmine)
5-methoxy-N, N-dimethyltryptamine (5-MeO-DMT)	Venomous secretions of the Sonoran Desert/Colorado River toad and certain plant species	Serotonin agonist
Ibogaine	*Tabernanthe iboga* and *Voacanga africana*, shrubs indigenous to West Africa	Poorly characterized; acts at multiple neurotransmitters
LSD (lysergic acid diethylamide)	First synthesized at Sandoz Laboratories (Switzerland) in 1943	Serotonin agonist
MDMA (3,4-methylenedioxymethamphetamine)	First synthesized at Merck Pharmaceuticals (Germany) in 1912	Promotes release of serotonin, (nor)epinephrine, and dopamine and may stimulate signaling of oxytocin and other hormones

Table 1. (Continued)

Substance	Derivation	Proposed Mechanism of Action
Mescaline (3,4,5-trimethoxyphenethylamine)	Peyote cactus, San Pedro cactus, and other cacti species indigenous to North and South America	Serotonin agonist
Psilocybin	*Psilocybe* and other mushroom species, found worldwide	Serotonin agonist

The effectiveness of psychedelics is thought to in part depend on the treatment intentions of the patient and the physical environment in which psychedelics are administered ("set" and "setting," respectively) [53]. In a clinical research setting, psychedelics are typically administered over a day-long dosing session in a monitored and controlled environment designed to promote relaxation and minimize disruption (eg, in a comfortable setting with the participant wearing eyeshades and listening to pre-selected music through headphones). In many cases, a specific number of structured psychotherapy sessions are delivered before and after psychedelic dosing. For example, treatment may involve 1–2 psychotherapy sessions before an extended 8–10-hour session in which the therapist or other health care personnel administers the psychedelic substance and monitors the participant for safety. The psychedelic session may then by followed by additional psychotherapy sessions to debrief and analyze the participant's psychedelic experience, often referred to as integration sessions. The cycle of psychedelic administration followed by post-psychedelic integration sessions may be repeated 2–3 times. Contemporary studies of psychedelic substances have used different treatment protocols for a range of disorders and have employed study designs with differing research aims (eg, safety, feasibility, efficacy, effectiveness, comparative effectiveness).

Given the prevalence of mental health and substance use disorders within the Veteran population, any novel or emerging treatments with the potential to improve clinical outcomes are of great interest to VA patients, researchers, and other stakeholders [54]. Although VA services include comprehensive care for mental health and substance use disorders in a range of settings including residential rehabilitation, [55] a proportion of Veterans may not experience improvement with existing treatment options [56]. Therefore, psychedelics and psychedelic-assisted psychotherapy represent a potential new option for those with mental health or substance use disorders who have not responded to available treatments. The aim of this review is to inform VHA program planning by synthesizing available evidence on the benefits and harms of psychedelics as primary or adjunct treatment for mental health and substance use disorders.

Methods

Protocol

A preregistered protocol for this review can be found on the PROSPERO international prospective register of systematic reviews (http://www.crd.york.ac.uk/PROSPERO/; registration number CRD42022330065).

Key Questions

The following key questions (KQs) were the focus of this review:

KQ1: What are the benefits and harms of psychedelic substances as primary or adjunct treatment for mental health and substance use disorders?

KQ1a: Do benefits or harms of psychedelic substances vary based on patient characteristics (eg, race/ethnicity, gender identity, age, comorbid mental health or substance use disorders, index trauma type), disorder type, or disorder severity?

Analytic Framework

The analytic framework shown in Figure 1 provides a conceptual overview of this review. The population of interest was adults with mental health and/or substance use disorders. Eligible outcomes included mental health and/or substance use disorder symptoms (Key Questions 1 and 1a) and treatment harms (Key Question 1). Whether benefits and/or risks of the intervention differ by patient characteristics (e. g., patient demographics, comorbidities, disease severity) or treatment protocol (e. g., number of sessions, dosage) was also of interest (Key Question 1a).

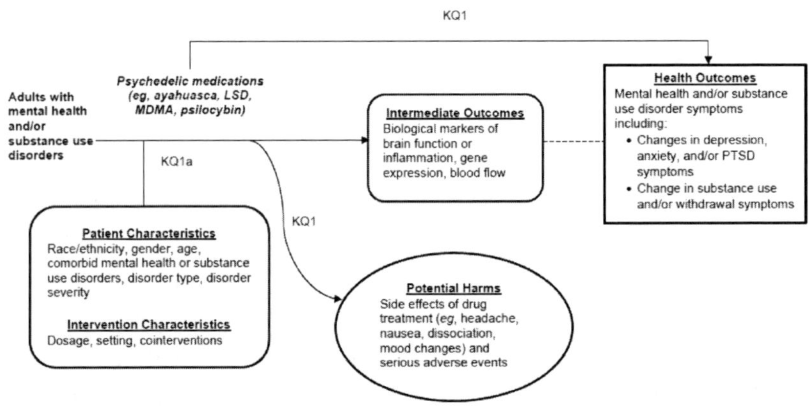

Abbreviations. LSD=lysergic acid; MDMA=3,4-methylenedioxymethamphetamine; PSTD=posttraumatic stress disorder.

Figure 1. Analytic Framework.

Eligibility Criteria

The ESP included studies that met the following criteria:

Population	Adults with mental health and/or substance use disorders (*eg*, depression, PTSD, opioid use disorder). Studies among adults with serious medical illness (*eg*, terminal cancer, end-stage renal disease) with mental health symptoms or substance use were excluded.
Intervention	Psychedelic substances (*eg*, ayahuasca/DMT, LSD, MDMA, psilocybin; excluding cannabinoids and ketamine) used as a primary treatment or as an adjunct to psychotherapy or another treatment (*ie*, psychedelic-assisted therapy)
Comparator	Any (*eg*, placebo, treatment as usual)
Outcomes	Disorder symptoms Quality of life/functioning Harms (eg, treatment-emergent adverse events)
Study Design	Systematic reviews, randomized controlled trials (RCTs), and concurrently controlled cohort studies. We considered

longitudinal studies without comparison groups (ie, pre-post studies) and case series (ie, N > 1) only to address gaps in evidence from studies with control groups. We excluded case reports (ie, N = 1).

Data Sources and Searches

To identify articles relevant to the key questions, a research librarian searched Ovid MEDLINE, Ovid PsycINFO, and ClinicalTrials.gov, as well as AHRQ, Cochrane Database of Systematic Reviews, and HSR&D through April 2022 using terms for hallucinogen, psychedelic, and mental disorders (see Appendix A in Supplemental Materials for complete search strategies). Additional citations were identified from hand-searching reference lists. We limited the search to published and indexed articles involving human subjects available in the English language. Study selection was based on the eligibility criteria described above. We excluded studies of cannabis and ketamine (a dissociative anesthetic) because these substances have distinct mechanisms of action compared to psychedelics and have been reviewed extensively elsewhere [57-59]. To ensure that study findings would be most applicable to contemporary diagnostic and management practices, we limited inclusion to studies published in 1994 or after to coincide with the publication of Diagnostic and Statistical Manual of Mental Disorders-4 [60].

Titles, abstracts, and full-text articles were independently reviewed by 2 investigators. All disagreements were resolved by consensus or discussion with a third investigator.

Data Abstraction and Assessment

Effect information and population, intervention, and comparator characteristics were abstracted from all included studies. The internal validity (risk of bias) of each included study was rated using the Cochrane risk of bias tools [61, 62]. All data abstraction and internal validity ratings were first completed by 1 investigator and then checked by another; disagreements were resolved by consensus or discussion with a third investigator.

We graded the strength of the evidence for each outcome based on the AHRQ Methods Guide for Comparative Effectiveness Reviews [63]. This approach provides a rating of confidence in reported findings based on study methodology (design, quality, and risk of bias), consistency (whether effects are in the same direction and have a consistent magnitude), directness (whether assessed outcomes are clinically important to patients and providers), and precision of findings (eg, confidence intervals). For this review, we applied the following general algorithm: high strength evidence consisted of multiple, large trials with low risk of bias, consistent and precise findings, and clinically relevant outcomes; moderate strength evidence consisted of multiple trials with low to unclear risk of bias, consistent and precise findings, and clinically relevant outcomes; low strength evidence consisted of a single trial or multiple small trials and/or multiple observational studies, with unclear to high risk of bias, consistent findings, and clinically relevant outcomes; and insufficient evidence consisted of a single or multiple small observational studies with unclear or high risk of bias, or no available studies.

Synthesis

We grouped studies by disorder and psychedelic type and described mean changes in symptoms, when possible including whether the psychedelic intervention led to a clinically meaningful improvement in symptom severity (as defined by the study) or disease remission. We focused synthesis on disorder-specific outcomes (eg, PTSD symptom severity) and did not describe outcomes related to the psychedelic experience itself or measures of mood or perception not directly relevant to the disorder being treated.

Trials of MDMA-assisted psychotherapy for PTSD used the Clinician-Administered PTSD Scale (CAPS) total severity score (CAPS-4 or CAPS-5, rated 0-136 or 0-80, respectively) to report mean changes in PTSD symptom severity from baseline for intervention and comparator groups. For these trials, we synthesized bias-adjusted standardized mean differences (SMDs; Hedges' g) in CAPS change scores between groups using random-effects meta-analysis. Precision of study- level and pooled mean differences is reported using 95% confidence intervals (CIs), which were also used to evaluate statistical significance at a significance level of .05. Heterogeneity in true study effects was estimated using restricted maximum-likelihood estimation and is presented as 95% prediction intervals (PIs). A PI encompassing values that substantively differ in direction and/or magnitude from the pooled MD indicates the presence of considerable heterogeneity [64, 65]. The Hartung-Knapp-Sidik-Jonkman method was used to better account for uncertainty in estimating the amount of heterogeneity [66]. Meta-analyses were conducted using the metafor [67] package for R (R Foundation for Statistical Computing, Vienna, Austria).

Results

Literature Flow

The literature flow diagram (Figure 2) summarizes the results of the study selection process (a full list of excluded studies is available in Appendix B in Supplemental Materials).

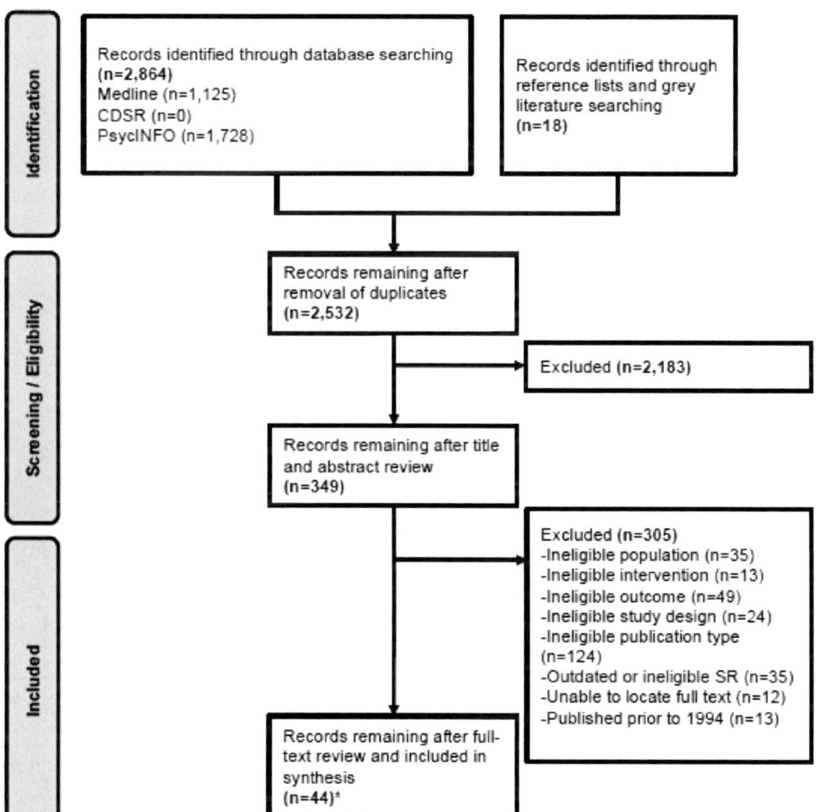

Notes. 38 studies in 44 publications.
Abbreviations. CDSR=Cochrane Database of Systematic Reviews; SR=systematic review.

Figure 2. Literature Flowchart.

Literature Overview

Our search identified 2,532 potentially relevant articles. We included 38 studies (in 44 publications), [1-36, 38-40, 68-71] which are summarized in Table 2. Additional study details are provided in each section below and in Appendix C in the Supplemental Materials. Fifteen studies were RCTs, 21 were pre-post studies, and 2 were cohorts compared to healthy, non-treated controls. Participants included adults with PTSD, depression, obsessive compulsive disorder (OCD), social anxiety, opioid use disorder (OUD), alcohol use disorder, tobacco use, and mixed substance use disorders and mood symptoms. In most cases, studies described participants as having moderate to severe disease who had not improved with past treatment trials (more detail is provided in each section below). Adults with a personal or family history of a psychotic disorder or bipolar I disorder were generally excluded from study participation, as were those with major medical comorbidities and pregnant individuals. Studies inconsistently reported whether participants had previously used psychedelics; in some cases, recent or past use was a reason for exclusion. Sample sizes ranged from 3–191; the largest study [37] (N = 191) was of adults seeking treatment for opioid or cocaine dependence with ibogaine.

Most studies (61%) were conducted exclusively outside the US, with Brazil and the United Kingdom being the most common locations. However, most studies did not report whether participants were local to the region or had travelled there for treatment purposes. Given the legal restrictions on psychedelic use in many locations, it is likely that some studies included participants from multiple countries. Participant mean age ranged from 25 to 51 in studies reporting this information. Among studies conducted completely or partially in the US, most participants were non-Hispanic white. Only 1 study exclusively enrolled US Veterans: a pre-post study of 51 Special Operations Forces Veterans who were treated for a range of mood symptoms with ibogaine and 5-MeO-DMT during a 3-day residential program in Mexico [40]. Three studies of MDMA-assisted psychotherapy for PTSD included Veterans (range: 14–85% of total sample) [1, 2, 11].

MDMA was the only psychedelic used in studies of adults with PTSD. Psilocybin and ayahuasca were used most often in studies of adults with depression or substance use. Ibogaine was used in studies of adults with OUD and mixed substance use disorders. No studies of LSD published after 1994 met our inclusion criteria. Most studies of MDMA and psilocybin included intensive psychotherapy as a co-intervention. In contrast, most studies of ayahuasca and ibogaine did not include a therapy co-intervention. Comparators in RCTs included 0mg placebo, low-dose placebo (a lower dose of the same psychedelic used in the intervention group), or another non-psychedelic medication (eg, escitalopram, diphenhydramine). Most studies of PTSD required participants to discontinue usual mental health treatments except for sedative hypnotics or anxiolytics used between MDMA sessions (2 trials did not clearly report whether discontinuation was required). In most studies of depression, participants were not on other medical treatments for depression or were required to discontinue their usual treatments (usually antidepressant medications including selective serotonin reuptake inhibitors) for at least 2 weeks prior to the study period. Detail on whether studies did or did not require participants to discontinue their usual treatment are in Appendix C of the Supplemental Materials.

Most trials of MDMA for PTSD and psilocybin for depression were designed to evaluate treatment efficacy, while studies of ayahuasca and ibogaine were more often designed to evaluate safety and feasibility. Common methodological limitations of RCTs were small sample sizes, unclear intervention adherence, and unclear handling and/or extent of missing data. Observational studies, which mostly used a pre-post design, were limited by the potential for selection bias and lack of control groups.

We identified 70 in-progress studies (see Appendix E in Supplemental Materials) examining psychedelic use in populations with mood disorders, anxiety disorders, and substance use disorders.

Posttraumatic Stress Disorder

In a clinical research setting, MDMA-assisted psychotherapy may reduce PTSD symptoms, resulting in a clinically meaningful improvement (defined as a reduction in CAPS score by at least 30%) and/or disease remission in the short term (1 month to 18 weeks). We have low confidence in these findings based on several small trials with consistent and direct results with some imprecision (wide confidence intervals). Few serious adverse events were reported across studies, and only 1 event was ultimately attributed to MDMA.

Table 2. Characteristics of included studies by treatment indication

Study	Location(s)	Study Design	Sample Size	Follow-up	Psychedelic(s)	Co-Intervention(s)	Comparator(s)	Risk of Bias Rating[a]
PTSD								
Bouso 2008 [69]	Spain	RCT	6	12 months	MDMA	Psychotherapy	0mg placebo	High
Mitchell 2021 [1]	US, Canada,	RCT	90	18 weeks	MDMA	Psychotherapy	0mg placebo	Some
	& Israel							concerns
Mithoefer 2011 [3]	US, Canada,	RCT	20	2 months –	MDMA	Psychotherapy	0mg placebo	Some
Mithoefer 2013 [8]	& Israel			mean 45 months				concerns
Mithoefer 2018 [2]	US	RCT	26	1 month	MDMA	Psychotherapy	Low-dose placebo	Low
Mithoefer 2019 [68][b]	US, Canada,	RCT	105	1–2	MDMA	Psychotherapy	0mg or low-dose	Low
	Switzerland,			months			placebo	
	& Israel							
Oehen 2013 [5]	Switzerland	RCT	12	12 months	MDMA	Psychotherapy	Low-dose placebo	Some
								concerns
Ot'alora 2018 [4]	US	RCT	28	1 month	MDMA	Psychotherapy	Low-dose placebo	Some
								concerns
NCT01689740 [6]	Israel	RCT	8	1 month	MDMA	Psychotherapy	Low-dose placebo	Not rated
NCT01958593 [7]	Canada	RCT	6	1 month	MDMA	Psychotherapy	0mg placebo	Not rated
Jardim 2021 [9]	Brazil	Pre-post	3	2 months	MDMA	Psychotherapy	NA	High
Monson 2020 [10]	US &	Pre-post	12	6 months	MDMA	Psychotherapy	NA	High
	Canada							
Wang 2021 [11]	US &	Pre-post	37	18 weeks	MDMA	Psychotherapy	NA	High
	Canada							
Major Depressive	*Disorder*							
Carhart-Harris 2021 [17]	UK	RCT	59	6 weeks	Psilocybin	Psychotherapy	Low-dose placebo and escitalopram	Some concerns

Study	Location(s)	Study Design	Sample Size	Follow-up	Psychedelic(s)	Co-Intervention(s)	Comparator(s)	Risk of Bias Rating[a]
Davis 2021 [12]	US	RCT	24	12 months	Psilocybin	Psychotherapy	Delayed treatment	Low
Gukasyan 2022 [70]							(wait list control)	
Palhano-Fontes 2019 [18]	Brazil	RCT	29	1 week	Ayahuasca	None	0mg placebo	Some concerns
Zeifman 2021 [22]								
Carhart-Harris 2016 [13]	UK	Pre-post	20	6 months	Psilocybin	Psychotherapy	NA	High
Carhart-Harris 2018 [14]								
Lyons 2018 [15]	UK	Cohort	30	1 week	Psilocybin	Psychotherapy	Healthy, non-	High
							treated controls	
Stroud 2018 [16]	UK	Cohort	32	1 month	Psilocybin	Psychotherapy	Healthy, non-	High
							treated controls	
Osorio 2015 [20]	Brazil	Pre-post	6	21 days	Ayahuasca	None	NA	High
Sanches 2016 [19]	Brazil	Pre-post	17	21 days	Ayahuasca	None	NA	High
Zeifman 2021 [22]								
Opioid Use								
Glue 2016 [23]	New Zealand	RCT	27	~9 days	Noribogainec	None	0mg placebo	Some
								concerns
Brown 2018 [24]	Mexico	Pre-post	30	12 months	Ibogaine	None	NA	High
Davis 2017 [25]	Mexico	Pre-post	88	3 months-3	Ibogaine	Detoxification	NA	High
				years		program		
Knuijver 2022 [27]	The	Pre-post	14	24 hours	Ibogaine	None	NA	High
	Netherlands							
Malcolm 2018 [28]	Mexico	Pre-post	50	48 hours	Ibogaine	Detoxification	NA	Unclear
						program		
Noller 2018 [26]	New Zealand	Pre-post	14	12 months	Ibogaine	Diazepam and	NA	High

Table 2. (Continued)

Study	Location(s)	Study Design	Sample Size	Follow-up	Psychedelic(s)	Co-Intervention(s)	Comparator(s)	Risk of Bias Rating[a]
						zopiclone		
Alcohol Use								
Bogenschutz 2022 [29]	US	RCT	95	36 weeks	Psilocybin	Psychotherapy	Diphenhydramine	Low
Bogenschutz 2015 [30]	US	Pre-post	10	36 weeks	Psilocybin	Psychotherapy	NA	High
Sessa 2021 [31]	UK	Pre-post	14	9 months	MDMA	Psychotherapy	NA	High
Tobacco Use								
Johnson 2014 [32]	US	Pre-post	15	6-16	Psilocybin	Psychotherapy	NA	High
Johnson 2017 [33]				months				
Cocaine and Cannabis Use								
Thomas 2013 [34]	Canada	Pre-post	12	6 months	Ayahuasca	Participation in 4-	NA	High
						day retreat		
Mash 2018 [37]	St. Kitts	Pre-post	191	1 month	Ibogaine	Inpatient	NA	High
						detoxification		
						program		
Mash 2001 [71]	St. Kitts	Pre-post	32	36 hours-	Ibogaine	Inpatient	NA	High
				10 days		detoxification		
						program		
Mash 2000 [36]	St. Kitts	Pre-post	27	1 month	Ibogaine	Inpatient	NA	High
						detoxification		
						program		
Schenberg 2014 [35]	Brazil	Pre-post	75	NR	Ibogaine	Psychotherapy	NA	High
Other Conditions								
Davis 2020 [40]	Mexico	Pre-post	51	1 month-2	Ibogaine	Group therapy	NA	High

Study	Location(s)	Study Design	Sample Size	Follow-up	Psychedelic(s)	Co-Intervention(s)	Comparator(s)	Risk of Bias Rating[a]
				years	5-MeO-DMT			
Dos Santos 2021 [38]	Brazil	RCT	17	3 weeks	Ayahuasca	None	0mg placebo	Some concerns
Moreno 2006 [39]	US	Pre-post	17	3 weeks	Psilocybin	None	NA	High

Notes.

[a] Full details of quality assessments are in Appendix C of Supplemental Materials;

[b] Pooled analysis of 6 studies: Mithoefer 2011, Mithoefer 2018, Oehen 2013, Otalora 2018, NCT01958593, and NCT01689740;

[c] Ibogaine active metabolite.

Abbreviations. PTSD=posttraumatic stress disorder; RCT=randomized controlled trial; UK=United Kingdom; US=United States.

We identified 7 unique RCTs [1-7] of MDMA-assisted psychotherapy compared to psychotherapy with a 0mg placebo or low-dose placebo, and 1 RCT [68] that pooled results from 6 of these trials. Studies used the CAPS total severity score (CAPS-4 or CAPS-5, rated 0–136 or 0–80, respectively) to report mean change from baseline in PTSD symptom severity for intervention and comparator groups. CAPS is conducted by a semi-structured interview that accesses an individual's trauma history as defined by the Diagnostic and Statistical Manual of Mental Disorders. All studies included participants with moderate (total severity score 40–59 on CAPS- 4 [72] and 23–34 on CAPS-51) or severe (≥ 60 on CAPS-4 and ≥35 on CAPS-5) symptoms at baseline (Table 3). Most studies included participants who had been experiencing PTSD symptoms for years and had previously undergone at least 1 medication or psychotherapy trial.

Participants assigned to intervention groups received MDMA 80–125mg with or without a 40–62.5mg supplemental dose. Three studies used a 0mg placebo, and 4 studies used a low-dose placebo (MDMA 25–40mg with or without a 15mg supplemental dose). Low-dose placebos were intended to maintain participant blinding by producing some sensations of having ingested a psychedelic but without the same therapeutic psychedelic effect as the active treatment dose. Intervention and control group participants underwent the same intensive psychotherapy protocol, which typically consisted of 2–3 preparatory sessions, 2–3 MDMA or placebo dosing sessions, and 4–6 follow-up sessions (integration sessions) which were all co-led by 2 mental health professionals. More information regarding the MDMA dosing sessions is available in Appendix C of the Supplemental Materials. All trials were conducted by researchers affiliated with the Multidisciplinary Association for Psychedelic Studies (MAPS) or were sponsored by this organization and all reported using the same standardized manual to guide psychotherapy sessions (publicly available at http://maps.org/treatment-manual). No study compared MDMA- assisted psychotherapy to another active treatment (I, e, psychotherapy paired with a different psychedelic at therapeutic dosages) or to no treatment. Follow-up duration in most trials was 1–2 months.

Table 3. Psychedelic-assisted psychotherapy for PTSD: study characteristics

Study Sample Size[a]	Patient Characteristics	(SD) CAPS Baseline[b]	Mean (SD) Symptom Duration	Past Treatment(s)	Psychedelic Dos	Psychotherapy Protocol[c] Total Number of Sessions and Duration (Hours	Comparator
RCTs							
Bouso, 2008 [69][d] N=6	Mean age: 36 % female: 100 % non-Hispanic White: 0%	NR	NR	At least 1 standard treatment (not further defined)	MDMA 50–75mg, 1 dosing session	3 90-min sessions before and after a single 8-hour MDMA session 7 sessions (17 hours)	0mg placebo
Mitchell, 2021 [1] N=79	Mean age: 41 % female: 66 % non-Hispanic White: 90	CAPS-5: 44.1 (6.04)	14 (12) years	NR	MDMA Session 1: 120mg Sessions 2-3: 180mg	3 90-min preparatory sessions, 3 8-hour MDMA sessions, and 9 90-min integration sessions 15 sessions (42 hours)	0mg placebo
Mithoefer, 20113 & Mithoefer, 2013 [8] N=20	Mean age: 40 % female: 85 % non-Hispanic White: 100	CAPS-4: 79.4 (22.4)	248 (173) months	At least 1 pharmacotherapy or psychotherap	MDMA Sessions 1-2: 125mg ±supplemental 62.5mg	2 90-min preparatory sessions, 2 all-day MDMA sessions and overnight clinic stays, 8 90-min integration sessions 12 sessions (~35 hours)	0mg placebo
Mithoefer, 2018 [2] N=19	Mean age: 37 % female: 27 % non-Hispanic White: 85	CAPS-4: 87.1 (16.4)[e]	85 (64) months	At least 3 months of SSRI or SNRI treatment and 6 months of psychotherapy	MDMA *Sessions 1-2: 75mg or 125mg ± supplemental half-dose*	3 90-min preparatory sessions, 2 8-hour MDMA sessions and overnight clinic stays, 6 90-min integration sessions *11 sessions (34-42 hours)*	

Table 3. (Continued)

Study Sample Size[a]	Patient Characteristics	(SD) CAPS Baseline[b]	Mean (SD) Symptom Duration	Past Treatment(s)	Psychedelic Dos	Psychotherapy Protocol[c] Total Number of Sessions and Duration (Hours	Comparator
Mithoefer 2019 [68][f] N=105	Mean age: 41 % female: 61 % non-Hispanic White: 92	CAPS-4: 84.5 (18.4)	215.3 (190) months	Pharmacotherapy or psychotherapy	MDMA Sessions 1-2: 75mg, 100mg, or 125 mg	2-3 90-min preparatory sessions, 2 8-hour MDMA sessions and overnight clinic stays, and 3-4 90-min integration sessions 7–9 sessions (24–27 hours)	0mg or lowdose placebo
Oehen, 2013 [5] N=12	Mean age: 41 % female: 83 Race/ethnicity NR	CAPS-4: 65.4 (11.7)[e]	18.3 (12) years	At least 3 months of SSRI treatment and 6 months of psychothera	MDMA Sessions 1-3: 125mg + 62.5mg supplemental dose	3 preparatory sessions, 3 8-hour MDMA sessions and overnight clinic stays, 12 integration sessions 18 sessions (NR)	Low-dose placebo
Ot'alora, 2018 [4] N=18	Mean age: 42 % female: 68 % non-Hispanic White: 93	CAPS-4: 91.9 (17.4)[e]	353 (232) months	At least 1 pharmacotherapy or psychotherapy	MDMA *Sessions 1-2: 100 or 125mg*	3 90-min preparatory sessions, 2 8-hour MDMA sessions, and 6 integration sessions *10 sessions (NR)*	Low-dose placebo
NCT01689740[6] N =8	Mean age: NR % female: 38 % non-Hispanic White: 87	Moderate - severe (CAPS NR)	> 6 months	NR	MDMA *Sessions 1-2: 125mg + 62.5mg supplemental dose*	3 preparatory sessions, 2 MDMA sessions, and 2 integration sessions *7 sessions (NR)*	Low - dose placebo

Study Sample Size[a]	Patient Characteristics	(SD) CAPS Baseline[b]	Mean (SD) Symptom Duration	Past Treatment(s)	Psychedelic Dos	Psychotherapy Protocol[c] Total Number of Sessions and Duration (Hours	Comparator
NCT01958593 [7] N=6	Mean age: 48 % female: 50 % non-Hispanic White: 83	Moderatesevere (CAPS NR)	> 6 months	NR	MDMA *Sessions 1-2: dose NR*	3 preparatory sessions, 2 MDMA sessions, and 2 integrative therapy sessions *7 sessions (NR)*	0mg placebo
Observational Studies							
Jardim, 2021 [9] N=3	Mean age: 40 % female: 67 % non-Hispanic White: 67	CAPS-4: 80 (7.5) [e]	NR	At least 1 pharmacotherapy or psychotherapy	MDMA Session 1 :112.5mg Sessions 2-3: 187.5mg	3 90-min preparatory sessions, 3 8-hour MDMA sessions, and 9 90-min integrative therapy sessions 15 sessions (42 hours)	None
Monson, 2020 [10] N=12 (6 couples)	Mean age: 47 % female: 50 % non-Hispanic White: 10	CAPS-5: 41.42 (5.76)	NR	Pharmacotherapy or psychotherapy	MDMA Session 1: 75mg Session 2: 100mg second session ± suppl. half-dose	5 preparatory CBCT sessions, 2 MDMA 6–8 hour MDMA sessions, 2 1.25 hour integration sessions, 8 post MDMA CBCT sessions 19 sessions (NR)	None
Wang, 2021 [11] N=37	Mean age: 36 % female: 60 % non-Hispanic White: 73	CAPS-5: 45.4 (7.2)	*10 (11) years*	Antidepressant (73%) or psychotherapy (52%)	MDMA *120–150mg in divided doses; 3 dosing sessions*	3 preparatory sessions, 3 6–8- hour MDMA sessions and overnight clinic stays, and 9 integration sessions *15 sessions (NR)*	None

Notes.

[a] Analytic sample;

[b] CAPS total severity score, range for CAPS-4 0-136 and range for CAPS-5 0-80;

[c] All sessions led by 2 co-therapists; Manualized therapy was conducted in accordance with the MDMA-assisted therapy treatment manual (http://maps.org/treatment-manual) unless otherwise specified.

[d] Study terminated early and not included in overall SOE rating;

[e] Weighted means calculated across intervention/comparator groups; f Pooled analysis of 6 studies: Mithoefer 2011, Mithoefer 2018, Oehen 2013, Otalora 2018, NCT01958593, and NCT01689740.

Abbreviations. CAPS=Clinician Administered PTSD Scale for Diagnostic and Statistical Manual of Mental Disorders; CBCT=cognitive behavioral conjoint therapy; MDMA=3,4-methylenedioxy-methamphetamine; NR=not reported; PTSD=posttraumatic stress disorder; RCT=randomized controlled trial; SSRI=selective serotonin reuptake inhibitor; SNRI=serotonin and norepinephrine reuptake inhibitor; UK=United Kingdom; US=United States.

Although all available trials reported mean changes in CAPS total severity scores, only 5 also reported the proportion of participants who no longer met criteria for PTSD (i. e, experienced disease remission) or the proportion who experienced a clinically meaningful improvement in symptoms (defined as ≥ 30-% decrease in CAPS total severity score compared to baseline).

Across these 5 trials, [1-5] a higher proportion of participants who received MDMA-assisted psychotherapy experienced PTSD remission and/or at least a 30% decrease in CAPS scores compared to comparison group participants (Table 4).

Table 4. Effects of MDMA-assisted psychotherapy on PTSD diagnosis and clinically meaningful improvement in CAPS total severity score

Study *Follow-up*	N[a]	Intervention and Comparator	PTSD Outcome Measures
Mitchell, 2021[1]	79	MDMA-assisted psychotherapy compared to	Participants no longer meeting PTSD diagnostic criteria = 33% MDMA group vs 5% placebo group
18 weeks		0mg placebo	
Mithoefer, 2011[3]	20	MDMA-assisted psychotherapy compared to	Participants no longer meeting PTSD diagnostic criteria = 83% MDMA group vs 25% placebo group
2 months		0mg placebo	CAPS response[b] = 83% MDMA group vs 25%
			placebo group
Mithoefer, 2018 [2]	19	MDMA-assisted psychotherapy compared to	Participants no longer meeting PTSD diagnostic criteria = 86% 75mg MDMA group and 58% 125mg
1 month		low-dose placebo	MDMA group vs 29% control group CAPS response[b] = 100% 75mg MDMA group and
			67% 125mg MDMA group vs 29% control group
Oehen, 2013 [5]	12	MDMA-assisted psychotherapy compared to	CAPS response[b] after all participants received full- dose MDMA = 75%
2 months		low-dose placebo	
Ot'alora, 2018 [4]	18	MDMA-assisted psychotherapy compared to	Participants no longer meeting PTSD diagnostic criteria = 44% 100mg MDMA group and 42%
1 month		low-dose placebo	125mg MDMA group vs 33% control group CAPS response[b] = 56% 100mg MDMA group and 50% 125mg MDMA group vs 17% control group

Notes.

[a] Analytic sample;

[b] Response was defined as >30% decrease in CAPS total severity score.

Abbreviations. CAPS=Clinician Administered PTSD Scale for Diagnostic and Statistical Manual of Mental Disorders; MDMA=3,4-methylenedioxy-methamphetamine; PTSD=posttraumatic stress disorder.

Results of a meta-analysis of 7 trials (Figure 3) indicate that participants receiving MDMA experienced significantly greater improvements in mean CAPS total severity scores compared with participants receiving 0mg or low-dose placebo (pooled standardized mean difference in change scores = -0.91, 95% CI [-1.33, -0.50]). Heterogeneity in true effects appeared to be minimal (95% PI [-1.33, -0.50]). No studies stratified results by patient characteristics or PTSD severity at baseline. These findings are consistent with results of a small RCT [69] conducted in Brazil that used a different assessment of PTSD symptomatology (Severity of Symptoms Scale for Post-traumatic Stress Disorder) and was terminated early due to reasons unrelated to trial conduct, as well as 3 observational studies [9-11].

Across most studies, control group participants also experienced symptom improvements regardless of the type of placebo used, although to a lesser degree than treatment group participants (median standardized symptom change of -0.90 and -1.54, respectively). Because both treatment and control group participants received psychotherapy in all studies, this observation suggests that treatment benefits are at least partially attributable to MDMA. Nonetheless, the small number and size of available studies limits the extent to which firm conclusions can be drawn about the relative contributions of receiving MDMA, undergoing intensive psychotherapy, and other factors (such as participation effects) to observed symptom improvement.

Additionally, the precise magnitude of benefit that could be expected from MDMA is difficult to determine from the available evidence, in part because very small RCTs are at risk of prognostic imbalance (a failure of randomization to balance groups on participants' responsiveness to treatment). The largest available RCT1 is less likely to be impacted by this bias, and provides an estimate of added treatment benefit due to MDMA that corresponds to an approximately 5 to 15- point greater reduction in PTSD symptom severity compared to psychotherapy only (unstandardized mean difference in CAPS-5 change scores = -10.5, 95% CI [-15.6, -5.4]). Like 2 other studies, however, this study used a 0mg placebo, which likely compromised participant blinding and may have led to biases in observed treatment effects.

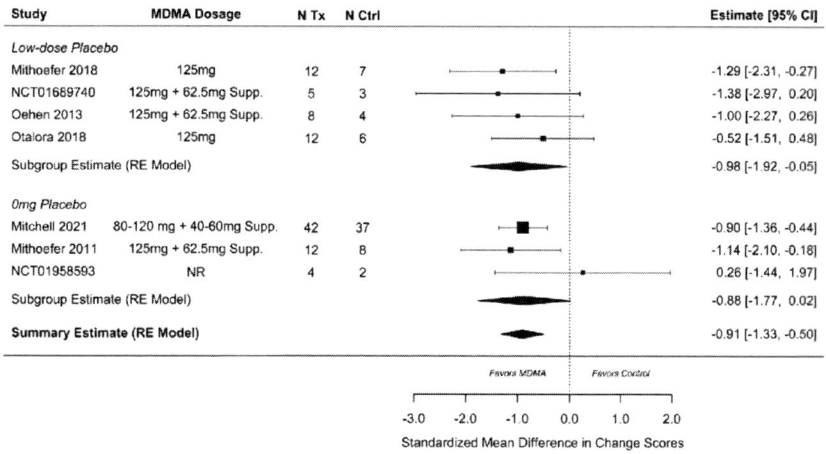

Abbreviations. Ctrl=control group; NR=not reported; Supp=supplemental dosage; RE=random-effects model; Tx=treatment group.

Figure 3. Change in Total CAPS Score Following MDMA-assisted Psychotherapy Compared to 0mg Placebo or Low-dose Placebo.

Major Depressive Disorder

Psilocybin-assisted psychotherapy may reduce depression severity and lead to a clinically significant improvement or sustained remission for some recipients at 12 months. Ayahuasca use may be associated with a short-term reduction in mean depression symptom scores and suicidality. Our confidence in these findings is low given study methodological limitations, inconsistency, and small sample sizes. No serious adverse events were reported for either intervention.

We identified 2 small RCTs [12, 17] of psilocybin-assisted psychotherapy and 3 small observational studies [13-16] in participants with moderate to severe depression (Table 5). The intervention in both trials consisted of 2 doses of psilocybin 20–30mg paired with pre-and post-treatment psychotherapy sessions led by 2 mental health professionals. In 1 of the trials, [12] conducted in the US among 24 adults with depression symptoms for a mean of 22 years, outcomes among the intervention group were compared to wait list controls who underwent the same treatment 8 weeks later. At baseline, participants had moderate depression according to the GRID-Hamilton Depression Rating Scale (GRID-HAMD; rated as no depression (0–7), mild depression (8–16), moderate depression (17–23), or severe depression (≥24)). If participants were taking antidepressants, they were required to refrain from using them prior to study screening and through completion of the primary outcome assessment but could start or restart antidepressant medication afterward. At 4-week and 3-, 6-, and 12-month follow-up, respectively, 0 (0%), 3 (12.5%), 5 (20.8%), and 8 (33.3%) of participants reported antidepressant use. Participants were allowed to continue psychotherapy throughout the trial if the type and frequency of psychotherapy had been stable and was expected to remain stable. At 4-week and 3-, 6-, and 12- month follow-up, respectively, 8 (33.3%), 9 (37.5%), 10 (41.7%), and 10 (41.7%) of participants reported receiving psychotherapy since receiving psilocybin.

Depression symptoms as measured by the GRID-HAMD significantly improved at 8 weeks compared to the delayed treatment group (standardized mean difference [SMD] = 2.6, 95% CI [1.5, 3.7]). In the immediate treatment group, the mean (SD) GRID-HAMD scores were 22.9 (3.6) at baseline, 8.0 (7.1) at week 5, and 8.5 (5.7) at week 8. Scores in the delayed treatment group remained stable: 22.5 (4.4) at baseline, 23.8 (5.4) at week 5, and 23.5 (6.0) at week 8. At 12 months, improvement on GRID-HAMD for all participants (immediate and delayed treatment groups) was also significant (SMD = 2.4, 95% CI [1.6, 3.2]) [70] At 12 months, 18/24 (75%) of participants experienced a clinically significant response, which was defined by the study as a decrease of 50% or more from their pre-treatment GRID-HAMD total score, and 14/24 (58%) met criteria for disease remission, defined as a GRID-HAMD total score of 7 or lower. GRID- HAMD scores at 12 months were not significantly different among participants who reported receiving psychotherapy during the follow-up period (the same analysis was not reported for antidepressant use). Suicidal ideation as measured by the Columbia Suicide Severity Rating Scale (CSSRS) severity of ideation subscale (score range of 0–5,with higher scores indicating presence of ideation with at least some intent to die) was 1.2 (1.2), 0.3 (0.7), 0.2 (0.7), 0.5 (1.0), 0.6 (1.1), 0.6 (1.1), respectively, at baseline, 1-week, 4-week and 3-, 6-, and 12-month follow-up (N = 23 due to missing data). No serious adverse events were reported and there were no reported suicide attempts or instances of self-harm at 12 months. The trial did not stratify results by patient characteristics or disease severity.

In a second trial [17] of psilocybin-assisted psychotherapy conducted in the UK that included 59 adults, the comparison group was treated with a low-dose placebo (psilocybin 1mg, presumed to have negligible activity) and escitalopram 10-20mg daily. The primary outcome measure was change from baseline scores on the Quick Inventory of Depressive Symptomatology-Self-

Report (QIDS-SR-16; rated as no depression (0–5), mild depression (6–10), moderate depression (11– 15), severe depression (16–20), or very severe depression (21–27)). At baseline, participants in the psilocybin group (N = 30) and escitalopram groups (N = 29), respectively, had mean QIDS- SR-16 scores (SD, range) of 14.5 (3.9; 7–23) and 16.4 (4.1; 6–22). Psilocybin group participants had depression for a mean of 22 years, had previously tried an average of 2 psychiatric medications, and 93% had previously undergone psychotherapy. Escitalopram group participants had depression for a mean of 15 years, had tried an average of 2 psychiatric medications, and 90% had previously undergone psychotherapy. Alcohol use was more common in the escitalopram group (average weekly use of 68 grams compared to 37 grams). Participants were required to stop any use of psychiatric medication at least 2 weeks before starting the trial and stop psychotherapy at least 3 weeks beforehand.

Both the psilocybin and escitalopram groups had reductions in mean QIDS-SR-16 scores. However, the change in mean scores from baseline to week 6 was not significantly different between the 2 groups (mean difference [MD] = -2.0, 95% CI [-5.0, 0.9]). A clinically meaningful response (defined as a decrease in QIDS-SR-16 by at least 50%) occurred in 21/30 (70%) of the psilocybin group and 14/29 (48%) in the escitalopram group. Remission (defined as QIDS-SR- 16 score <5) occurred in 17/30 (57%) in the psilocybin group and 8/29 (28%) in the escitalopram group. Neither response nor remission rates were significantly different between groups (Table 5). Changes in suicidal ideation as measured by the Suicidal Ideation Attributes Scale (SIDAS) were also not significantly different. No serious adverse events occurred. The trial did not stratify results by patient characteristics or disease severity.

The same group of researchers who conducted the UK trial also published 4 small observational studies on an intervention consisting of 2 doses of psilocybin (10mg followed by 25mg) combined with psychological support before, during, and after psilocybin treatments [13-16]. The number of participants who were exposed to this intervention ranged from 12–20 in each study, but importantly, some participants overlapped between studies. Results consistently showed a reduction in depression severity (as measured by QIDS-16 and the Beck Depression Inventory) at 1–8 weeks following the intervention. In the study with the longest duration, the change in QIDS-SR-16 from baseline to 6 months among 20 participants was significant (within-group SMD = 1.4, $p < 0.001$) [14]. These observational studies aimed to test the feasibility of studying psilocybin-assisted psychotherapy and explore associations of psilocybin use with factors related to depression such as future life event forecasting and emotional face recognition (both outcomes are outside the scope of this review). Although necessary to establish a basis for further study, results of these observational studies did not weigh heavily in our assessment of the evidence compared with findings from RCTs.

We identified 1 small RCT18 (N = 29) on ayahuasca for treatment of depression and 2 small pre- post studies (Table 6). In the trial conducted in Brazil, participants had moderate to severe depression as defined by mean Hamilton Depression Rating (HAM-D; rated as mild (10–13), mild to moderate (14–17), or moderate to severe (>17)) with a mean (SD) baseline score of 21.83 (5.35), had tried at least 2 antidepressant medications, and most (80%) had previously tried psychotherapy. Participants in the intervention group received 1 dose of ayahuasca without additional co-interventions aside from supervision during the dosing session and follow-up study assessments. The control group received an 0mg placebo designed to mimic the taste and color of ayahuasca. Mean HAM-D scores 1 week after treatment were significantly different between groups and favored ayahuasca (SMD = 0.98, 95% CI [0.21, 1.75]). A higher proportion of participants in the ayahuasca group met criteria for a clinically meaningful response (reduction in HAM-D score by at least 50%) and remission (HAM-D ≤7) (Table 6). This trial did not follow participants longer than 1 week, so the durability of these responses is unknown. Suicidal ideation decreased in both groups, but between-group differences were not significant. It is notable that 76% of participants had a comorbid personality disorder, 31% had comorbid anxiety disorder, and all were under regular use of benzodiazepines during the trial. Whether these factors influenced results is unclear, and the trial did not stratify results by patient characteristics.

Table 5. Study characteristics and outcomes of psilocybin-assisted psychotherapy for depression

Study Sample Size	Patient Characteristics	Mean (SD) Baseline Severity and Symptom Duration Past Treatment	Psychedelic Dose	Psychotherapy Protocol[a] Total # Sessions and Duration (Hours)	Comparator	Outcomes
RCTs						
Carhart- Harris 2021 [17] N=59	Mean age: 41 % female: 34 % non-Hispanic White: 88	HAMD: 18.8 (2.8)[b] 19 (11) years Average of 2 previous medication trials; 92% previously tried psychotherapy	Psilocybin Sessions 1-2: 25mg	1 preparatory session, 2 dosing sessions, 3 debriefing sessions 6 sessions (NR)	Psilocybin 1mg dosed twice and escitalopram 10–20mg daily	MD change in QIDS-SR-16 from baseline to week 6 = -2.0, 95% CI [−5.0, 0.9] 6-week QIDS-SR-16 response[c] 21/30 (70%) of the psilocybin group and 14/29 (48%) in the escitalopram group (difference, 22 percentage points; 95% CI [−3, 48]) 6-week remission[d] 17/30 (57%) in the psilocybin group and 8/29 (28%) in the escitalopram group (difference, 28.1

Table 5. (Continued)

Study Sample Size	Patient Characteristics	Mean (SD) Baseline Severity and Symptom Duration Past Treatment	Psychedelic Dose	Psychotherapy Protocol[a] Total # Sessions and Duration (Hours)	Comparator	Outcomes
						percentage points; 95% CI [2.3, 53.8]). MD change in SIDAS score from baseline to week 6 = -1.3, 95% CI [-6.5, -0.3]
Davis 2021 [12] & Gukasyan 2022 [70] N=24	Mean age: 40 % female: 67 % non-Hispanic White: 92	HAMD: 22.7 (4.0)[b] 22 (12) years NR	Psilocybin *Session 1: 20mg/70kg Session 2: 30mg/70 kg*	Preparatory visits (8 hrs total), support during 2 day-long psilocybin sessions, and follow-up visits (2–3 hrs total) *At least 18 in-person visits (~11 hours psychotherapy)*	Delayed treatment (wait list control)	SMD GRID-HAMD at 8 weeks (between group difference) = 2.6, 95% CI [1.5, 3.7] SMD GRID-HAMD at 12 months (all participants) = 2.4, 95% CI [1.6, 3.2] 12-month GRID-HAMD response[c] 18/24 (75%) 12-month remission[e] 14/24 (58%) CSSRS low overall and not

Study Sample Size	Patient Characteristics	Mean (SD) Baseline Severity and Symptom Duration Past Treatment	Psychedelic Dose	Psychotherapy Protocol[a] Total # Sessions and Duration (Hours)	Comparator	Outcomes
						significantly different between groups at 8 weeks
Observational Studies						
Carhart- Harris 2016 [13] & 2018 [14] N=20	Age: 27–64 % female: 30 % white: 75	HAMD: 21.5 (4.2) 18 (8) years *Psychotherapy (92%)*	Psilocybin *Session 1: 10mg Session 2: 25mg*	1 preparatory session (4 hrs), 2 dosing sessions (6–7 hrs each), and 2 integration sessions *5 sessions (NR)*	NA	SMD in QIDS-SR-16 from baseline to 6 months = 1.4, $p < 0.001$ MD in suicidality scores on QIDS-SR-16 from baseline to 5 weeks = -0.7, 95% CI [-0.22, -1.2] Relapse rate (QIDS score of 6+ or above) at 6 months among responders: 3/9 (33%)
Lyons 2018 [15] [f] N=30	Mean age: 42 % female: 27 % non-Hispanic White: 93	BDI: 19.2 (1.5) NR	Psilocybin *Session 1: 10mg Session 2: 25mg*	1 preparatory session (4 hrs), 2 dosing sessions (6-7 hrs each), and 2 integration sessions *5 sessions (NR)*	Healthy, nontreated controls	Mean BDI = 34.33 at baseline vs 12.13 at 1 week among depressive patients ($p < 0.001$) No significant difference found in baseline vs follow-

Table 5. (Continued)

Study Sample Size	Patient Characteristics	Mean (SD) Baseline Severity and Symptom Duration Past Treatment	Psychedelic Dose	Psychotherapy Protocol[a] Total # Sessions and Duration (Hours)	Comparator	Outcomes
						up BDI scores among the healthy comparison group.
Stroud 2018 [16] [f] N=33	Mean age: 45 % female: 47 % non-Hispanic White: NR	QIDS: 11.7 (3.0) [b] NR	Psilocybin *Session 1: 10mg Session 2: 25mg*	1 preparatory session (4 hrs), 2 dosing sessions (6-7 hrs each), and 2 integration sessions *5 sessions (NR)*	Healthy, nontreated controls	Mean QIDS-16 = 18.88 at baseline vs 7.65 at 1 week after psilocybin sessions, ($p < .001$) No significant difference found in baseline vs follow-up QIDS- 16 scores among the healthy comparison group

Notes.

[a] All sessions led by 2 psychiatrists;

[b] Weighted mean calculated across intervention and control groups;

[c] Response defined by the study as a decrease of 50% or more from their pre-treatment total score;

[d] Defined as <5 on QIDS-SR; [e] Defined as a GRID-HAMD total score of 7 or lower;

[f] Intervention group also formed part of the sample in Carhart-Harris 2016 and Carhart-Harris 2018.

Abbreviations. BDI=Beck Depression Inventory; CI=confidence interval; CSSRS=Columbia Suicide Severity Rating Scale; GRID-HAMD=GRID-Hamilton Depression Rating Scale; HAM-D=Hamilton Rating Scale for Depression; MADRS= Montgomery-Asberg Depression Rating Scale; MD=mean difference; NR=not reported; QIDS-SR-16=16-item Quick Inventory of Depressive Symptomatology Self Report; RCT=randomized controlled trial; SD=standard deviation; SI=suicidal ideation; SMD=standardized mean difference; SIDAS=Suicidal Ideation Attributes Scale.

Table 7. Study characteristics and outcomes of psychedelic treatment for OUD

Study *Sample Size Country Follow-Up*	Patient Characteristics	Psychedelic *Dose*	Co-intervention(s)	Comparator	Withdrawal and/or Opioid Use Outcomes
RCT					
Glue 2016 [23] N=27 *New Zealand ~9 days*	Mean age: 41 % female: 22 % non-Hispanic White: 74	Noribogaine[a] *60mg, 120mg, or 180mg, 1 dosing session*	None	0mg placebo	Mean time to opioid substitution treatment = 8.6 hrs in 60mg group vs 22.5 hrs in 120mg group vs 11.4 hrs in 180mg group vs 13.9 hrs in placebo group
Brown 2018 [24] N=30 *Mexico 12 months*	Mean age: 29 % female: 17 % non-Hispanic White: 90	Ibogaine *1,540 ± 920mg*	None	NA	MD SOWS at mean time interval of 76.5 hrs = 17.0 points ($p < .001$) ASI for drug use = 0.40 at baseline vs 0.17 at 12 months # participants with opioid-free days in the previous 30 days at 12 months = 8.8
Davis 2017 [25] N=88 *Mexico 3 months-3 years*	Age: 41% 25-34 years old, 39% 35-54 years old % female: 27 %non-Hispanic White: 89	Ibogaine *15 mg/kg ±5, 1 dosing session*	Participation in detoxification program	NA	% participants with reduction in cravings = 50% at 1 week; 35% at 3 or more months Opioid use post-treatment: 30% abstinent, 48% returned to use, 17% no change, 6% use increased
Knuijver 2022 [27] N=14 *The Netherlands 24 hours*	Age (median): 48 % female: 14 % non-Hispanic White: NR	Ibogaine *10 mg/kg, 1 dosing session*	None	NA	Return to morphine use within 24 hrs = 79% Median COWS among 5 not on morphine after 24 hrs = 0

Table 7. (Continued)

Study *Sample Size Country Follow-Up*	Patient Characteristics	Psychedelic *Dose*	Co-intervention(s)	Comparator	Withdrawal and/or Opioid Use Outcomes
Malcolm 2018 [28] N=50 *Mexico 48 hours*	Mean age: 31 % female: 39 % non-Hispanic White: 78	Ibogaine *18–20 mg/kg, 1 dosing session*	Participation in detoxification program	NA	Mean COWS before ibogaine = 8.2 at 48 hrs and 7.64 at 24 hrs vs mean COWS after ibogaine = 5.26 at 24 hrs and 3.30 at 48 hrs Mean SOWS before ibogaine = 20.51 at 48 hrs and 17.09 at 24 hrs vs Mean SOWS after ibogaine = 12.63 at 24 hrs and 10.04 at 48 hrs Mean BSCS before ibogaine = 6.58 at 48 hrs and 5.98 at 24 hrs vs mean BCBS after ibogaine = 2.69 at 24 hrs and 1.92 at 48 hrs
Noller 2018 [26] N=14 *New Zealand 12 months*	Mean age: 38 % female: 50 % non-Hispanic White: 100	Ibogaine *25–55 mg/kg (mean 31.4, SD 7.6), 1 dosing session*	Diazepam 5- 30mg and zopiclone 7.5–15mg	NA	Mean SOWS = 25.21 at baseline vs 14.21 at 12-24 hrs (p = 0.015) Mean SOWS = 24 at baseline vs 8.5 at 42-84 hrs (p = 0.070) ASI = 0.32 at baseline vs 0.06 at 12 months ($p <$ 0.01) Negative urine drug screen at 12 months = 6/8, 75%

Notes.

[a] An ibogaine active metabolite.

Abbreviations. ASI=Addiction Severity Index; BSCS=Brief Substance Craving Scale; COWS=Clinical Opioid Withdrawal Scale; hrs=hours; OOWS=Objective Opiate Withdrawal Scale; OP-SCL=Opiate-Symptom Checklist; SD=standard deviation; SOWS=Subjective Opioid Withdrawal Scale.

The same researchers who conducted this RCT also conducted 2 small observational studies [19, 20, 22] that identified similar reductions in depression symptom severity in the 3 weeks following use of ayahuasca by 23 adults with recurrent depression. Among 15 patients with suicidality at baseline, ayahuasca use was associated with a reduction in suicidality as measured by Montgomery-Åsberg Depression Rating Scale-Suicidality Item (MADRS-SI) in the acute period (up to 180 minutes after ayahuasca administration) and for the next 21 days. These observational studies contributed little to our assessment of the evidence given that RCT data are available. No serious adverse events were reported for any studies of ayahuasca.

Opioid Use

Ibogaine may not reduce short-term opioid withdrawal symptoms compared to placebo. Our confidence in this finding is low based on the small number of studies available, study methodologic limitations, and inconsistent findings. Although several pre-post studies [24-28] found that ibogaine use was associated with a reduction in opioid withdrawal symptoms, this finding was not replicated in an RCT (Table 7) [23] Whether ibogaine use is associated with long-term opioid use reduction is unclear. Only 3 small uncontrolled observational studies with high attrition have evaluated long-term outcomes. Available evidence is therefore insufficient to draw conclusions about the long-term efficacy of ibogaine. Importantly, ibogaine has been associated with serious adverse events, namely prolonged QTc interval on an electrocardiogram (ECG) and cardiac arrhythmia. Across studies, 1 death occurred during treatment.

Only 1 small RCT has been conducted on ibogaine use to treat opioid withdrawal symptoms. In this trial [23] (which was conducted in New Zealand and designed to evaluate ibogaine safety), 27 participants on methadone treatment for OUD were randomized to receive 1 of 3 doses of noribogaine (an ibogaine active metabolite at 60mg, 120mg, or 240mg) or placebo in the immediate time period following their last use of an opioid. In the week before receiving noribogaine, participants stopped methadone and received long-acting morphine for 6 days followed by short-acting morphine for 1 day. Approximately 2 hours after their last dose of short-acting morphine, participants received noribogaine or placebo and were monitored for withdrawal symptoms. The study's primary efficacy outcome was the time in hours before participants requested a dose of morphine or methadone. The trial found that noribogaine at any dose did not result in a longer time to resuming opioid use (and did not significantly reduce withdrawal symptoms) compared to placebo, noting that participants in both groups were treated in the same physical space and could have influenced each other. None of the participants experienced serious adverse effects. Norigobaine was associated with dose-dependent effect on QTc interval prolongation on electrocardiogram, which is a risk factor for life-threatening cardiac arrhythmias. The trial did not follow participants long term.

In a small uncontrolled observational study [27] in the Netherlands with similar research aims as the New Zealand trial, 14 adults on methadone treatment for OUD who were transitioned to morphine received ibogaine 10mg/kg and were monitored for withdrawal. Most participants (11/14, 79%) did not restart morphine within 24 hours, and among these participants the median Clinical Opiate Withdrawal Scale (COWS) score was 0, indicating no or mild withdrawal symptoms. Half of participants had a prolonged QTc > 500ms during the treatment period (a change from baseline) and received magnesium infusions as a result, without any adverse consequences. All participants experienced ataxia with an inability to walk without support, which reversed within 48 hours. Like the New Zealand trial, this study did not follow participants long term.

Four additional uncontrolled observational studies [24-26, 28] of adults receiving ibogaine with the intent of opioid detoxification (N = 14–88) found that participants had lower measures of opioid withdrawal and/or opioid craving post-ibogaine compared to pre-ibogaine use. In a small observational study [26] conducted in New Zealand, 14 adults completed treatment for opioid withdrawal with ibogaine 25–55mg/kg, diazepam 5–30mg, and zopiclone 7.5–15mg. On average, participants reported having fewer withdrawal symptoms 12–24 hours after receiving ibogaine compared to baseline. One participant (not included in the analysis) died during treatment under circumstances that are not well described. In a report by New Zealand officials, the death was deemed very likely "related to ibogaine ingestion and most probably related to a cardiac arrhythmia." A subset of participants (8/14, 57%) were followed for 12 months. Among these participants, the Addiction Severity Index Lite (ASI-Lite) for drug use was significantly lower at 12 months compared with baseline, and most participants (6/8, 75%) had negative drug screens at 12 months. Only 1 other study reported on long-term opioid use. In a retrospective study of 88 adults who received ibogaine at a treatment center in Mexico with a history of heroin (51%) or prescription opioid use

(49%), 30% of participants reported never using opioids again, while 48% said that their opioid use was reduced compared to the period before ibogaine treatment, 17% reported no change, and 6% increased their use [25].

Alcohol Use

Psilocybin-assisted psychotherapy may reduce heavy drinking days and average alcohol consumption per day among adults with alcohol use disorder. Although results are consistent and direct, our confidence in these findings is low due to study methodologic limitations and small sample sizes. MDMA-assisted psychotherapy for alcohol use has been less studied and evidence is currently insufficient to draw conclusions.

One RCT [29] has been conducted on psilocybin-assisted psychotherapy for alcohol disorder (Table 8). In this US trial, 95 adults with an average of 14 years of alcohol dependence were randomized to receive 12 psychotherapy sessions with 2 psilocybin dosing sessions or diphenhydramine 50–100mg. At baseline, participants in the psilocybin group consumed a mean (SD) of 7.52 (4.58) standard drinks per day (defined as 14 grams of ethanol) compared to 7.10 (4.05) in the diphenhydramine group. The study did not report whether participants had previous experience with treatment for alcohol dependence. Participants receiving psilocybin experienced a significantly greater reduction in the percent of heavy drinking days and number of drinks per day compared to the diphenhydramine group at 32-week follow-up. Reduction in the percent of drinking days also favored psilocybin, but this finding was nonsignificant, and improvements on all outcomes were observed in both groups. No serious adverse events occurred among participants who received psilocybin.

In a small uncontrolled observational study conducted by the same group as the trial, [30] 10 adults were administered a 14-week psilocybin-assisted psychotherapy program that included 1–2 psilocybin dosing sessions starting in week 4. In the period after dosing (weeks 5–12), the percent of heavy drinking days and any drinking days were decreased compared with baseline and with the period prior to the initial dosing of psilocybin. At the study endpoint of 36 weeks, percent heavy drinking days and any drinking days were trending upward but still below baseline.

MDMA-assisted psychotherapy was evaluated as a treatment for alcohol use disorder in a UK study [31] of 14 adults with mostly moderate to severe alcohol use disorder. Participants were enrolled in an 8-week treatment program consisting of 10 psychotherapy sessions, in 2 of which they received

MDMA. At 9 months post-treatment, 9 participants were abstinent from alcohol and 2 had reduced their use to fewer than 14 units of alcohol per week.

Table 8. Study characteristics and outcomes of psychedelic-assisted psychotherapy for AUD

Study Sample Size Country Follow-up	Patient Characteristic	Psychedelic Dose	Co-intervention(s)	Comparator	Outcomes
RCT					
Bogenschutz 2022 [29] N=95 US 36 weeks	Mean age: 46 % female: 44 % non-Hispanic White: 79	Psilocybin Session 1: 25mg/70kg Session 2: 30–40mg/70kg	12 sessions of psychotherapy using motivational enhancement therapy and cognitive behavioral therapy	Diphenhydramine Session 1: 50mg Session 2: 100mg	MD % heavy drinking days = 13.86, 95% CI [3.00, 24.72] MD % drinking days at baseline = 13.44, 95% CI [–0.18, 27.05] MD drinks per day = 1.09, 95% CI [0.27, 1.92]
Pre-post Observational Studies					
Bogenschutz 2015 [30] N=10 US 36 weeks	Mean age: 40 % female: 40 % non-Hispanic White: 30	Psilocybin 0.3–0.4mg/kg	12 psychotherapy sessions	NA	MD % heavy drinking days weeks 5–12 relative to baseline = 26.0, 95% CI [8.7, 43.2] and relative weeks 1–4 = 18.2, 95% CI [2.8, 33.5] MD % drinking days weeks 5–12 relative to baseline = 27.2, 95% CI [9.0, 45.4] and relative weeks 1–4 = 21.9, 95% CI [5.1, 38.6]
Sessa 2021 [31] N=14 *UK 9 months*	Mean age: 48 % female: 43 %non-Hispanic White: NR	MDMA 125mg initial dose, followed by 62.5mg booster dose	10 psychotherapy sessions	NA	9 participants were abstinent from alcohol and 2 reduced use to <14 units of alcohol per week at 9 months follow-up.

Abbreviations. AUD=alcohol use disorder; CI=confidence interval; MD=mean difference; MDMA=3,4-methylenedioxymethamphetamine; NR=not reported.

Tobacco Use

Evidence regarding psychedelic-assisted psychotherapy for tobacco use is limited to 1 small uncontrolled observational study of psilocybin use, which is insufficient to make conclusions about efficacy. The average participant in this US study [32, 33] (N = 15) was aged 51, smoked 19 cigarettes per day for a 31 years, and had 6 previous lifetime quit attempts (see Appendix C in the Supplemental Materials for additional study characteristics). The intervention consisted of intensive cognitive behavioral therapy delivered in 19 in-person sessions, with 3 sessions of psilocybin administration as well as brief daily phone calls for 2 weeks following participants' target quit dates. At 12 months, 10/15 (67%) adults were abstinent from smoking as measured by smoking timeline follow-back assessments and verified by exhaled carbon monoxide and urinary cotinine levels. Among those who participated in longer-term follow-up (range: 16–57 months), 9/12 (60%) were abstinent from smoking by the same measures. No serious adverse events were reported.

In addition to its small sample size, a limitation of this study is the potential for selection bias. Although participants were typical of those seeking medical care for tobacco cessation in terms of tobacco use history and the number of quit attempts, most (10/15, 67%) reported past use of hallucinogens. It is possible that the participants with past hallucinogen use had different expectations regarding the potential of this treatment compared to those without past hallucinogen use.

Cocaine and Cannabis Use

Psychedelics, specifically ayahuasca and ibogaine, have also been evaluated in uncontrolled observational studies as treatment for other substance use including cocaine and cannabis. Due to study methodologic limitations, small sample sizes, indirectness, and inconsistency, this evidence is insufficient to draw conclusions about the effects of ayahuasca and ibogaine on use of cocaine and cannabis. See Appendix C in the Supplemental Materials for detailed study characteristics.

One observational study [34] evaluated the use of ayahuasca among participants with mixed forms of substance use. In this Canadian pre-post study [34] of 12 adults participating in a 4-day "Working with Addiction and Stress" retreat that incorporated ayahuasca ceremonies, the proportion of participants who reported using alcohol, tobacco, and cocaine declined. No change was observed for opiate or cannabis use, and no serious adverse events were reported.

Three observational studies [36, 37, 71] of ibogaine have also been conducted among individuals with cocaine or opioid dependence who self-referred to a treatment program on St. Kitts in the West Indies. The largest and most recent study [37] of this treatment program included 102 adults with opioid dependence and 89 with cocaine dependence who underwent 1 ibogaine dosing session during a 12-day inpatient detoxification program. Self-reported cravings as measured by the Heroin (HCQ-29) and Cocaine (CCQ-45) Craving Questionnaires were lower at the time of discharge compared to before treatment, and remained lower among 37 participants with opioid dependence and 32 with cocaine dependence who completed follow-up at 1 month. No serious adverse events were reported, though orthostatic hypotension occurred in 5% of participants and transient nausea, vomiting, and ataxia were reported as common side effects shortly after ibogaine administration.

In a retrospective study [35] of 75 adults in Brazil who underwent 1–9 ibogaine dosing sessions in conjunction with outpatient psychotherapy, 61% of participants reported abstinence. The duration of reported abstinence was longer for participants who underwent multiple ibogaine dosing sessions compared to 1 dosing session (median 8.4 months compared to median 5.5 months). No serious adverse events were reported.

Other Conditions

Psychedelic substances have been investigated as treatment for social anxiety, OCD, and for non-specific mood and anxiety symptoms in a single RCT and 2 uncontrolled observational studies. This evidence is insufficient to draw any conclusions about the effectiveness of psychedelics for these disorders. See Appendix C in the Supplemental Materials for detailed study characteristics.

An RCT [38] of 17 adults with clinical symptoms of social anxiety disorder (SAD) found that Beck Anxiety Inventory scores were not significantly different after a single ayahuasca dosing session compared to 0mg placebo.[38] However, ayahuasca was associated with a significant improvement in self-perception of speech performance as measured by the Self-Statements During Public Speaking Scale. In a pre-post study[39] of 9 adults with OCD in the US who received variable doses of psilocybin for up to 4 total treatments, all participants experienced a decrease in OCD symptoms as measured by the Yale-Brown Obsessive Compulsive Scale (23–100% reduction in YBOCS scores).

Lastly, ibogaine plus 5-MeO-DMT has been used as treatment for US Special Forces Veterans with a range of mood and anxiety symptoms. A retrospective study[40] of 51 Veterans who participated in a psychedelic clinical program in Mexico during which they received 1 dose of ibogaine and 3 doses of 5-MeO-DMT found significant reductions in PTSD symptoms (SMD PTSD Checklist-5 = -3.6, $p < 0.001$), depression (SMD Patient Health Questionnaire-2 = -3.7, $p < 0.001$), anxiety (SMD Generalized Anxiety Disorder 2-Item = -3.1, $p < 0.001$), and suicidal ideation (SMD Depressive Symptom Index Suicidality Subscale = -1.9, $p < 0.001$) 30-days post- treatment.

Harms

Transient side effects were commonly reported and may occur before, during, or after a psychedelic session (for full list of observed harms see Supplemental Materials Appendix C).

Ibogaine has been associated with serious adverse events, including death in 1 study [26]. Several studies found a dose-dependent effect of ibogaine on QTc interval prolongation on ECG, which is a risk factor for cardiac arrhythmia [23, 27]. Other common side effects of ibogaine include headache, nausea, imbalance, and visual impairment.

MDMA may also be associated with cardiac risks. Only 1 study reported a serious adverse event attributed to MDMA, a participant with premature ventricular contractions (PVCs) at baseline experienced an increase in PVCs requiring an overnight hospital stay for observation [2]. Other transient side effects of MDMA include symptoms related to mood (eg, anxiety, irritability, restlessness), sleep (eg, fatigue, insomnia), sensation (eg, dizziness, impaired balance), pain (eg headache, muscle tension), and gastrointestinal systems (eg, nausea, vomiting, low appetite).

Psilocybin was associated with transient effects on heart rate (eg, tachycardia, palpitations) and elevated blood pressure, but these events were not described as serious. Common side effects of psilocybin include anxiety, fear, headache, and nausea. Ayahuasca was not associated with serious adverse events in included studies. Common side effects of ayahuasca include headache, nausea, and vomiting.

Discussion

The aim of this review was to synthesize evidence on the benefits and harms of psychedelics as primary or adjunct treatment for mental health and substance use disorders. Given the prevalence of mental health and substance use disorders with the Veteran population, any novel or emerging treatments with the potential to improve clinical outcomes are of great interest.

MDMA-assisted psychotherapy for PTSD is the most extensively studied intervention involving psychedelics. In a clinical research setting, MDMA paired with intensive psychotherapy co-led by 2 mental health professionals may reduce PTSD symptom severity and lead to clinically meaningful improvement and/or disease remission for some participants in the short term.

Although results are fairly consistent and direct, trial sample sizes are small and at risk of prognostic imbalance (a failure of randomization to balance groups on participants' responsiveness to treatment). Common side effects of MDMA include anxiety, restlessness, headache, and nausea but serious adverse events appear to be rare.

Although promising, our confidence in these findings is low. The evidence on MDMA-assisted psychotherapy remains preliminary and several important research questions have yet to be addressed. Among these is whether outcomes vary by patient characteristics, index trauma type, disorder severity, or the number or types of past treatments tried. Available evidence also has unclear applicability to Veteran populations, as most studies did not include Veterans and none have been conducted in a VHA setting. Moreover, the psychotherapy component of studied interventions—typically requiring 30 hours or more of psychotherapy co-led by 2 mental health professionals—is more intensive than typically occurs in clinical practice. Researchers are beginning to study whether treatment protocols can be reproduced at scale [11], but this evidence is preliminary. Whether this level of treatment is feasible in everyday practice and whether treatment benefits may still be observed with lower intensity psychotherapy are questions for future research.

Other interventions involving psychedelics have been less extensively studied. Psilocybin- assisted psychotherapy for depression may reduce symptom severity and lead to sustained remission at 12 months for a proportion of recipients compared to wait list controls, but these same benefits were not observed (in a separate trial) when psilocybin-assisted psychotherapy was compared with psychotherapy and daily escitalopram. We have low confidence in these findings, which are based on 1 small trial for each comparator. Ayahuasca use for depression may be associated with a reduction in short-term symptoms and suicidality. However, our confidence in these findings is also low due to a smaller number of trials with small sample sizes and some inconsistency in results.

Among treatments evaluated for substance use disorders, psilocybin-assisted psychotherapy for alcohol use disorder may reduce alcohol consumption (heavy drinking days and the number of drinks per day), but we have low confidence is this finding (which is based on results of 1 small trial). MDMA-assisted psychotherapy has also been studied for treatment of alcohol use disorder, but results are limited to 1 small observational study and are insufficient to make conclusions.

Similarly, evidence on psilocybin as an adjunct to psychotherapy to reduce tobacco use and ayahuasca as treatment for cocaine, cannabis, and other forms of substance use is limited to 1 or a small number of observational studies and is insufficient to make conclusions.

Ibogaine may not reduce opioid-related withdrawal symptoms or reduce long-term opioid use. We have low confidence in these findings, which are drawn from a small number of studies with small sample sizes, study methodologic limitations, and inconsistent findings. Ibogaine had also been studied as a treatment to reduce cocaine use and to reduce problematic general substance use, but results are limited to a small number of observational studies with mixed populations and evidence is insufficient to draw conclusions. Ibogaine plus 5-MeO-DMT was found to improve a range of mood and anxiety symptoms in a retrospective study of US Special Forces Veterans participating in a treatment program in Mexico. However, this study had a high risk of bias and results have not been replicated in other studies. Given safety concerns associated with ibogaine use, particularly the documented risk of QTc prolongation, cardiac arrhythmias, and death, treatment should only be undertaken in the context of a clinical trial with appropriate safety monitoring.

Finally, most available studies on psychedelics required participants to discontinue their usual mental health medications, most often for a least 2 weeks before the study start. Risk of harms arising from medication discontinuation may have been minimal in the research context (due to presumably close patient contact and oversight), but conceivably could be greater in real-world settings. If the recommendation to discontinue medication becomes accepted practice as psychedelics move through the FDA drug development pathway, the risks of doing so must be taken into consideration when assessing the overall balance of risks and benefits of psychedelic treatments.

Limitations

Limitations of our review methods include our use of sequential review (rather than dual independent review) for data abstraction and risk of bias assessment. Additionally, both statistical precision and heterogeneity can be poorly estimated in small meta-analyses. We took steps to ameliorate these concerns, including use of corrections to better account for uncertainty in the estimation of heterogeneity, but some caution should be used in interpreting reported meta-analytic confidence intervals and prediction intervals.

The available evidence on psychedelics as primary or adjunct treatment for mental health disorders and substance use also has several limitations. First, psychedelics have been studied in a limited number of populations and settings by a relatively small number of researchers and institutions, which has partly been in response to legal and regulatory restrictions. Despite broad recruitment efforts, it is possible that participants of studies to date are not representative of general adult populations with mental health or substance use disorders. For example, US studies have been predominantly conducted among young, mostly non-Hispanic white populations with moderate to severe disease and access to a clinical research center or treatment program.

Whether treatment effects can be replicated in a broader array of populations and treatment settings is unclear. Similarly, little is known about the durability of psychedelic treatment effects, as most studies followed participants for no longer than a year. Whether exposure to psychedelics changes the long-term symptomatology of adults diagnosed with PTSD or depression, for example, is largely unknown.

Second, despite the use of low-dose placebos in some trials (*eg*, use of low-dose placebo MDMA in studies of MDMA-assisted psychotherapy for PTSD), many participants were able to correctly guess whether they were in the intervention or comparison groups (among trials that reported this information). Participant blinding was likely largely ineffective in studies that used a 0mg placebo, which may have biased observed treatment effects.

Lastly, because research on psychedelics is still in an early phase, whether and how psychedelic treatments could fit into usual care pathways is unclear. Even for areas with some promise, such as MDMA-assisted psychotherapy for PTSD, several clinical questions remain including whether benefits are limited to those with moderate to severe disease, whether adults should try more established treatments before considering psychedelic treatment, and if not, which criteria should be met to recommend psychedelics as primary treatment. Available evidence has also not addressed whether those who improve with psychedelic treatments should start or restart other therapies to maintain benefits long term. Additionally, the extent to which psychotherapy protocols employed in interventions involving psychedelics are consistent with current VA/Department of Defense (DoD) guidelines is also unclear. For example, studies of MDMA- assisted psychotherapy for PTSD used the MAPS standard treatment manual to guide psychotherapy sessions, but it is unclear to what degree the MAPS approach overlaps with currently recommended trauma-focused psychotherapies such as Prolonged Exposure as outlined in the applicable VA/DoD guideline (https://www.healthquality.va.gov/guidelines/mh/ptsd/).

Future Research

Recommendations for future research on psychedelics as primary or adjunct treatment for mental health and substance use disorders include:

- Inclusion of Veteran populations, particularly those with combat-related trauma, with detailed reporting of treatment histories and disease severity at baseline.
- Inclusion of more diverse populations, particularly with respect to race/ethnicity, socioeconomic status, and rurality, to better understand variability in treatment effectiveness, safety, and acceptability.
- Evaluation of the clinical implications of discontinuing mental health medications prior to undergoing psychedelic treatments and whether the benefits of doing so outweigh potential harms.
- Use of low-dose placebo rather than 0mg placebo to improve the adequacy of blinding, and improved reporting of blinding effectiveness.

Questions to be addressed at the health system level include:

- How could and should interventions involving psychedelics be incorporated into current standard of care and usual care pathways?
- Are psychedelic treatment protocols scalable and reproducible across a broad range of regions and settings?

- What are best practices for implementation of psychedelic treatment programs?
- If implemented, how can access to these resource-intensive treatments be distributed equitably?

A large number of underway studies were identified (see Appendix C in the Supplemental Materials for full details) in a wide range of populations (eg, adults with PTSD, mood disorders, and substance use). However, most are feasibility or pilot trials that may not fully address these research gaps.

Conclusion

Novel approaches to treatment of adults with mental health and substance use disorders are needed given the limitations of existing therapies. MDMA-assisted psychotherapy for PTSD, the most extensively studied intervention to date, may reduce PTSD symptom severity and lead to disease remission in a proportion of cases. Psilocybin-assisted psychotherapy and ayahuasca use for depression and psilocybin for alcohol use disorder may also be effective. However, our confidence in these findings is low, mainly due to the small number of trials available and the small sample sizes of these studies. Treatments that utilize psychedelics are still in an early phase of development and many gaps in the evidence need to be addressed. The most critical gaps include whether treatment effects are durable and consistent across patient characteristics and disease severity, whether the benefits of discontinuing mental health medications to undergo psychedelic treatments outweigh risks, and whether psychedelic treatment protocols are reproducible and scalable in everyday practice, including in VHA settings.

References

[1] Mitchell J M, Bogenschutz M, Lilienstein A, et al. MDMA-assisted therapy for severe PTSD: a randomized, double-blind, placebo-controlled phase 3 study. *Nature Medicine.* 2021;27(6):1025-1033.

[2] Mithoefer M C, Mithoefer A T, Feduccia A A, et al. 3,4-methylenedioxymethamphetamine (MDMA)-assisted psychotherapy for post-traumatic stress disorder in military veterans, firefighters, and police officers: a randomised, double-blind, dose-response, phase 2 clinical trial. *The Lancet*

Psychiatry. 2018;5(6):486-497.

[3] Mithoefer M C, Wagner M T, Mithoefer A T, Jerome L, Doblin R. The safety and efficacy of {+/-}3,4-methylenedioxymethamphetamine-assisted psychotherapy in subjects with chronic, treatment-resistant posttraumatic stress disorder: the first randomized controlled pilot study. *Journal of Psychopharmacology.* 2011;25(4):439-452.

[4] Ot'alora G M, Grigsby J, Poulter B, et al. 3,4-Methylenedioxymethamphetamine-assisted psychotherapy for treatment of chronic posttraumatic stress disorder: A randomized phase 2 controlled trial. *Journal of Psychopharmacology.* 2018;32(12):1295-1307.

[5] Oehen P, Traber R, Widmer V, Schnyder U. A randomized, controlled pilot study of MDMA (+/- 3,4-Methylenedioxymethamphetamine)-assisted psychotherapy for treatment of resistant, chronic Post-Traumatic Stress Disorder (PTSD). *Journal of Psychopharmacology.* 2013;27(1):40-52.

[6] Kotler M. A Randomized, Double-Blind, Active Placebo-Controlled Phase 2 Pilot Study of MDMA-assisted Psychotherapy in People With Chronic, Treatment-Resistant Posttraumatic Stress Disorder (PTSD). NCT01689740. Multidisplinary Association for Psychedelic Studies. https://clinicaltrials.gov/ct2/show/record/NCT01689740?term=NCT01689740&draw=2& rank=1. Published 2017. Accessed August 22, 2022.

[7] Pacey I. A Randomized, Double-Blind, Controlled Phase 2 Pilot Study of Manualized 3,4-methylenedioxymethamphetamine (MDMA)-Assisted Psychotherapy in 12 Subjects With Treatment-Resistant Posttraumatic Stress Disorder (PTSD) - Canada. NCT01958593. Multidisciplinary Association for Psychedelic Studies. https://clinicaltrials.gov/ct2/show/record/NCT01958593?term=NCT01958593&draw=2& rank=1. Published 2017. Accessed August 22, 2022.

[8] Mithoefer M C, Wagner M T, Mithoefer A T, et al. Durability of improvement in post- traumatic stress disorder symptoms and absence of harmful effects or drug dependency after 3,4-methylenedioxymethamphetamine-assisted psychotherapy: a prospective long- term follow-up study. *Journal of Psychopharmacology.* 2013;27(1):28-39.

[9] Jardim A V, Jardim D V, Chaves BR, et al. 3,4-methylenedioxymethamphetamine (MDMA)-assisted psychotherapy for victims of sexual abuse with severe post-traumatic stress disorder: an open label pilot study in Brazil. *Revista Brasileira de Psiquiatria.* 2021;43(2):181-185.

[10] Monson C M, Wagner A C, Mithoefer A T, et al. MDMA-facilitated cognitive-behavioural conjoint therapy for posttraumatic stress disorder: An uncontrolled trial. *European Journal of Psychotraumatology.* 2020;11(1):1840123.

[11] Wang J B, Lin J, Bedrosian L, et al. Scaling Up: Multisite Open-Label Clinical Trials of MDMA-Assisted Therapy for Severe Posttraumatic Stress Disorder. *Journal of Humanistic Psychology.* 2021;0(0):00221678211023663.

[12] Davis A K, Barrett F S, May D G, et al. Effects of Psilocybin-Assisted Therapy on Major Depressive Disorder: A Randomized Clinical Trial. *JAMA Psychiatry.* 2021;78(5):481- 489.

[13] Carhart-Harris RL, Bolstridge M, Rucker J, et al. Psilocybin with psychological

support for treatment-resistant depression: an open-label feasibility study. *The Lancet Psychiatry.* 2016;3(7):619-627.

[14] Carhart-Harris R L, Bolstridge M, Day CMJ, et al. Psilocybin with psychological support for treatment-resistant depression: six-month follow-up. *Psychopharmacology.* 2018;235(2):399-408.

[15] Lyons T, Carhart-Harris RL. More realistic forecasting of future life events after psilocybin for treatment-resistant depression. *Frontiers in Psychology.* 2018;9.

[16] Stroud JB, Freeman TP, Leech R, et al. Psilocybin with psychological support improves emotional face recognition in treatment-resistant depression. *Psychopharmacology.* 2018;235(2):459-466.

[17] Carhart-Harris R, Giribaldi B, Watts R, et al. Trial of Psilocybin versus Escitalopram for Depression. *New England Journal of Medicine.* 2021;384(15):1402-1411.

[18] Palhano-Fontes F, Barreto D, Onias H, et al. Rapid antidepressant effects of the psychedelic ayahuasca in treatment-resistant depression: a randomized placebo-controlled trial. *Psychological Medicine.* 2019;49(4):655-663.

[19] Sanches R F, de Lima Osorio F, Dos Santos RG, et al. Antidepressant Effects of a Single Dose of Ayahuasca in Patients With Recurrent Depression: A SPECT Study. *Journal of Clinical Psychopharmacology.* 2016;36(1):77-81.

[20] Osorio L, Sanches R F, Macedo LR, et al. Antidepressant effects of a single dose of ayahuasca in patients with recurrent depression: a preliminary report. *Revista Brasileira de Psiquiatria.* 2015;37(1):13-20.

[21] Zeifman R J, Palhano-Fontes F, Hallak J, Arcoverde E, Maia-Oliveira JP, Araujo DB. The Impact of Ayahuasca on Suicidality: Results From a Randomized Controlled Trial. *Frontiers in Pharmacology.* 2019;10.

[22] Zeifman R J, Singhal N, Dos Santos R G, et al. Rapid and sustained decreases in suicidality following a single dose of ayahuasca among individuals with recurrent major depressive disorder: results from an open-label trial. *Psychopharmacology.* 2021;238(2):453-459.

[23] Glue P, Cape G, Tunnicliff D, et al. Ascending Single-Dose, Double-Blind, Placebo-Controlled Safety Study of Noribogaine in Opioid-Dependent Patients. *Clinical Pharmacology in Drug Development.* 2016;5(6):460-468.

[24] Brown T K, Alper K. Treatment of opioid use disorder with ibogaine: detoxification and drug use outcomes. *American Journal of Drug & Alcohol Abuse.* 2018;44(1):24-36.

[25] Davis A K, Barsuglia J P, Windham-Herman A-M, Lynch M, Polanco M. Subjective effectiveness of ibogaine treatment for problematic opioid consumption: Short- and long- term outcomes and current psychological functioning. *Journal of Psychedelic Studies.* 2017;1(2):65-73.

[26] Noller G E, Frampton C M, Yazar-Klosinski B. Ibogaine treatment outcomes for opioid dependence from a twelve-month follow-up observational study. *American Journal of Drug & Alcohol Abuse.* 2018;44(1):37-46.

[27] Knuijver T, Schellekens A, Belgers M, et al. Safety of ibogaine administration in detoxification of opioid-dependent individuals: a descriptive open-label observational study. *Addiction.* 2022;117(1):118-128.

[28] Malcolm BJ, Polanco M, Barsuglia JP. Changes in Withdrawal and Craving Scores

in Participants Undergoing Opioid Detoxification Utilizing Ibogaine. *Journal of Psychoactive Drugs.* 2018;50(3):256-265.

[29] Bogenschutz M P, Ross S, Bhatt S, et al. Percentage of Heavy Drinking Days Following Psilocybin-Assisted Psychotherapy vs Placebo in the Treatment of Adult Patients With Alcohol Use Disorder: A Randomized Clinical Trial. *JAMA Psychiatry.* 2022.

[30] Bogenschutz M P, Forcehimes A A, Pommy J A, Wilcox CE, Barbosa PC, Strassman RJ. Psilocybin-assisted treatment for alcohol dependence: a proof-of-concept study. *Journal of Psychopharmacology.* 2015;29(3):289-299.

[31] Sessa B, Higbed L, O'Brien S, et al. First study of safety and tolerability of 3,4-methylenedioxymethamphetamine-assisted psychotherapy in patients with alcohol use disorder. *Journal of Psychopharmacology.* 2021;35(4):375-383.

[32] Johnson M W, Garcia-Romeu A, Cosimano MP, Griffiths RR. Pilot study of the 5-HT2AR agonist psilocybin in the treatment of tobacco addiction. *Journal of Psychopharmacology.* 2014;28(11):983-992.

[33] Johnson M W, Garcia-Romeu A, Griffiths RR. Long-term follow-up of psilocybin-facilitated smoking cessation. *The American Journal of Drug and Alcohol Abuse.* 2017;43(1):55-60.

[34] Thomas G, Lucas P, Capler N R, Tupper K W, Martin G. Ayahuasca-assisted therapy for addiction: results from a preliminary observational study in Canada. *Current Drug Abuse Reviews.* 2013;6(1):30-42.

[35] Schenberg E E, de Castro Comis M A, Chaves BR, da Silveira DX. Treating drug dependence with the aid of ibogaine: a retrospective study. *Journal of Psychopharmacology.* 2014;28(11):993-1000.

[36] Mash D C, Kovera C A, Pablo J, et al. Ibogaine: complex pharmacokinetics, concerns for safety, and preliminary efficacy measures. *Annals of the New York Academy of Sciences.* 2000;914:394-401.

[37] Mash D C, Duque L, Page B, Allen-Ferdinand K. Ibogaine Detoxification Transitions Opioid and Cocaine Abusers Between Dependence and Abstinence: Clinical Observations and Treatment Outcomes. *Front Pharmacol.* 2018;9:529.

[38] Dos Santos R G, Osorio F L, Rocha J M, et al. Ayahuasca Improves Self-perception of Speech Performance in Subjects With Social Anxiety Disorder: A Pilot, Proof-of- Concept, Randomized, Placebo-Controlled Trial. *Journal of Clinical Psychopharmacology.* 2021;41(5):540-550.

[39] Moreno F A, Wiegand C B, Taitano E K, Delgado P L. Safety, tolerability, and efficacy of psilocybin in 9 patients with obsessive-compulsive disorder. *Journal of Clinical Psychiatry.* 2006;67(11):1735-1740.

[40] Davis A K, Averill L A, Sepeda N D, Barsuglia J P, Amoroso T. Psychedelic treatment for trauma-related psychological and cognitive impairment among US Special Operations Forces Veterans. *Chronic Stress.* 2020;4:2470547020939564.

[41] Nichols D E. Psychedelics. *Pharmacol. Rev.* 2016;68(2):264-355.

[42] Garcia-Romeu A, Kersgaard B, Addy PH. Clinical applications of hallucinogens: A review. *Exp Clin Psychopharmacol.* 2016;24(4):229-268.

[43] Tupper K W, Wood E, Yensen R, Johnson MW. Psychedelic medicine: a re-emerging therapeutic paradigm. *CMAJ Canadian Medical Association Journal.*

2015;187(14):1054-1059.

[44] Nichols D E. Entactogens: How the Name for a Novel Class of Psychoactive Agents Originated. *Front Psychiatry.* 2022;13:863088.

[45] Sessa B. The History of Psychedelics in Medicine. *Handbuch Psychoaktive Substanzen,*2016.

[46] Nichols D E, Walter H. The History of Psychedelics in Psychiatry. *Pharmacopsychiatry.* 2021;54(4):151-166.

[47] Psychotropic Substances Act of 1978. In. *Public Law 95-633.* Vol Statute 92: Senate and House of Representatives of the United States of America; 1978.

[48] Marks M. Psychedelic medicine for mental illness and substance use disorders: overcoming social and legal obstacles. *NYUJ Legis & Pub Pol'y.* 2018;21:69.

[49] Compass Pathways. COMPASS Pathways Receives FDA Breakthrough Therapy Designation for Psilocybin Therapy for Treatment-Resistant Depression. Cision PR Newswire. https://www.prnewswire.com/news-releases/compass-pathways-receives-fda-breakthrough-therapy-designation-for-psilocybin-therapy-for-treatment-resistant- depression-834088100.html. Published 2018. Accessed August 2018.

[50] Multidisciplinary Association for Psychedelic Studies. FDA Grants MAPS Breakthrough Therapy Designation for Phase 3 Trials of MDMA-Assisted Therapy for PTSD. Multidisciplinary Association for Psychedelic Studies. Newsletter: August 2017 Web site. https://maps.org/2017/08/16/fda-grants-maps-breakthrough-therapy-designation-for- phase-3-trials-of-mdma-assisted-psychotherapy-for-ptsd/. Published 2017. Accessed August 2022.

[51] An Act: Ballot Measure 109. In: Elections Division Secretary of State, ed: Oregon Secretary of State; 2020.

[52] Feduccia AA, Mithoefer MC. MDMA-assisted psychotherapy for PTSD: Are memory reconsolidation and fear extinction underlying mechanisms? *Progress in Neuro- Psychopharmacology & Biological Psychiatry.* 2018;84(Pt A):221-228.

[53] Carhart-Harris RL, Roseman L, Haijen E, et al. Psychedelics and the essential importance of context. *J Psychopharmacol.* 2018;32(7):725-731.

[54] Averill LA, Abdallah CG. Investigational drugs for assisting psychotherapy for posttraumatic stress disorder (PTSD): emerging approaches and shifting paradigms in the era of psychedelic medicine. *Expert Opinion on Investigational Drugs.* 2022;31(2):133- 137.

[55] National Academies of Sciences Engineering and Medicine. In: *Evaluation of the Department of Veterans Affairs Mental Health Services.* Washington (DC): National Academies Press (US); 2018.

[56] Gaynes B N. Identifying difficult-to-treat depression: differential diagnosis, subtypes, and comorbidities. *J Clin Psychiatry.* 2009;70 Suppl 6:10-15.

[57] Goldberg S B, Shechet B, Nicholas C R, et al. Post-acute psychological effects of classical serotonergic psychedelics: a systematic review and meta-analysis. *Psychological Medicine.* 2020;50(16):2655-2666.

[58] Wheeler S W, Dyer N L. A systematic review of psychedelic-assisted psychotherapy for mental health: An evaluation of the current wave of research and suggestions for the future. *Psychology of Consciousness: Theory, Research, and Practice.* 2020;7(3):279- 315.

[59] Romeo B, Karila L, Martelli C, Benyamina A. Efficacy of psychedelic treatments on depressive symptoms: A meta-analysis. *Journal of Psychopharmacology.* 2020;34(10):1079-1085.

[60] *Diagnostic and Statistical Manual of Mental Disorders.* 4th ed. Washington D.C.: American Psychiatric Association; 1994.

[61] Sterne J A, Hernán M A, Reeves B C, et al. ROBINS-I: a tool for assessing risk of bias in non-randomised studies of interventions. *BMJ.* 2016;355:i4919.

[62] Sterne JAC, Savović J, Page MJ, et al. RoB 2: a revised tool for assessing risk of bias in randomised trials. *BMJ.* 2019;366:l4898.

[63] Berkman N D, Lohr K N, Ansari M, et al. AHRQ Methods for Effective Health Care Grading the Strength of a Body of Evidence When Assessing Health Care Interventions for the Effective Health Care Program of the Agency for Healthcare Research and Quality: An Update. In: *Methods Guide for Effectiveness and Comparative Effectiveness Reviews.* Rockville (MD): Agency for Healthcare Research and Quality (US); 2008.

[64] Borenstein M, Higgins J P, Hedges L V, Rothstein H R. Basics of meta-analysis: I(2) is not an absolute measure of heterogeneity. *Res Synth Methods.* 2017;8(1):5-18.

[65] Parr N J, Schweer-Collins M L, Darlington T M, Tanner-Smith E E. Meta-analytic approaches for examining complexity and heterogeneity in studies of adolescent development. *J Adolesc.* 2019;77:168-178.

[66] Knapp G, Hartung J. Improved tests for a random effects meta-regression with a single covariate. *Stat Med.* 2003;22(17):2693-2710.

[67] Viechtbauer W. metafor: Meta-analysis package for R. The Comprehensive R Archive Network. https://cran.r-project.org/web/packages/metafor/index.html. Published 2020. Accessed August 2022.

[68] Mithoefer M C, Feduccia A A, Jerome L, et al. MDMA-assisted psychotherapy for treatment of PTSD: study design and rationale for phase 3 trials based on pooled analysis of six phase 2 randomized controlled trials. *Psychopharmacology.* 2019;236(9):2735- 2745.

[69] Bouso J C, Doblin R, Farre M, Alcazar MA, Gomez-Jarabo G. MDMA-assisted psychotherapy using low doses in a small sample of women with chronic posttraumatic stress disorder. *Journal of Psychoactive Drugs.* 2008;40(3):225-236.

[70] Gukasyan N, Davis AK, Barrett FS, et al. Efficacy and safety of psilocybin-assisted treatment for major depressive disorder: Prospective 12-month follow-up. *Journal of Psychopharmacology.* 2022;36(2):151-158.

[71] Mash D C, Kovera C A, Pablo J, et al. Ibogaine in the treatment of heroin withdrawal. *The Alkaloids Chemistry & Biology.* 2001;56:155-171.

[72] Weathers F, Keane T, Davidson J. Clinician-Administered PTSD Scale: A Review of the First Ten Years of Research. *Depression & Anxiety.* 2001;13:132-156.

Chapter 4

Evidence Brief: Psychedelic Medications for Mental Health and Substance Use Disorders: Supplemental Materials*

U.S. Department of Veterans Affairs

Appendix A: Search Strategy

Systematic Reviews

Search for current systematic reviews (limited to last 7 years) Date Searched: 04-26-22			
A. Bibliographic Databases:	#	Search Statement	Results
MEDLINE:		exp Hallucinogens/ad, ae, pd, tu, th, to [Administration & Dosage,	17439
Systematic	1	Adverse Effects, Pharmacology, Therapeutic Use, Therapy,	
Reviews		Toxicity]	
Ovid MEDLINE(R)	2	(MDMA or LSD or DMT or ayahuasca or psilocybin or psychedelic*). ti,ab.	14393
ALL 1946 to April 25, 2022	3	exp Mental Disorders/dt, pc, rh, tu, th [Drug Therapy, Prevention & Control, Rehabilitation, Therapeutic Use, Therapy]	450492
	4	exp Cannabinoids/ or exp Cannabis/	24987
	5	1 or 2	26925

* This is an edited, reformatted and augmented version of Department of Veterans Affairs Evidence Synthesis Program, Health Services Research and Development Service, Office of Research and Development Publication No. VA ESP Project #09-199; 2022, dated October 2022.

In: The Psychedelic Landscape
Editor: James P. Macintosh
ISBN: 979-8-89530-991-9

Search for current systematic reviews (limited to last 7 years) Date Searched: 04-26-22			
	6	3 and 5	1813
	7	6 not 4	1468
	8	limit 7 to (english language and humans)	1078
		(systematic review.ti. or meta-analysis.pt. or meta-analysis.ti. or	514028
		systematic literature review.ti. or this systematic review.tw. or	
		pooling project.tw. or (systematic review. ti,ab. and review.pt.) or	
		meta synthesis.ti. or meta-analy*.ti. or integrative review.tw. or	
		integrative research review.tw. or rapid review.tw. or umbrella	
		review.tw. or consensus development conference.pt. or practice	
		guideline.pt. or drug class reviews.ti. or cochrane database syst	
		rev.jn. or acp journal club.jn. or health technol assess.jn. or evid	
		rep technol assess summ.jn. or jbi database system rev	
		implement rep.jn. or (clinical guideline and management).tw. or	
		((evidence based.ti. or evidence-based medicine/ or best	
	9	practice*.ti. or evidence synthesis. ti,ab.) and (((review.pt. or	
		diseases category/ or behavior.mp.) and behavior mechanisms/)	
		or therapeutics/ or evaluation studies.pt. or validation studies.pt.	
		or guideline.pt. or pmcbook.mp.)) or (((systematic or systematically).tw. or critical. ti,ab. or study selection.tw. or	
		((predetermined or inclusion) and criteri*).tw. or exclusion	
		criteri*.tw. or main outcome measures.tw. or standard of care.tw.	
		or standards of care.tw.) and ((survey or surveys).ti,ab. or	
		overview*.tw. or review. ti,ab. or reviews.ti,ab. or search*.tw. or	
		handsearch.tw. or analysis.ti. or critique. ti,ab. or appraisal.tw. or	

Search for current systematic reviews (limited to last 7 years) Date Searched: 04-26-22			
		(reduction.tw. and (risk/ or risk.tw.) and (death or	
		recurrence).mp.)) and ((literature or articles or publications or	
		publication or bibliography or bibliographies or published). ti,ab. or	
		pooled data.tw. or unpublished.tw. or citation.tw. or citations.tw. or	
		database. ti,ab. or internet.ti,ab. or textbooks.ti,ab. or	
		references.tw. or scales.tw. or papers.tw. or datasets.tw. or	
		trials.ti,ab. or meta-analy*.tw. or (clinical and studies). ti,ab. or	
		treatment outcome/ or treatment outcome.tw. or pmcbook.mp.)))	
		not (letter or newspaper article). pt.	
	10	8 AND 9	47
CDSR: Protocols and Reviews	1	hallucinogen*. ti,ab.	1
	2	(MDMA or LSD or DMT or ayahuasca or psilocybin or	7
EBM Reviews -		psychedelic*). ti,ab.	
	3	mental disorder.ti,ab.	16
Cochrane			
	4	Cannabinoids or Cannabis. ti,ab.	57
Database of			
Systematic	5	1 or 2	8
Reviews 2005 to			
	6	3 and 5	0
April 20, 2022			
	7	6 not 4	0
	8	limit 7 to (english language and humans)	0

Search for current systematic reviews (limited to last 7 years) Date Searched: 04-26-22		
B. Non-bibliographic databases	Evidence	Results
AHRQ: evidence reports, technology assessments, U.S	http://www.ahrq.gov/research/findings/evidence-based-reports/search.html Search: (mental disorders OR substance use) AND (MDMA or LSD or DMT or ayahuasca or psilocybin or psychedelic)	2

Search for current systematic reviews (limited to last 7 years) Date Searched: 04-26-22		
Preventative Services Task Force Evidence Synthesis	AHRQ. 2020. Pharmacologic and Nonpharmacologic Treatments for Posttraumatic Stress Disorder: An Update of the PTSD Repository Evidence Base. https://effectivehealthcare.ahrq.gov/products/ptsd- repository-update/protocol AHRQ. 2020. Pharmacologic and Nonpharmacologic Treatments for Posttraumatic Stress Disorder. https://effectivehealthcare.ahrq.gov/products/ptsd-repository-expanded/research	
CADTH	https://www.cadth.ca Search: (mental disorders OR substance use) AND (MDMA or LSD or DMT or ayahuasca or psilocybin or psychedelic) CADTH. 2021. Psychedelic-Assisted Psychotherapy for Post-Traumatic Stress Disorder, Anxiety Disorders, Mood Disorders, or Substance Use Disorders. https://www.cadth.ca/psychedelic-assisted-psychotherapy-post- traumatic-stress-disorder-anxiety-disorders-mood-disorders	1
ECRI Institute	https://guidelines.ecri.org/ Search: (mental disorders OR substance use) AND (MDMA or LSD or DMT or ayahuasca or psilocybin or psychedelic)	0
HTA: Health Technology Assessments (UP TO 2016)	http://www.ohsu.edu/xd/education/library/ See CDSR search above	0
EPPI-Centre	http://eppi.ioe.ac.uk/cms/Default.aspx?tabid=62 Use browser search function [CNTL + F] for keyword search Search: MDMA or LSD or DMT or ayahuasca or psilocybin or psychedelic	0
NLM	http://www.ncbi.nlm.nih.gov/books Search: (mental disorders OR substance use) AND (MDMA or LSD or DMT or ayahuasca or psilocybin or psychedelic)	0
VA Products - VATAP, PBM and HSR&D publications	A. http://www.hsrd.research.va.gov/research/default.cfm Search: (mental disorders OR substance use) AND (MDMA or LSD or DMT or ayahuasca or psilocybin or psychedelic)	0

Primary Studies

Search for primary literature Date searched: 04-26-22		
MEDLINE [Ovid MEDLINE(R) ALL 1946 to April 25, 2022]		
#	Search Statement	Results
1	exp Hallucinogens/ad, ae, pd, tu, th, to [Administration & Dosage, Adverse Effects, Pharmacology, Therapeutic Use, Therapy, Toxicity]	17439
2	(MDMA or LSD or DMT or ayahuasca or psilocybin or psychedelic*).ti,ab.	14393
3	exp Mental Disorders/dt, pc, rh, tu, th [Drug Therapy, Prevention & Control, Rehabilitation, Therapeutic Use, Therapy]	450492
4	exp Cannabinoids/ or exp Cannabis/	24987
5	1 or 2	26925
6	3 and 5	1813
7	6 not 4	1468
8	limit 7 to (english language and humans)	1078
PsycINFO [APA PsycInfo 1806 to April Week 3 2022]		
#	Search Statement	Results
1	exp Hallucinogenic Drugs/	4238
2	(MDMA or LSD or DMT or ayahuasca or psilocybin or psychedelic*). ti,ab.	6788
3	exp Mental Disorders/	929175
4	exp Cannabinoids/ or exp Cannabis/	15155
5	1 or 2	8737
6	3 and 5	2513
7	6 not 4	2333
8	limit 7 to (english language and humans)	1728

Appendix B: Excluded Studies

Exclude reasons: 1=Ineligible population, 2=Ineligible intervention, 3=Ineligible comparator, 4=Ineligible outcome, 5=Ineligible timing, 6=Ineligible study design, 7=Ineligible publication type, 8=Outdated or ineligible systematic review, 9=non-English language, 10=unable to retrieve full-text, 11=study published before 1994.

Citation	Exclude Reason
Abramson HA. LSD in psychotherapy and alcoholism. *American Journal of Psychotherapy*. 1966;20(3):415-438.	E7

Citation	Exclude Reason
Abramson HA. Lysergic acid diethylamide (LSD 25). XXXXI. The use of LSD as an adjunct to psychotherapy: fact and fiction. *Journal of Asthma Research*. 1973;10(4):227-235.	E7
Abuzzahab FS, Sr., Anderson BJ. A review of LSD treatment in alcoholism. *International Pharmacopsychiatry*. 1971;6(4):223-235.	E7
Aday JS, Mitzkovitz CM, Bloesch EK, Davoli CC, Davis AK. Long-term effects of psychedelic drugs: A systematic review. *Neuroscience and Biobehavioral Reviews*. 2020;113:179-189.	E8
Agin-Liebes G. The role of self-compassion in psilocybin-assisted motivational enhancement therapy to treat alcohol dependence: A randomized controlled trial. *Dissertation Abstracts International: Section B: The Sciences and Engineering*. 2021;82(9-B).	E10
Albaugh BJ, Anderson PO. Peyote in the treatment of alcoholism among American Indians. *American Journal of Psychiatry*. 1974;131(11):1247-1250.	E7
Alexander L. Mind and body in biological psychiatry. *Biological Psychiatry*. 1973;5(3):225-238.	E10
Almond K, Allan R. Incorporating MDMA as an adjunct in emotionally focused couples therapy with clients impacted by trauma or PTSD. *The Family Journal*. 2019;27(3):293-299.	E7
Alper KR. Ibogaine: a review. *The Alkaloids Chemistry & Biology*. 2001;56:1-38.	E7
Alper KR, Glick SD. Psychotropic complementary medicines. *British Journal of Psychiatry*. 2006;188:587; author reply 587-588.	E7
Alper KR, Lotsof HS, Frenken GM, Luciano DJ, Bastiaans J. Treatment of acute opioid withdrawal with ibogaine. American Journal on Addictions. 1999;8(3):234- 242.	E11
Amoroso T. The Psychopharmacology of +/-3,4 Methylenedioxymethamphetamine and its Role in the Treatment of Posttraumatic Stress Disorder. *Journal of Psychoactive Drugs*. 2015;47(5):337-344.	E7
Amoroso T, Workman M. Treating posttraumatic stress disorder with MDMA-assisted psychotherapy: A preliminary meta-analysis and comparison to prolonged exposure therapy. *Journal of Psychopharmacology*. 2016;30(7):595-600.	E8
Andersen KAA, Carhart-Harris R, Nutt DJ, Erritzoe D. Therapeutic effects of classic serotonergic psychedelics: A systematic review of modern-era clinical studies. *Acta Psychiatrica Scandinavica*. 2021;143(2):101-118.	E8
Anonymous. LSD: the search for definite conclusions. *JAMA*. 1966;196(4):Suppl:32-33.	E7
Anonymous. Dependence on LSD and other hallucinogenic drugs. *JAMA*. 1967;202(1):141-144.	E7

Citation	Exclude Reason
Anonymous. Preventing misuse of L.S.D. *Lancet*. 1967;1(7483):202.	E7
Anonymous. Control of amphetamines and L.S.D. *Lancet*. 1970;1(7649):708.	E7
Anonymous. L.S.D. in psychiatry. *Lancet*. 1970;2(7678):877-878.	E7
Anonymous. Treatment of alcoholism. II. *Maryland State Medical Journal*. 1973;22(4):17-19.	E7
Anonymous. Think harder about ecstasy. *Nature*. 2004;429(6988):113.	E7
Anonymous. Magic mushroom compound is a potential treatment for patients with major depression. *Nursing Standard*. 2016;30(41):15.	E7
Apud Pelaez IE. Personality Traits in Former Spanish Substance Users Recovered with Ayahuasca. *Journal of Psychoactive Drugs*. 2020;52(3):264-272.	E4
Argento E, Capler R, Thomas G, Lucas P, Tupper KW. Exploring ayahuasca- assisted therapy for addiction: A qualitative analysis of preliminary findings among an Indigenous community in Canada. *Drug & Alcohol Review*. 2019;38(7):781-789.	E6
Argento E, Tupper KW, Socias ME. The tripping point: The potential role of psychedelic-assisted therapy in the response to the opioid crisis. *International Journal of Drug Policy*. 2019;66:80-81.	E7
Modeling Study. *Clinical Drug Investigation*. 2022;42(3):243-252.	E6
Averill LA, Abdallah CG. Investigational drugs for assisting psychotherapy for posttraumatic stress disorder (PTSD): emerging approaches and shifting paradigms in the era of psychedelic medicine. *Expert Opinion on Investigational Drugs*. 2022;31(2):133-137.	E7
Bahji A, Forsyth A, Groll D, Hawken ER. Efficacy of 3,4-methylenedioxymethamphetamine (MDMA)-assisted psychotherapy for posttraumatic stress disorder: A systematic review and meta-analysis. *Progress in Neuro-Psychopharmacology & Biological Psychiatry*. 2020;96:109735.	E8
Barabasz-Gembczyk A, Kucia K. Ayahuasca - potential therapeutic properties in psychiatry. Research review. *Psychiatria Polska*. 2020;54(2):381-389.	E7
Barker ET, Buck MF. LSD in a coercive milieu therapy program. *Canadian Psychiatric Association Journal*. 1977;22(6):311-314.	E4
Barnett BS, Greer GR. Psychedelic psychiatry and the consult-liaison psychiatrist: A primer. *Journal of the Academy of Consultation Liaison Psychiatry*. 2021;62(4):460-471.	E7
Barrios AA. An explanation of the behavioral and therapeutic effects of the hallucinogens. *International Journal of Neuropsychiatry*. 1965;1(6):574-592.	E7

Citation	Exclude Reason
Basky G. Policy in focus: Is psilocybin the next cannabis? *CMAJ Canadian*	E7
Medical Association Journal. 2021;193(45):E1741-E1742.	
Bateman C. Ibogaine may help drug addicts live the 'never again'. *South African Medical Journal Suid-Afrikaanse Tydskrif Vir Geneeskunde*. 2006;96(7):580, 582.	E7
Bedi G. 3,4-Methylenedioxymethamphetamine as a Psychiatric Treatment. *JAMA Psychiatry*. 2018;75(5):419-420.	E7
Bergman RL. Navajo peyote use: its apparent safety. *American Journal of Psychiatry*. 1971;128(6):695-699.	E1
Bienemann B, Ruschel NS, Campos ML, Negreiros MA, Mograbi DC. Self- reported negative outcomes of psilocybin users: A quantitative textual analysis. *PLoS ONE*. 2020;15(2).	E1
Bird CIV, Modlin NL, Rucker JJH. Psilocybin and MDMA for the treatment of trauma-related psychopathology. International Review of Psychiatry. 2021;33(3):229-249.	E7
Boer AP, Sipprelle CN. Induced anxiety in the treatment for LSD effects. Psychotherapy & Psychosomatics. 1969;17(2):108-113.	E6
Bogenschutz MP, Johnson MW. Classic hallucinogens in the treatment of addictions. Progress in Neuro-Psychopharmacology & Biological Psychiatry. 2016; 64:250-258.	E7
Bonny HL, Pahnke WN. The use of music in psychedelic (LSD) psychotherapy. *Journal of Music Therapy*. 1972;9(2):64-87.	E7
Bouso JC, Ryan C. Using MDMA in the treatment of post-traumatic stress disorder. Holland, Julie [Ed] (2001). 2001; Ecstasy: The complete guide: A comprehensive look at the risks and benefits of MDMA. (pp. 248-260). x.	E7
Bowen WT, Soskin RA, Chotlos JW. Lysergic acid diethylamide as a variable in the hospital treatment of alcoholism. Journal of Nervous and Mental Disease. 1970;150(2):111-118.	E11
Bramble FB. Dependency needs in chronic hallucinogenic drug abusers. Dissertation Abstracts International. 1974;34(7-B).	E4
Breeksema JJ, Niemeijer AR, Krediet E, Vermetten E, Schoevers RA. Psychedelic Treatments for Psychiatric Disorders: A Systematic Review and Thematic Synthesis of Patient Experiences in Qualitative Studies. CNS Drugs. 2020;34(9):925-946.	E6
Brewerton TD, Lafrance A, Mithoefer MC. The potential use of N-methyl-3,4-methylenedioxyamphetamine (MDMA) assisted psychotherapy in the treatment of*eating disorders comorbid with PTSD. Medical Hypotheses. 2021;146:110367.*	E6
Brewerton TD, Wang JB, Lafrance A, et al. MDMA-assisted therapy significantly reduces eating disorder symptoms in a randomized	E4

Citation	Exclude Reason
placebo-controlled trial of *adults with severe PTSD. Journal of Psychiatric Research. 2022;149:128-135.*	
Brown TK, Noller GE, Denenberg JO. Ibogaine and Subjective Experience: Transformative States and Psychopharmacotherapy in the Treatment of Opioid Use Disorder. Journal of Psychoactive Drugs. 2019;51(2):155-165.	E4
Bryce JC. An evaluation of LSD in the treatment of chronic alcoholism. *Canadian Psychiatric Association Journal.* 1970;15(1):77-78.	E7
Buckman J. Theoretical aspects of L.S.D. therapy. International Journal of Social Psychiatry. 1967;13(2):126-138.	E7
Carbonaro TM, Gatch MB. Neuropharmacology of N, N-dimethyltryptamine. Brain Research Bulletin. 2016;126(Pt 1):74-88.	E7
Chabrol H. MDMA assisted psychotherapy found to have a large effect for chronic post-traumatic stress disorder. *Journal of Psychopharmacology.* 2013;27(9):865-866.	E7
Chang AF, Caldwell AB, Moss T. The stability of personality traits in alcoholics during and after treatment as measured by the MMPI: A one year follow-up study. *Proceedings of the Annual Convention of the American Psychological Association.* 1973:389-390.	E11
Check E. Psychedelic drugs: the ups and downs of ecstasy. *Nature.* 2004;429(6988):126-128.	E7
Cheek FE, Osmond H, Sarett M. Observations regarding the use of LSD-25 in the treatment of alcoholism. Journal of Psychopharmacology. 1966;1(2):56-74.	E10
Chessick RD, Haertzen CA, Wikler A. Tolerance to LSD-25 in schizophrenic subjects. Archives of General Psychiatry. 1964;10(6):653-658.	E4
Chi T, Gold JA. A review of emerging therapeutic potential of psychedelic drugs in the treatment of psychiatric illnesses. *Journal of the Neurological Sciences.* 2020;411:116715.	E7
Cholden LS, Kurland A, Savage C. Clinical reactions and tolerance to LSD in chronic schizophrenia. Journal of Nervous & Mental Disease. 1955;122(3):211-221.	E1
Cipriani A, Cowen PJ. 3,4-methylenedioxymethamphetamine (MDMA)-assisted *psychotherapy for post-traumatic stress disorder in service personnel. The Lancet Psychiatry. 2018;5(6):453-455.*	E7
Cline HS, Freeman H. Resistance to lysergic acid in schizophrenic patients. *Psychiatric Quarterly. 1956;30(4):676-683.*	E11
Clyman RC. LSD psychotherapy: a review of the literature and some proposals for future research. *Rhode Island Medical Journal.* 1972;55(9):282-286.	E7

Citation	Exclude Reason
Cohen RS. Adverse symptomatology and suicide associated with the use of methylenedioxymethamphetamine (MDMA; "Ecstasy"). *Biological Psychiatry. 1996;39(9):819-820.*	E1
Corey VR, Pisano VD, Halpern JH. Effects of 3,4-Methylenedioxymethamphetamine on Patient Utterances in a Psychotherapeutic *Setting. Journal of Nervous & Mental Disease. 2016;204(7):519-523.*	E4
Corkery JM. Ibogaine as a treatment for substance misuse: Potential benefits and practical dangers. *Progress in Brain Research. 2018;242:217-257.*	E7
Cox DJ, Garcia-Romeu A, Johnson MW. Predicting changes in substance use following psychedelic experiences: natural language processing of psychedelic session narratives. *American Journal of Drug & Alcohol Abuse. 2021;47(4):444-454.*	E10
Crowley N. A role for psychedelics in psychiatry? *British Journal of Psychiatry. 2005;187:483; author reply 484-485.*	E7
Curran HV, Nutt D, de Wit H. Psychedelics and related drugs: therapeutic possibilities, mechanisms and regulation. *Psychopharmacology. 2018;235(2):373-375.*	E7
Curry AE. Elixir of anguish: The phenomenology of the alcoholic's perennial quest. *Psychiatric Quarterly Supplement. 1964;38(1):13-20.*	E4
Danforth AL, Grob CS, Struble C, et al. Reduction in social anxiety after MDMA-assisted psychotherapy with autistic adults: a randomized, double-blind, placebo-controlled pilot study. *Psychopharmacology. 2018;235(11):3137-3148.*	E1
Danforth AL, Struble CM, Yazar-Klosinski B, Grob CS. MDMA-assisted therapy: A new treatment model for social anxiety in autistic adults. *Progress in Neuro-Psychopharmacology & Biological Psychiatry. 2016;64:237-249.*	E7
Davey CG. Out of the night-time and into the day: Ketamine and MDMA as therapies for mental disorders. *Australian & New Zealand Journal of Psychiatry. 2021;55(8):741-743.*	E7
Davis AK, Barrett FS, Griffiths RR. Psychological flexibility mediates the relations between acute psychedelic effects and subjective decreases in depression and anxiety. *Journal of Contextual Behavioral Science. 2020;15:39-45.*	E1
Davis AK, Griffiths RR. Errors in a response rate and in effect sizes in study of psilocybin-assisted therapy for major depressive disorder. *JAMA Psychiatry. 2021;78(5):569.*	E7
Davis AK, Renn E, Windham-Herman AM, Polanco M, Barsuglia JP. A Mixed- Method Analysis of Persisting Effects Associated with	E4

Citation	Exclude Reason
Positive Outcomes Following Ibogaine Detoxification. Journal of Psychoactive Drugs. 2018;50(4):287- 297.	
Davis AK, So S, Lancelotta R, Barsuglia JP, Griffiths RR. 5-methoxy-N,N- dimethyltryptamine (5-MeO-DMT) used in a naturalistic group setting is associated with unintended improvements in depression and anxiety. American Journal of Drug & Alcohol Abuse. 2019;45(2):161-169.	E1
Daws RE, Timmermann C, Giribaldi B, et al. Increased global integration in the brain after psilocybin therapy for depression. *Nature Medicine.* 2022;28(4):844- 851.	E4
Day J. The role and reaction of the psychiatrist in LSD therapy. *Journal of Nervous & Mental Disease.* 1957;125(3):437-438.	E7
de Almeida RN, de Menezes Galvao AC, da Silva FS, et al. Modulation of serum brain-derived neurotrophic factor by a single dose of ayahuasca: Observation from a randomized controlled trial. *Frontiers in Psychology.* 2019;10.	E4
De Gregorio D, Aguilar-Valles A, Preller KH, et al. Hallucinogens in Mental Health: Preclinical and Clinical Studies on LSD, Psilocybin, MDMA, and Ketamine. *Journal of Neuroscience.* 2021;41(5):891-900.	E7
de Kleine RA, Rothbaum BO, van Minnen A. Pharmacological enhancement of exposure-based treatment in PTSD: A qualitative review. *European Journal of Psychotraumatology.* 2013;4:21626.	E8
de Veen BT, Schellekens AF, Verheij MM, Homberg JR. Psilocybin for treating substance use disorders? *Expert Review of Neurotherapeutics.* 2017;17(2):203- 212.	E7
Denber HC. Studies with mescaline. *Rivista di Neurobiologia.* 1964;10(4):Suppl:1157-1168.	E7
Denber HC. Mescaline and lysergic acid diethylamide: therapeutic implications of the drug-induced state. *Diseases of the Nervous System.* 1969;30(2):Suppl:23-27.	E10
Denson R. Dissociative delirium after treatment with lysergide. *Canadian Medical Association Journal.* 1967;97(20):1222-1224.	E6
Denson R. Lysergide therapy and the mauve factor. *Acta Psychiatrica Scandinavica.* 1968;44(3):280-288.	E11
Denson R. Complications of therapy with lysergide. *Canadian Medical Association Journal.* 1969;101(11):53-57.	E11
Denson R, Sydiaha D. A controlled study of LSD treatment in alcoholism and neurosis. *British Journal of Psychiatry.* 1970;116(533):443-445.	E1
Ditman KS, et al. Psychological and drug variables in the LSD experiences of alcoholics. *Psychotherapy and Psychosomatics.* 1967;15(1):15.	E10

Citation	Exclude Reason
DiVito AJ, Leger RF. Psychedelics as an emerging novel intervention in the treatment of substance use disorder: a review. *Molecular Biology Reports*. 2020;47(12):9791-9799.	E7
Dominguez-Clave E, Soler J, Pascual JC, et al. Ayahuasca improves emotion dysregulation in a community sample and in individuals with borderline-like traits. *Psychopharmacology*. 2019;236(2):573-580.	E1
Donnelly JR. The need for ibogaine in drug and alcohol addiction treatment. *Journal of Legal Medicine*. 2011;32(1):93-114.	E7
Dos Santos RG, Balthazar FM, Bouso JC, Hallak JE. The current state of research on ayahuasca: A systematic review of human studies assessing psychiatric symptoms, neuropsychological functioning, and neuroimaging. *Journal of Psychopharmacology*. 2016;30(12):1230-1247.	E1
Dos Santos RG, Bouso JC, Alcazar-Corcoles MA, Hallak JEC. Efficacy, tolerability, and safety of serotonergic psychedelics for the management of mood, anxiety, and substance-use disorders: a systematic review of systematic reviews. *Expert Review of Clinical Pharmacology*. 2018;11(9):889-902.	E8
Dos Santos RG, Hallak JE, Baker G, Dursun S. Hallucinogenic/psychedelic 5HT2A receptor agonists as rapid antidepressant therapeutics: Evidence and mechanisms of action. *Journal of Psychopharmacology*. 2021;35(4):453-458.	*E7*
Dos Santos RG, Osorio FL, Crippa JA, Hallak JE. Antidepressive and anxiolytic effects of ayahuasca: a systematic literature review of animal and human studies. *Revista Brasileira de Psiquiatria*. 2016;38(1):65-72.	*E8*
dos Santos RG, Osorio FL, Crippa JAS, Bouso JC, Hallak JEC. The therapeutic potential of ayahuasca and other serotonergic hallucinogens in the treatment of social anxiety. *Osorio, Flavia de Lima [Ed]; Donadon, Mariana Fortunata [Ed] (2018)*. 2018;Social anxiety disorder:Recognition.	E7
Doss MK, Povazan M, Rosenberg MD, et al. Psilocybin therapy increases cognitive and neural flexibility in patients with major depressive disorder. *Transl Psychiatry Psychiatry*. 2021;11(1):574.	*E4*
Eagle CT. Music and LSD: An empirical study. *Journal of Music Therapy*. 1972;9(1):23-36.	E6
Erritzoe D, Roseman L, Nour MM, et al. Effects of psilocybin therapy on personality structure. *Acta Psychiatrica Scandinavica*. 2018;138(5):368-378.	E4
Fadiman J, Korb S. Might microdosing psychedelics be safe and beneficial? An initial exploration. *Journal of Psychoactive Drugs*. 2019;51(2):118-122.	E6

Citation	Exclude Reason
Faillace LA. Clinical use of psychotomimetic drugs. *Comprehensive Psychiatry*. 1966;7(1):13-20.	E7
Faillace LA, Vourlekis A, Szara S. Clinical evaluation of some hallucinogenic tryptamine derivatives. *Journal of Nervous & Mental Disease*. 1967;145(4):306- 313.	E4
Faillace LA, Vourlekis A, Szara S. Hallucinogenic drugs in the treatment of alcoholism: a two-year follow-up. *Comprehensive Psychiatry*. 1970;11(1):51-56.	E11
Fauvel B, Strika-Bruneau L, Piolino P. Changes in self-rumination and self- compassion mediate the effect of psychedelic experiences on decreases in depression, anxiety, and stress. *Psychology of Consciousness: Theory, Research, and Practice*. 2021(Pagination).	E1
Feduccia AA, Jerome L, Mithoefer MC, Holland J. Discontinuation of medications classified as reuptake inhibitors affects treatment response of MDMA-assisted psychotherapy. *Psychopharmacology*. 2021;238(2):581-588.	*E4*
Feduccia AA, Jerome L, Yazar-Klosinski B, Emerson A, Mithoefer MC, Doblin R. Breakthrough for trauma treatment: Safety and efficacy of mdma-assisted psychotherapy compared to paroxetine and sertraline. *Frontiers in Psychiatry*. 2019;10:650.	*E8*
Fink M, Simeon J, Haque W, Itil T. Prolonged adverse reactions to LSD in psychotic subjects. *Archives of General Psychiatry*. 1966;15(5):450-454.	E6
Frenken G. From the roots up: ibogaine and addict self-help. *The Alkaloids Chemistry & Biology*. 2001;56:283-292.	E7
Fuentes JJ, Fonseca F, Elices M, Farre M, Torrens M. Therapeutic use of LSD in psychiatry: A systematic review of randomized-controlled clinical trials. Frontiers in Psychiatry. 2020;10:943.	E8
Galvao-Coelho NL, Marx W, Gonzalez M, et al. Classic serotonergic psychedelics for mood and depressive symptoms: a meta-analysis of mood disorder patients and healthy participants. *Psychopharmacology*. 2021;238(2):341-354.	E8
Garcia-Romeu A, Barrett FS, Carbonaro TM, Johnson MW, Griffiths RR. Optimal dosing for psilocybin pharmacotherapy: Considering weight-adjusted and fixed dosing approaches. *Journal of Psychopharmacology*. 2021;35(4):353-361.	E4
Garcia-Romeu A, Davis AK, Erowid F, Erowid E, Griffiths RR, Johnson MW. Cessation and reduction in alcohol consumption and misuse after psychedelic use. *Journal of Psychopharmacology*. 2019;33(9):1088-1101.	E2
Garcia-Romeu A, Griffiths RR, Johnson MW. Psilocybin-occasioned mystical experiences in the treatment of tobacco addiction. *Current Drug Abuse Reviews*. 2014;7(3):157-164.	E4

Citation	Exclude Reason
Gilbert CS, Earleywine M, Mian MN, Altman BR. Symptom specificity of ayahuasca's effect on depressive symptoms. *Journal of Psychedelic Studies*. 2021;5(1):37-43.	E1
Gill H, Gill B, Chen-Li D, et al. The emerging role of psilocybin and MDMA in the treatment of mental illness. *Expert Review of Neurotherapeutics*. 2020;20(12):1263-1273.	E7
Giovannetti C, Garcia Arce S, Rush B, Mendive F. Pilot Evaluation of a Residential Drug Addiction Treatment Combining Traditional Amazonian Medicine, Ayahuasca and Psychotherapy on Depression and Anxiety. *Journal of Psychoactive Drugs*. 2020;52(5):472-481.	E4
Goldberg SB, Pace BT, Nicholas CR, Raison CL, Hutson PR. The experimental effects of psilocybin on symptoms of anxiety and depression: A meta-analysis. *Psychiatry Research*. 2020;284:112749.	E8
Goldberg SB, Shechet B, Nicholas CR, et al. Post-acute psychological effects of classical serotonergic psychedelics: a systematic review and meta-analysis. *Psychological Medicine*. 2020;50(16):2655-2666.	E8
Gomez-Busto FJ, Ortiz MI. Virtual reality and psychedelics for the treatment of psychiatric disease: A systematic literature review. Clinical Neuropsychiatry: *Journal of Treatment Evaluation*. 2020;17(6):365-380.	E8
Gorman I, Belser AB, Jerome L, et al. Posttraumatic Growth After MDMA-Assisted Psychotherapy for Posttraumatic Stress Disorder. *Journal of Traumatic Stress*. 2020;33(2):161-170.	E8
Greenway KT, Garel N, Jerome L, Feduccia AA. Integrating psychotherapy and psychopharmacology: psychedelic-assisted psychotherapy and other combined treatments. *Expert Review of Clinical Pharmacology*. 2020;13(6):655-670.	E7
Greer GR, Tolbert R. A method of conducting therapeutic sessions with MDMA. *Journal of Psychoactive Drugs*. 1998;30(4):371-379.	E6
Grinspoon L, Bakalar JB. The psychedelic drug therapies. *Current Psychiatric Therapies. 1981*;20:275-283.	E10
Grof S, Soskin RA, Richards WA, Kurland AA. DPT as an adjunct in psychotherapy of alcoholics. *International Pharmacopsychiatry*. 1973;8(1):104-115.	E11
Halpern JH, Sherwood AR, Hudson JI, Yurgelun-Todd D, Pope HG, Jr. Psychological and Cognitive Effects of Long-Term Peyote Use Among Native Americans. *Biological Psychiatry*. 2005;58(8):624-631.	E1

Citation	Exclude Reason
Hamill J, Hallak J, Dursun SM, Baker G. Ayahuasca: Psychological and Physiologic Effects, Pharmacology and Potential Uses in Addiction and Mental Illness. *Current Neuropharmacology.* 2019;17(2):108-128.	E7
Harris R, Gurel L. A study of ayahuasca use in North America. *Journal of Psychoactive Drugs.* 2012;44(3):209-215.	E1
Hatrick JA, Dewhurst K. Delayed psychosis due to L.S.D. *Lancet.* 1970;2(7676):742-744.	E1
Hausner M, Dolezal V. Follow-up studies in group and individual LSD psychotherapy. *Activitas Nervosa Superior.* 1966;8(1):87-95.	E1
Hausner M, Dolezal V. Follow-up evaluation of LSD psychotherapy of inpatients. *Activitas Nervosa Superior.* 1968;10(3):282-283.	E1
Heal DJ, Gosden J, Smith SL. Evaluating the abuse potential of psychedelic drugs as part of the safety pharmacology assessment for medical use in humans. *Neuropharmacology.* 2018;142:89-115.	E7
Heink A, Katsikas S, Lange-Altman T. Examination of the Phenomenology of the Ibogaine Treatment Experience: Role of Altered States of Consciousness and Psychedelic Experiences. Journal of Psychoactive Drugs. 2017;49(3):201-208.	E1
Heink AL. Examination of the phenomeonology of the ibogaine treatment experience on change: Role of altered states of consciousness and psychedelic experiences. Dissertation Abstracts International: Section B: *The Sciences and Engineering.* 2016;76(11-B(E).	E10
Hendricks PS. Back to the future: a return to psychedelic treatment models for addiction. *Journal of Psychopharmacology.* 2014;28(11):981-982.	E7
Hendricks PS, Clark CB, Johnson MW, Fontaine KR, Cropsey KL. Hallucinogen use predicts reduced recidivism among substance-involved offenders under community corrections supervision. *Journal of Psychopharmacology.* 2014;28(1):62-66.	E4
Hendricks PS, Thorne CB, Clark CB, Coombs DW, Johnson MW. Classic psychedelic use is associated with reduced psychological distress and suicidality in the United States adult population. *Journal of Psychopharmacology.* 2015;29(3):280-288.	E1
Heuschkel K, Kuypers KPC. Depression, mindfulness, and psilocybin: Possible complementary effects of mindfulness meditation and psilocybin in the treatment of depression. A review. *Frontiers in Psychiatry.* 2020;11:224.	E8
Hittner JB, Quello SB. Combating substance abuse with ibogaine: pre- and posttreatment recommendations and an example of	E6

Citation	Exclude Reason
successive model fitting analyses. *Journal of Psychoactive Drugs*. 2004;36(2):191-199.	
Hoch PH. Remarks on LSD and mescaline. Journal of Nervous & Mental Disease. 1957;125(3):442-444.	E7
Hoelen DW, Spiering W, Valk GD. Long-QT syndrome induced by the antiaddiction drug ibogaine. *New England Journal of Medicine*. 2009;360(3):308-309.	E6
Hofling CK, Winslow WW, Stone WN. Drug therapy. *Progress in Neurology & Psychiatry*. 1969;24:478-497.	E7
Hollister LE, Shelton J, Krieger G. A controlled comparison of lysergic acid diethylamide (LSD) and dextroamphetmine in alcoholics. *American Journal of Psychiatry*. 1969;125(10):1352-1357.	E11
Holoyda B. Psychedelic Psychiatry: Preparing for Novel Treatments Involving Altered States of Consciousness. *Psychiatric Services*. 2020;71(12):1297-1299.	E7
Hosanagar A, Cusimano J, Radhakrishnan R. Therapeutic Potential of Psychedelics in Treatment of Psychiatric Disorders, Part 2: Review of the Evidence. *Journal of Clinical Psychiatry*. 2021;82(3):23.	E7
Hosanagar A, Cusimano J, Radhakrishnan R. Therapeutic Potential of Psychedelics in the Treatment of Psychiatric Disorders, Part 1: Psychopharmacology and Neurobiological Effects. *Journal of Clinical Psychiatry*. 2021;82(2):23.	E7
Hoskins MD, Sinnerton R, Nakamura A, et al. Pharmacological-assisted psychotherapy for post-traumatic stress disorder: A systematic review and meta- analysis. *European Journal of Psychotraumatology*. 2021;12(1):1853379.	E8
Hostiuc S, Buda O, Ion DA. Harmine for catatonic schizophrenia. A forgotten experiment. *Schizophrenia Research*. 2014;159(1):249-250.	E7
Hrdina PD, Bakish D, Ravindran A, Chudzik J, Cavazzoni P, Lapierre YD. Platelet serotonergic indices in major depression: up-regulation of 5-HT2A receptors unchanged by antidepressant treatment. *Psychiatry Research*. 1997;66(2-3):73- 85.	E4
Huang DS. The efficacy of psychedelic-assisted psychotherapy. *Dissertation Abstracts International: Section B: The Sciences and Engineering*. 2020;81(12-B).	E10
Hungerford DA, Taylor KM, Shagass C, LaBadie GU, Balaban GB, Paton GR. Cytogenetic effects of LSD 25 therapy in man. *JAMA*. 1968;206(10):2287-2291.	E4

Citation	Exclude Reason
Hutchison CA, Bressi SK. MDMA-assisted psychotherapy for posttraumatic stress disorder: Implications for social work practice and research. *Clinical Social Work Journal*. 2020;48(4):421-430.	E7
Hutten NRPW, Mason NL, Dolder PC, Kuypers KPC. Self-rated effectiveness of microdosing with psychedelics for mental and physical health problems among microdosers. *Frontiers in Psychiatry*. 2019;10:672.	E2
Illingworth BJ, Lewis DJ, Lambarth AT, et al. A comparison of MDMA-assisted psychotherapy to non-assisted psychotherapy in treatment-resistant PTSD: A systematic review and meta-analysis. *Journal of Psychopharmacology*. 2021;35(5):501-511.	E8
Itil TM, Keskiner S, Holden JM. The use of LSD and ditran in the treatment of therapy resistant schizophrenics (symptom provocation approach). *Diseases of the Nervous System*. 1969;30(2): Suppl:93-103.	E4
Jerome L, Feduccia AA, Wang JB, et al. Long-term follow-up outcomes of MDMA- assisted psychotherapy for treatment of PTSD: a longitudinal pooled analysis of six phase 2 trials. *Psychopharmacology*. 2020;237(8):2485-2497.	E8
Jerome L, Schuster S, Yazar-Klosinski BB. Can MDMA play a role in the treatment of substance abuse? *Current Drug Abuse Reviews*. 2013;6(1):54-62.	E7
Johnson FG. LSD in the treatment of alcoholism. *American Journal of Psychiatry*. 1969;126(4):481-487.	E11
Johnson FG. A comparison of short-term treatment effects of intravenous sodium amytal-methedrine and LSD in the alcoholic. *Canadian Psychiatric Association Journal*. 1970;15(5):493-497.	E4
Johnson MW, Garcia-Romeu A, Johnson PS, Griffiths RR. An online survey of tobacco smoking cessation associated with naturalistic psychedelic use. *Journal of Psychopharmacology*. 2017;31(7):841-850.	E2
Johnson MW, Griffiths RR. Potential Therapeutic Effects of Psilocybin. *Neurotherapeutics*. 2017;14(3):734-740.	E7
Johnson MW, Griffiths RR, Hendricks PS, Henningfield JE. The abuse potential of medical psilocybin according to the 8 factors of the Controlled Substances Act. *Neuropharmacology*. 2018;142:143-166.	E7
Johnstad PG. A dangerous method? Psychedelic therapy at Modum Bad, Norway, 1961-76. *History of Psychiatry*. 2020;31(2):217-226.	E7
Jones G, Ricard JA, Lipson J, Nock MK. Associations between classic psychedelics and opioid use disorder in a nationally-	E2

Citation	Exclude Reason
representative U.S. adult sample. *Scientific Reports.* 2022;12(1):4099.	
Jones GM, Nock MK. Lifetime use of MDMA/ecstasy and psilocybin is associated with reduced odds of major depressive episodes. *Journal of Psychopharmacology.* 2022;36(1):57-65.	E2
Kadriu B, Greenwald M, Henter ID, et al. Ketamine and Serotonergic Psychedelics: Common Mechanisms Underlying the Effects of Rapid-Acting Antidepressants. International Journal of Neuropsychopharmacology. 2021;24(1):8-21.	E7
Kalechstein AD, De La Garza R, II, Mahoney JJ, III, Fantegrossi WE, Newton TF.	E1
MDMA use and neurocognition: A meta-analytic review. *Psychopharmacology.* 2007;189(4):531-537.	
Knuijver T, Belgers M, Markus W, Verkes RJ, van Oosteren T, Schellekens A. Hallucinogen Persisting Perception Disorder After Ibogaine Treatment for Opioid Dependence. *Journal of Clinical Psychopharmacology.* 2018;38(6):646-648.	E6
Krebs TS, Johansen P-O. Psychedelics and mental health: A population study. *PLoS ONE.* 2013;8(8).	E2
Krebs TS, Johansen PO. Lysergic acid diethylamide (LSD) for alcoholism: meta-analysis of randomized controlled trials. *Journal of Psychopharmacology.* 2012;26(7):994-1002.	E8
Krediet E, Bostoen T, Breeksema J, van Schagen A, Passie T, Vermetten E. Reviewing the Potential of Psychedelics for the Treatment of PTSD. *International Journal of Neuropsychopharmacology.* 2020;23(6):385-400.	E7
Krystal JH, Kelmendi B, Petrakis IL. Psychotherapy-supported MDMA treatment for PTSD. *Cell Reports Medicine.* 2021;2(8):100378.	E7
Kupferschmidt K. Can ecstasy treat the agony of PTSD? Science. 2014;345(6192):22-23.	E7
Kurland AA, Unger S, Shaffer JW, Savage C. Psychedelic therapy utilizing LSD in the treatment of the alcoholic patient: a preliminary report. *American Journal of Psychiatry.* 1967;123(10):1202-1209.	E4
Kverno KS, Mangano E. Treatment-Resistant Depression: Approaches to Treatment. *Journal of Psychosocial Nursing & Mental Health Services.* 2021;59(9):7-11.	E7
Lajoie M. Can ayahuasca enhance the treatment of addiction? A comprehensive literature review. Dissertation Abstracts International: Section B: *The Sciences and Engineering.* 2018;79(1-B(E).	E10
Lappin JM, Sara GE. Psychostimulant use and the brain. *Addiction.* 2019;114(11):2065-2077.	E7

Citation	Exclude Reason
Larova V. The evolution of posttraumatic stress disorder treatment: Lessons learned from MDMA-assisted psychotherapy. *Dissertation Abstracts International: Section B: The Sciences and Engineering*. 2021;82(2-B).	E8
Larsen JK. LSD treatment in Scandinavia: emphasizing indications and short-term treatment outcomes of 151 patients in Denmark. *Nordic Journal of Psychiatry*. 2017;71(7):489-495.	E1
Larsen JK. Early LSD treatment in Denmark from 1960 to 1974: An analysis of possible and long-lasting changes in the adult personality following psychedelic treatment. A historical retrospective cohort study. *Medicine*. 2021;100(23):e26300.	E1
Latimer D, Stocker MD, Sayers K, et al. MDMA to Treat PTSD in Adults. *Psychopharmacology Bulletin*. 2021;51(3):125-149.	E7
Lea T, Amada N, Jungaberle H, Schecke H, Scherbaum N, Klein M. Perceived outcomes of psychedelic microdosing as self-managed therapies for mental and substance use disorders. *Psychopharmacology*. 2020;237(5):1521-1532.	E2
Ledermann EK. Existential psychotherapy. *Israel Annals of Psychiatry & Related Disciplines*. 1970;8(3):255-262.	E7
Leger RF, Unterwald EM. Assessing the effects of methodological differences on outcomes in the use of psychedelics in the treatment of anxiety and depressive disorders: A systematic review and meta-analysis. *Journal of Psychopharmacology*. 2022;36(1):20-30.	E8
Li N-X, Hu Y-R, Chen W-N, Zhang B. Dose effect of psilocybin on primary and secondary depression: A preliminary systematic review and meta-analysis. *Journal of Affective Disorders*. 2022;296:26-34.	E8
Liechti ME. Modern Clinical Research on LSD. *Neuropsychopharmacology*. 2017;42(11):2114-2127.	E7
Loizaga-Velder A, Verres R. Therapeutic effects of ritual ayahuasca use in the treatment of substance dependence--qualitative results. *Journal of Psychoactive Drugs*. 2014;46(1):63-72.	E6
Lotsof HS, Alexander NE. Case studies of ibogaine treatment: implications for patient management strategies. *The Alkaloids Chemistry & Biology*. 2001;56:293- 313.	E7
Luciano D. Observations on treatment with ibogaine. *American Journal on Addictions*. 1998;7(1):89-90.	E11
Ludwig A, Levine J, Stark L, Lazar R. A clinical study of LSD treatment in alcoholism. *American Journal of Psychiatry*. 1969;126(1):59-69.	E4
Luz M, Mash DC. Evaluating the toxicity and therapeutic potential of ibogaine in the treatment of chronic opioid abuse. *Expert Opinion On Drug Metabolism & Toxicology*. 2021;17(9):1019-1022.	E4

Citation	Exclude Reason
Lyons T, Carhart-Harris RL. Increased nature relatedness and decreased authoritarian political views after psilocybin for treatment-resistant depression. *Journal of Psychopharmacology.* 2018;32(7):811-819.	E1
Maciulaitis R, Kontrimaviciute V, Bressolle FM, Briedis V. Ibogaine, an anti- addictive drug: pharmacology and time to go further in development. A narrative review. *Human & Experimental Toxicology*. 2008;27(3):181-194.	E1
Madsen JD, Hoffart A. Psychotherapy with the aid of LSD. Nordic Journal of Psychiatry. 1996;50(6):477-486.	E4
Madsen JD, Oyslebo T, Hoffart A. A follow-up study of psycholytic therapy with the aid of LSD. *Nordic Journal of Psychiatry.* 1996;50(6):487-494.	E4
Malitz S. The role of mescaline and D-lysergic acid in psychiatric treatment. *Diseases of the Nervous System.* 1966;7 Suppl(7):39-42.	E7
Malleson N. Acute adverse reactions to LSD in clinical and experimental use in the United Kingdom. British Journal of Psychiatry. 1971;118(543):229-230.	E4
Marks M, Cohen IG. Psychedelic therapy: a roadmap for wider acceptance and utilization. *Nature Medicine.* 2021;27(10):1669-1671.	E7
Marschall J, Fejer G, Lempe P, et al. Psilocybin microdosing does not affect emotion-related symptoms and processing: A preregistered field and lab-based study. *Journal of Psychopharmacology*. 2022;36(1):97-113.	E1
Marseille E, Kahn JG, Yazar-Klosinski B, Doblin R. The cost-effectiveness of MDMA-assisted psychotherapy for the treatment of chronic, treatment-resistant PTSD. *PLoS ONE* [Electronic Resource]. 2020;15(10):e0239997.	E6
Marseille E, Mitchell JM, Kahn JG. Updated cost-effectiveness of MDMA-assisted therapy for the treatment of posttraumatic stress disorder in the United States: Findings from a phase 3 trial. *PLoS ONE* [Electronic Resource]. 2022;17(2):e0263252.	E6
Martin AJ. A case of early paranoiac psychosis treated by Lysergic Acid Diethylamide (LSD). *Acta Psychotherapeutica.* 1964;12(2):119-130.	E6
Mash DC, Kovera CA, Buck BE, et al. Medication development of ibogaine as a pharmacotherapy for drug dependence. *Annals of the New York Academy of Sciences.* 1998;844:274-292.	E7
McCabe OL, Savage C, Kurland A, Unger S. Psychedelic (LSD) therapy of neurotic disorders: Short term effects. *Journal of Psychedelic Drugs.* 1972;5(1):18-28.	E4

Citation	Exclude Reason
Mechaneck R, Feldstein S, Dahlberg CC, Jaffe J. Experimental investigation of LSD as a psychotherapeutic adjunct. Comprehensive Psychiatry. 1968;9(5):490-498.	E7
Merlis S. The effects of mescaline sulfate in chronic schizophrenia. *Journal of Nervous & Mental Disease.* 1957;125(3):432-434.	E4
Mertens LJ, Preller KH. Classical Psychedelics as Therapeutics in Psychiatry - Current Clinical Evidence and Potential Therapeutic Mechanisms in Substance Use and Mood Disorders. *Pharmacopsychiatry*. 2021;54(4):176-190.	E7
Mertens LJ, Wall MB, Roseman L, Demetriou L, Nutt DJ, Carhart-Harris RL. Therapeutic mechanisms of psilocybin: Changes in amygdala and prefrontal functional connectivity during emotional processing after psilocybin for treatment-resistant depression. *Journal of Psychopharmacology*. 2020;34(2):167-180.	E4
Mian MN, Altman BR, Earleywine M. Ayahuasca's antidepressant effects covary with behavioral activation as well as mindfulness. Journal of Psychoactive Drugs. 2020;52(2):130-137.	E2
Mithoefer M. MDMA-assisted psychotherapy for the treatment of post-traumatic stress disorder. Winkelman, Michael J [Ed]; Roberts, Thomas B [Ed] (2007). 2007; Psychedelic medicine: New evidence for hallucinogenic substances as treatments.	E10
Mithoefer MC, Feduccia AA, Jerome L, et al. MDMA-assisted psychotherapy for treatment of PTSD: study design and rationale for phase 3 trials based on pooled analysis of six phase 2 randomized controlled trials. *Psychopharmacology*. 2019;236(9):2735-2745.	E8
Molla S. The personal experiences of ayahuasca brew users as a therapeutic E2 catalyst for substance dependence: A qualitative exploratory approach. *Dissertation Abstracts International: Section B: The Sciences and Engineering*. 2021;82(9-B).	E2
Moreno FA, Delgado PL. Hallucinogen-induced relief of obsessions and compulsions. *American Journal of Psychiatry*. 1997;154(7):1037-1038.	E6
Motta RW. MDMA ("Ecstasy") for PTSD. *Motta, Robert W (2020)*. 2020;Alternative E7 therapies for PTSD:The science of mind-body treatments. (pp. 163-178). 229 pp. Washington.	E7
Mottin JL. Drug-induced attenuation of alcohol consumption. A review and evaluation of claimed, potential or current therapies. *Quarterly Journal of Studies on Alcohol*. 1973;34(2):444-472.	E7
Mullard A. Will psychedelics be 'a revolution in psychiatry'? *Nature Reviews Drug Discovery*. 2021;20(6):418-419.	E7
Muthukumaraswamy SD, Forsyth A, Lumley T. Blinding and expectancy confounds in psychedelic randomized controlled trials. *Expert Review of Clinical Pharmacology*. 2021;14(9):1133-1152.	E7

Citation	Exclude Reason
Muttoni S, Ardissino M, John C. Classical psychedelics for the treatment of depression and anxiety: A systematic review. *Journal of Affective Disorders.*	E8
Nafees T, Wase HA, Amir Malik MF. Is the 3,4-Methylenedioxymethamphetamine assisted psychotherapy a novel approach to managing post-traumatic stress disorder? *JPMA - Journal of the Pakistan Medical Association*. 2019;69(8):1229	E7
Nayak SM, Gukasyan N, Barrett FS, Erowid E, Erowid F, Griffiths RR. Classic psychedelic coadministration with lithium, but not lamotrigine, is associated with seizures: *An analysis of online psychedelic experience reports.*	E1
Nicholas CR, Wang JB, Coker A, et al. The effects of MDMA-assisted therapy on alcohol and substance use in a phase 3 trial for treatment of severe PTSD. *Drug & Alcohol Dependence*. 2022;233:109356.	E4
Noorani T, Garcia-Romeu A, Swift TC, Griffiths RR, Johnson MW. Psychedelic therapy for smoking cessation: Qualitative analysis of participant accounts. *Journal of Psychopharmacology.* 2018;32(7):756-769.	E4
Nour MM, Krzanowski J. Therapeutic potential of psychedelic agents. *British Journal of Psychiatry.* 2015;206(5):433-434.	E7
Nunes AA, dos Santos RG, Osorio FL, Sanches RF, Crippa JAS, Hallak JEC. Effects of ayahuasca and its alkaloids on drug dependence: A systematic literature review of quantitative studies in animals and humans. *Journal of Psychoactive Drugs.* 2016;48(3):195-205.	E8
O'Shea B, Fagan J. Lysergic acid diethylamide. Irish Medical Journal. 2001;94(7):217.	E7
Pahnke WN, Kurland AA, Unger S, Savage C, Grof S. The experimental use of psychedelic (LSD) psychotherapy. *Internationale Zeitschrift fur Klinische Pharmakologie, Therapie und Toxikologie*. 1971;4(4):446-454.	E1
Palladino L. Vine of soul: A phenomenological study of ayahuasca and its effect on depression. Dissertation Abstracts International: Section B: *The Sciences and Engineering.* 2010;71(1-B):668.	E2
Parashos AJ. The psilocybin-induced "state of drunkenness" in normal volunteers and schizophrenics. *Behavioral Neuropsychiatry.* 1976;8(1-12):1976-1977.	E4
Parker LA, Siegel S. Modulation of the effects of rewarding drugs by ibogaine. *The Alkaloids Chemistry & Biology*. 2001;56:211-225.	E7
Parrott AC. The psychotherapeutic potential of MDMA (3,4-methylenedioxymethamphetamine): an evidence-based review. *Psychopharmacology*. 2007;191(2):181-193.	E7

Citation	Exclude Reason
Pearson C, Siegel J, Gold JA. Psilocybin-assisted psychotherapy for depression: Emerging research on a psychedelic compound with a rich history. *Journal of the Neurological Sciences*. 2022;434:120096.	*E7*
Perrine DM. Hallucinogens and obsessive-compulsive disorder. *American Journal of Psychiatry*. 1999;156(7):1123.	E7
Ponte L, Jerome L, Hamilton S, et al. Sleep Quality Improvements After MDMA- Assisted Psychotherapy for the Treatment of Posttraumatic Stress Disorder. *Journal of Traumatic Stress*. 2021;34(4):851-863.	E4
Popik P, Layer RT, Skolnick P. 100 years of ibogaine: neurochemical and pharmacological actions of a putative anti-addictive drug. *Pharmacological Reviews*. 1995;47(2):235-253.	E7
Pos R. LSD-25 as an adjunct to long-term psychotherapy. *Canadian Psychiatric Association Journal*. 1966;11(4):330-342.	E4
Prue RE. King alcohol to chief peyote: A grounded theory investigation of the supportive factors of the native American church for drug and alcohol abuse recovery. *Dissertation Abstracts International Section A: Humanities and Social Sciences*. 2009;69(11-A).	E2
Reiff CM, McDonald WM. MDMA-assisted psychotherapy for the treatment of PTSD. *Revista Brasileira de Psiquiatria*. 2021;43(2):123-124.	E7
Reiff CM, Richman EE, Nemeroff CB, et al. Psychedelics and Psychedelic- Assisted Psychotherapy. *American Journal of Psychiatry*. 2020;177(5):391-410.	E8
Renelli M, Fletcher J, Tupper KW, Files N, Loizaga-Velder A, Lafrance A. An exploratory study of experiences with conventional eating disorder treatment and ceremonial ayahuasca for the healing of eating disorders. *Eating & Weight Disorders: EWD*. 2020;25(2):437-444.	E2
Rhead JC, Soskin RA, Turek I, et al. Psychedelic drug (DPT)-assisted psychotherapy with alcoholics: A controlled study. *Journal of Psychedelic Drugs*. 1977;9(4):287-300.	*E10*
Rodrigues AV, Almeida FJ, Vieira-Coelho MA. Dimethyltryptamine: Endogenous Role and Therapeutic Potential. *Journal of Psychoactive Drugs*. 2019;51(4):299- 310.	*E7*
Romeo B, Hermand M, Petillion A, Karila L, Benyamina A. Clinical and biological predictors of psychedelic response in the treatment of psychiatric and addictive disorders: A systematic review. *Journal of Psychiatric Research*. 2021;137:273- 282.	*E8*
Romeo B, Karila L, Martelli C, Benyamina A. Efficacy of psychedelic treatments on depressive symptoms: A meta-analysis. *Journal of Psychopharmacology*. 2020;34(10):1079-1085	*E8*

Citation	Exclude Reason
Roseman L, Demetriou L, Wall MB, Nutt DJ, Carhart-Harris RL. Increased amygdala responses to emotional faces after psilocybin for treatment-resistant depression. *Neuropharmacology*. 2018;142:263-269.	E4
Rucker J, Jafari H, Mantingh T, et al. Psilocybin-assisted therapy for the treatment of resistant major depressive disorder (PsiDeR): protocol for a randomised, placebo-controlled feasibility trial. *BMJ Open*. 2021;11(12):e056091.	E7
Rucker JJ, Jelen LA, Flynn S, Frowde KD, Young AH. Psychedelics in the treatment of unipolar mood disorders: a systematic review. *Journal of Psychopharmacology*. 2016;30(12):1220-1229.	E8
Rydzynski Z, Gruszczynski W. Treatment of alcoholism with psychotomimetic drugs. A follow-up study. *Activitas Nervosa Superior*. 1978;20(1):81-82.	E4
Sandison RA. Psychological aspects of the LSD treatment of the neuroses. *Journal of Mental Science*. 1954;100(419):508-515.	E4
Sandison RA, Whitelaw JD. Further studies in the therapeutic value of lysergic acid diethylamide in mental illness. *Journal of Mental Science*. 1957;103(431):332- 343.	E1
Sarett M, Cheek F, Osmond H. Reports of wives of alcoholics of effects of LSD-25 treatment of their husbands. *Archives of General Psychiatry*. 1966;14(2):171-178.	E1
Sarris J, Pinzon Rubiano D, Day K, Galvao-Coelho NL, Perkins D. Psychedelic medicines for mood disorders: current evidence and clinical considerations. *Current Opinion in Psychiatry*. 2022;35(1):22-29.	E7
Sartori SB, Singewald N. Novel pharmacological targets in drug development for the treatment of anxiety and anxiety-related disorders. *Pharmacology & Therapeutics*. 2019;204:107402.	E7
Savage C, Fadiman J, Mogar R, Allen MH. The effects of psychedelic (LSD) therapy on values, personality, and behavior. *International Journal of Neuropsychiatry*. 1966;2(3):241-254.	E4
Savage C, McCabe OL. Residential psychedelic (LSD) therapy for the narcotic addict. A controlled study. *Archives of General Psychiatry*. 1973;28(6):808-814.	E1
Savage C, McCabe OL, Kurland AA, Hanlon T. LSD-assisted psychotherapy in the treatment of severe chronic neurosis. *Journal of Altered States of Consciousness*. 1973;1(1):31-47.	E4
Schenberg EE. Psychedelic drugs as new tools in psychiatric therapeutics. *Revista Brasileira de Psiquiatria*. 2021;43(2):121-122.	E7
Schenk S, Newcombe D. Methylenedioxymethamphetamine (MDMA) in Psychiatry: Pros, Cons, and Suggestions. *Journal of Clinical Psychopharmacology*. 2018;38(6):632-638.	E7

Citation	Exclude Reason
Schep LJ, Slaughter RJ, Galea S, Newcombe D. Ibogaine for treating drug dependence. What is a safe dose? *Drug & Alcohol Dependence*. 2016;166:1-5.	E7
Schmid Y, Gasser P, Oehen P, Liechti ME. Acute subjective effects in LSD- and MDMA-assisted psychotherapy. *Journal of Psychopharmacology*. 2021;35(4):362-374.	E4
Sessa B. Self-medication of LSD and MDMA to treat mental disorders: A case series. *Merrick, Joav [Ed]*. 2012.	E2
Sessa B, Aday JS, O'Brien S, et al. Debunking the myth of 'Blue Mondays': No evidence of affect drop after taking clinical MDMA. *Journal of Psychopharmacology*. 2022;36(3):360-367.	E4
Sessa B, Johnson MW. Can psychedelic compounds play a part in drug dependence therapy? *British Journal of Psychiatry*. 2015;206(1):1-3.	E7
Sessa B, Sakal C, O'Brien S, Nutt D. First study of safety and tolerability of 3,4-methylenedioxymethamphetamine (MDMA)-assisted psychotherapy in patients with alcohol use disorder: preliminary data on the first four participants. *BMJ Case Reports*. 2019;12(7):15.	E4
Shagass C, Bittle RM. Therapeutic effects of LSD: a follow-up study. *Journal of Nervous & Mental Disease*. 1967;144(6):471-478.	E1
Sheppard SG. A preliminary investigation of ibogaine: case reports and recommendations for further study. *Journal of Substance Abuse Treatment*. 1994;11(4):379-385	E6
Sherwood AM, Prisinzano TE. Novel psychotherapeutics - a cautiously optimistic focus on Hallucinogens. *Expert Review of Clinical Pharmacology*. 2018;11(1):1-3.	E7
Shirvaikar RV, Kelkar YW. Therapeutic trial of lysergic Acid diethylamide (LSD) and thioridazine in chronic schizophrenia. *Neurology India*. 1966;14(2):97-101.	E4
Siegel AN, Meshkat S, Benitah K, et al. Registered clinical studies investigating psychedelic drugs for psychiatric disorders. *Journal of Psychiatric Research*. 2021;139:71-81.	E8
Skolnick P. Ibogaine as a glutamate antagonist: relevance to its putative antiaddictive properties. *The Alkaloids Chemistry & Biology*. 2001;56:55-62.	E7
Smith CG. Gilles De La Tourette syndrome treated with LSD. *Irish Journal of Medical Science*. 1969;8(6):269-271.	E6
Smith CM. A new adjunct to the treatment of alcoholism: the hallucinogenic drugs. *Quarterly Journal of Studies on Alcohol*. 1958;19(3):406-417.	E4

Citation	Exclude Reason
Smith CM. Some reflections on the possible therapeutic effects of thehallucinogens; with special reference to alcoholism. *Quarterly Journal of Studies on Alcohol.* 1959;20(2):292-301.	E7
Smith KW, Sicignano DJ, Hernandez AV, White CM. MDMA-Assisted E8 Psychotherapy for Treatment of Posttraumatic Stress Disorder: A Systematic Review with Meta-Analysis. *Journal of Clinical Pharmacology*. 2022;62(4):463- 471.	E8
Sola EM. MDMA-assisted psychotherapy for PTSD: A thematic analysis of transformation in combat veterans. *Dissertation Abstracts International: Section B: The Sciences and Engineering.* 2018;79(10-B(E).	E6
Solursh LP. The use of LSD-25 in psychotherapy: An evaluation. *International Journal of Neuropsychiatry*. 1966;2(6):651-656.	E4
Soskin RA. Personality and attitude change after two alcoholism treatment programs. Comparative contributions of lysergide and Human Relations Training. *Quarterly Journal of Studies on Alcohol.* 1970;31(4):920-931.	E4
Soskin RA. The use of LSD in time-limited psychotherapy. *Journal of Nervous & Mental Disease*. 1973;157(6):410-419.	E1
Soskin RA. Dipropyltryptamine in psychotherapy. *Current Psychiatric Therapies*. 1975;15:147-156.	E7
Spriggs MJ, Kettner H, Carhart-Harris RL. Positive effects of psychedelics on depression and wellbeing scores in individuals reporting an eating disorder. *Eating & Weight Disorders: EWD.* 2021;26(4):1265-1270.	E1
Strauss N. Psilocybin-assisted therapy for anxiety and depression: implications for euthanasia. *Medical Journal of Australia.* 2017;206(11):468-469.	E7
Suzuki J, Dekker MA, Valenti ES, et al. Toxicities associated with NBOMe ingestion-A novel class of potent hallucinogens: A review of the literature. *Psychosomatics: Journal of Consultation and Liaison Psychiatry*. 2015;56(2):129- 139.	E7
Teixeira PJ, Johnson MW, Timmermann C, et al. Psychedelics and health behaviour change. *Journal of Psychopharmacology*. 2022;36(1):12-19.	E7
Thomas K, Malcolm B, Lastra D. Psilocybin-Assisted Therapy: A Review of a Novel Treatment for Psychiatric Disorders. *Journal of Psychoactive Drugs*.	E7
Tomsovic M, Edwards RV. Lysergide treatment of schizophrenic and nonschizophrenic alcoholics: a controlled evaluation. *Quarterly Journal of Studies on Alcohol*. 1970;31(4):932-949.	E11

Citation	Exclude Reason
Tupper KW, Wood E, Yensen R, Johnson MW. Psychedelic medicine: a re- emerging therapeutic paradigm. *CMAJ Canadian Medical Association Journal*. 2015;187(14):1054-1059.	E7
Uthaug MV, Mason NL, Toennes SW, et al. A placebo-controlled study of the effects of ayahuasca, set and setting on mental health of participants in ayahuasca group retreats. *Psychopharmacology*. 2021;238(7):1899-1910.	E1
Van Dusen W, Wilson W, Miners W, Hook H. Treatment of alcoholism with lysergide. *Quarterly Journal of Studies on Alcohol*. 1967;28(2):295-304.	E11
Vargas-Perez H, Doblin R. The potential of psychedelics as a preventative and auxiliary therapy for drug abuse. *Current Drug Abuse Reviews*. 2013;6(1):1.	E7
Varker T, Watson L, Gibson K, Forbes D, O'Donnell ML. Efficacy of Psychoactive Drugs for the Treatment of Posttraumatic Stress Disorder: A Systematic Review of MDMA, Ketamine, LSD and Psilocybin. *Journal of Psychoactive Drugs*. 2021;53(1):85-95.	E8
Vastag B. Addiction research. Ibogaine therapy: a 'vast, uncontrolled experiment'. *Science*. 2005;308(5720):345-346	E7
Vermetten E, Yehuda R. MDMA-assisted psychotherapy for posttraumatic stress disorder: A promising novel approach to treatment. *Neuropsychopharmacology*. 2020;45(1):231-232.	E7
Viamontes JA. Review of drug effectiveness in the treatment of alcoholism. *American Journal of Psychiatry*. 1972;128(12):1570-1571.	E7
Voineskos D, Daskalakis ZJ, Blumberger DM. Management of treatment-resistant depression: Challenges and strategies. *Neuropsychiatric Disease and Treatment*. 2020;16:221-234.	E7
Wagner AC, Mithoefer MC, Mithoefer AT, Monson CM. Combining Cognitive- Behavioral Conjoint Therapy for PTSD with 3,4-Methylenedioxymethamphetamine (MDMA): A Case Example. *Journal of Psychoactive Drugs*. 2019;51(2):166-173.	E6
Wagner MT, Mithoefer MC, Mithoefer AT, et al. Therapeutic effect of increased openness: Investigating mechanism of action in MDMA-assisted psychotherapy. *Journal of Psychopharmacology*. 2017;31(8):967-974.	E4
Watts R, Day C, Krzanowski J, Nutt D, Carhart-Harris R. Patients' accounts of increased "connectedness" and "acceptance" after psilocybin for treatment- resistant depression. *Journal of Humanistic Psychology*. 2017;57(5):520-564.	E6
Weston NM, Gibbs D, Bird CIV, et al. Historic psychedelic drug trials and the treatment of anxiety disorders. *Depression & Anxiety*. 2020;37(12):1261-1279.	E8

Citation	Exclude Reason
Wheeler SW, Dyer NL. A systematic review of psychedelic-assisted psychotherapy for mental health: An evaluation of the current wave of research and suggestions for the future. *Psychology of Consciousness: Theory, Research, and Practice*. 2020;7(3):279-315.	E8
Williams MT, Reed S, Aggarwal R. Culturally informed research design issues in a study for MDMA-assisted psychotherapy for posttraumatic stress disorder. *Journal of Psychedelic Studies*. 2020;4(1):40-50.	E7
Yaden DB, Yaden ME, Griffiths RR. Psychedelics in Psychiatry-Keeping the Renaissance From Going Off the Rails. *JAMA Psychiatry*. 2021;78(5):469-470.	E7
Yensen R, Di Leo FB, Rhead JC, et al. MDA-assisted psychotherapy with neurotic outpatients: A pilot study. *Journal of Nervous and Mental Disease*. 1976;163(4):233-245.	E1
Young AH. The age of psychedelics. *Journal of Psychopharmacology*. 2022;36(1):3-5.	E7
Zeifman RJ, Yu D, Singhal N, Wang G, Nayak SM, Weissman CR. Decreases in Suicidality Following Psychedelic Therapy: A Meta-Analysis of Individual Patient Data Across Clinical Trials. *Journal of Clinical Psychiatry*. 2022;83(2):18.	E8

Appendix C: Evidence Tables Characteristics of Included Primary Studies

RCTs

Author Year	Psychedelic Medication	Participant Characteristics	Dose Sessions	Co-intervention	Comparator	Medication Discontinued Prior to Intervention?
N	Follow-up					
Alcohol Use Disorder						
Bogenschutz 2022 [1] N=95	Psilocybin 36 weeks	Mean age: 45.7 % female: 42 % non-Hispanic White: NR	Session 1: 25 mg/kg Session 2: 30-40 mg/kg based on session 1 experience 2 sessions, 8 hours	12 psychotherapy sessions	Diphenhydramine: 50mg	NR
Major Depressive Disorder						
Carhart-Harris 2021 [2] N=59	Psilocybin 6 weeks	Mean age: 41 % female: 34 % non-Hispanic White: 88	25 mg 3 weeks apart + 6 weeks of daily placebo 2 sessions	1 preparatory session, 2 dosing sessions, 3 debriefing sessions	Escitalopram	Yes
Davis 2021 [3] & Gukasyan 2022 [4] N=27	Psilocybin *1 month, 12 months*	Mean age: 40 % female: 67 % non-Hispanic White: 92	Session 1: 20mg/70 kg Session 2:	2 prep meetings (8 hours total) and	8-week delay group	Yes

Author Year	Psychedelic Medication	Participant Characteristics	Dose Sessions	Co-intervention	Comparator	Medication Discontinued Prior to Intervention?
			30mg/70kg *2 sessions*	follow-up (2–3 hours total)		
Palhano- Fontes 2019 [5] & Zeifman 2019 [6] N=29	Ayahuasca 7 days	Mean age: 42 % female: 72 % non-Hispanic White: 59	1ml/kg ayahuasca containing 0.36mg/kg N, N-DMT One 8hr session	None	Placebo (0mg)	Yes
Opioid Use Disorder						
Glue 2016 [7] N=27	Ibogaine (Noribogaine) 72 hours + 120 hours, 168, 216 hours after dose	Mean age: 41 % female: 22 % non-Hispanic White: 74	60mg, 120mg, 180mg (ascending dose) 1 session	None	Placebo (0mg)	NR
Posttraumatic Stress Disorder						
Bouso 2008 [8] [a] N=6	MDMA 12 months	Mean age: 36 % female: 100 % non-Hispanic White: 0 (100% Spanish)	50 mg-75mg 1 session	Three 90-min sessions before and after a single 8- hour MDMA session	Placebo	Yes
Mitchell 2021 [9] N=90	MDMA 18 weeks after baseline	Mean age: 41 % female: 66 %	80-120mg + 40-60mg supplement	Three 90-min preparatory sessions, 3 8-	Placebo (0mg)	Yes

Author Year	Psychedelic Medication	Participant Characteristics	Dose Sessions	Co-intervention	Comparator	Medication Discontinued Prior to Intervention?
		non-Hispanic White: 90	Three 8hr sessions, 4 weeks apart	hour MDMA sessions, and 9 90-min integration sessions		
Mithoefer 2011 [10] & Mithoefer 2013 [11] N=20	MDMA 2 months	Mean age: 40 % female: 85 % non-Hispanic White: 100	125mg + 62.5mg optional supplement 2 experimental sessions 3–5 weeks apart	Two 90-min preparatory sessions, 2 all-day MDMA sessions and overnight clinic stays, 8 90-min integration sessions	Placebo (0mg)	Yes
Mithoefer 2018 [12] N=26	MDMA 1 month after second experimental session	Mean age: 37 % female: 27 % non-Hispanic White: 85	75mg or 125mg MDMA Two 8hr sessions	Two 90-min preparatory sessions, two 8-hour MDMA sessions and overnight clinic stays, six 90-min integration sessions	Active control (30mg)	Yes

Author Year	Psychedelic Medication	Participant Characteristics	Dose Sessions	Co-intervention	Comparator	Medication Discontinued Prior to Intervention?
Mithoefer 2019 [13] [b] N=105	MDMA 3 weeks, 2 months, 12 months	Mean age: 41 % female: 83 Race/ethnicity: NR	125mg + 62.5mg supplemental dose 3 sessions, 8hr each	3 preparatory sessions, three 8-hour MDMA sessions and overnight clinic stays, 12 integration sessions	Active control (25 mg + 12.5mg)	Yes
Oehen 2013 [14] N=12	MDMA *3 weeks, 2 months, 12 months*	Mean age: 41 % female: 83 Race/ethnicity: NR	125mg + 62.5mg supplemental dose *3 sessions, 8hr each*	3 preparatory sessions, three 8- hour MDMA sessions and overnight clinic stays, 12 integration sessions	Active control (25 mg + 12.5mg)	Yes
Ot'alora 2018 [15] N=28	MDMA 1 month	Mean age: 42 % female: 68 % non-Hispanic White: 93	125 or 100mg Two 8hr sessions, 1 month apart	Three 90-min preparatory sessions, two 8-hour MDMA sessions, and 6	Active control (40mg)	Yes

Author Year	Psychedelic Medication	Participant Characteristics	Dose Sessions	Co-intervention	Comparator	Medication Discontinued Prior to Intervention?
				integration sessions		
NCT0195859 3 N=6	MDMA 1 month after second experimental session	Mean age: 48 % female: 50 % non-Hispanic White: 83	Dose NR 2 sessions	3 preparatory sessions, 2 MDMA sessions, and 2 integrative therapy sessions	Placebo (0mg)	NR
NCT0168974 0 N=8	MDMA 1 month after second experimental session	Mean age: NR % female: 38 % non-Hispanic White: 87	125mg + 62.5mg supplemental dose Two 6–8hr sessions	3 preparatory sessions, 2 MDMA sessions, and 2 integration sessions	Active control (25 mg + 12.5mg)	NR
Social Anxiety Disorder						
Dos Santos 2021 [16] N=17	Ayahuasca 1 week, 2 weeks, 3 weeks	Age: 25 % female: 88 Race: NR	2 mL/kg 1 session	None	Placebo (0mg)	NR

Notes.

[a] Bouso 2008 study terminated early due to "political pressure."

[b] Mithoefer 2019 is a pooled analysis of Mithoefer 2011, Mithoefer 2018, Oehen 2013, Otalora 2018, NCT0195893, and NCT01689740.

Abbreviations. hr=hour; MDMA=3,4-methylenedioxy-methamphetamine; N, N-DMT=N, N-Dimethyltryptamine; mg=milligram; NR=not reported.

Observational Studies

Author Year *N*	Psychedelic Medication *Follow-up*	Participant Characteristics	Dose *Sessions*	Co-intervention	Medication Tapered Prior to Intervention?
Alcohol Use Disorder					
Bogenschutz 2015 [17] N=10	Psilocybin *36 weeks*	Mean age: 40 % female: 40 % non-Hispanic White: 30	Session 1: 0.3 mg/kg Session 2: 0.4 mg/kg dependent on initial experience *2 sessions, 8 hours*	7 sessions of Motivational Enhancement Therapy, 3 preparation sessions, and 2 debriefing sessions	NR
Sessa 2021 [18] N=14	MDMA *8 weeks, 3, 6, and 9 months*	Mean age: 48 % female: 43 Race/ethnicity: NR	125mg + 62.5mg booster dose *2 sessions,* *6-8 hours*	10 psychotherapy sessions	Yes
Major Depressive Disorder					
Carhart-Harris 2016 [19] & 2018 [20] N=20	Psilocybin *1 week - 6 months*	Age: 27-64 % female: 70 % non-Hispanic White: 75	10mg, 25 mg *2 sessions, 1 week apart*	None	Yes
Lyons 2018 [21] [a] N=30	Psilocybin *1 week - 30 days*	Mean age: 42 % female: 27 % non-Hispanic White: 93	10mg, 25 mg (1 week apart) *2 sessions, 1 week apart*	Psychological support consisting of a preparation session and integration sessions led by 2 clinical psychiatrists	Yes

Author Year *N*	Psychedelic Medication *Follow-up*	Participant Characteristics	Dose *Sessions*	Co-intervention	Medication Tapered Prior to Intervention?
Osorio 2015 [22] N=6	Ayahuasca *40 min – 21 days post ingestion*	Mean age: 44 % female: 66 % non-Hispanic White: NR	120-200ml (2.2ml/kg), with 0.8mg/ml DMT and 0.21 mg/ml harmine *1 session, 4 hrs*	None	Yes
Sanches 2016 [23] & Zeifman 2021 [24] N=17	Ayahuasca *1–21 days after treatment*	Mean age: 42.71 % female: NR % non-Hispanic White: NR	120–200ml (2.2ml/kg), with 0.8mg/ml DMT and 0.21 mg/ml harmine *1 session, 4 hours*	None	Yes
Stroud 2018 [25] [a] N=17	Psilocybin *1 month*	Mean age:44.94 % female: 47 % non-Hispanic White: NR	10mg 1st dose, 25mg 2nd dose *2 sessions*	Integrative therapy	Yes
Obsessive Compulsive Disorder					
Moreno 2006 [26] N=9	Psilocybin *24 hours*	Mean age: 40.9 % female: 22.2 % non-Hispanic White: NR	Varying dose 100ug/kg, 200 ug/kg, or 300 ug/kg with 25 ug/kg dose during 1 of the treatment sessions *4 sessions, 1 week apart, lasting 8 hours*	None	Yes
Opioid Use Disorder					

Author Year *N*	Psychedelic Medication *Follow-up*	Participant Characteristics	Dose *Sessions*	Co-intervention	Medication Tapered Prior to Intervention?
Brown 2018 [27] N=30	Ibogaine *1–12 months*	Mean age: 29 % female: 17 % non-Hispanic White: 90	1540 mg ± 920 mg *NR*	None	Yes
Davis 2017 [28] *N=88*	Ibogaine 3 years	Age: 9% 18–24 years old, 41% 25–34 years old, 39% 35–54 years old, 10% 55+ years old % female: 27 % non-Hispanic White: 89	10–20mg/kg *1 session*	Participation in detoxification program	Yes
Knuijver 2022 [29] N=14	Ibogaine *2–24 hours after treatment*	Age (median): 48 % female: 14 % non-Hispanic White: NR	10mg/kg *1 session*	None	Yes
Malcolm 2018 [30] N=50	Ibogaine *24 and 48 hours*	Mean age: 31 % female: 39 % non-Hispanic White: 78	18–20mg/kg *1 session*	3-part treatment program: coaching, medical screening, detoxification treatment, optional residential aftercare program	Yes
Noller 2018 [31] N=14	Ibogaine *12 months*	Mean age: 38 % female: 50 % non-Hispanic White: 100	25–55 mg/kg (mean 31.4, SD 7.6) *1 session*	Diazepam 5–30mg and zopiclone 7.5–15mg	NR
Posttraumatic Stress Disorder					

Author Year *N*	Psychedelic Medication *Follow-up*	Participant Characteristics	Dose *Sessions*	Co-intervention	Medication Tapered Prior to Intervention?
Jardim 2021 [32] N=3	MDMA *2 months*	Mean age: 40 % female: 67 % non-Hispanic White: 67	Session 1 :112.5mg Sessions 2–3: 187.5mg *3 sessions, 8 hours*	Three 90-min preparatory sessions, three 8-hour MDMA sessions, and nine 90- min integrative therapy sessions	Yes
Monson 2020 [33] N=12	MDMA *3- and 6-months post-treatment*	Mean age: 47 % female: 40 % non-Hispanic White: 100	75mg 1st session, 100mg 2nd session *2 sessions*	5 preparatory CBCT sessions, 2 MDMA 6-8 hour MDMA sessions, two 1.25-hour integration sessions, 8 post MDMA CBCT sessions	Yes
Wang 2021 [34] N=37	MDMA *18 weeks after baseline*	Mean age: 36 % female: 60 % White: 73 % not Hispanic/Latino: 94.6	80–100mg + 40–50mg supplement 1st session, 120–25mg + 60– 62.5mg supplement 2nd and 3rd session *Three 6-8 hour sessions, 3-5 weeks apart*	3 preparatory sessions, three 6–8-hour MDMA sessions and overnight clinic stays, and 9 integration sessions	Yes
Substance Use Disorder					

Author Year *N*	Psychedelic Medication *Follow-up*	Participant Characteristics	Dose *Sessions*	Co-intervention	Medication Tapered Prior to Intervention?
Thomas 2013 [35] N=12	Ayahuasca *6 months*	NR	Dose NR *2 sessions*	Participation in 4-day "Working with Addiction and Stress" retreats	NR
Mash 2000 [36] N=27	Ibogaine *1 month*	Mean age: 35 for opioid group, 38 for cocaine group % female: 17 % non-Hispanic White: NR	500, 600, or 800mg *1 session*	Participation in inpatient detoxification program	NR
Mash 2001 [37] N=32	Ibogaine *36 hours–10 days*	Mean age: 34 % female: 31 % non-Hispanic White: 82	800 mg *1 dosing session*	NR	NR
Mash 2018 [38] N=191	Ibogaine *1 month*	Mean age: 35.9 % female: 24.6 % non-Hispanic White: 87.4	8–12 mg/kg *1 dosing session*	Psychological support	NR
Schenberg 2014 [39]	Ibogaine *NR*	Mean age: NR % female: 11 % non-Hispanic White: NR	7.5–20mg/kg *1–9 sessions, 1 dosing session with optional additional sessions as appropriate*	Psychological therapy	NR
Tobacco Use					
Johnson 2014 [40] & 2017 [41] N=15	Psilocybin 6 months	Mean age: 51 % female: 33.3 % non-Hispanic White: 93%	Moderate dose: 20mg/70kg High dose: 30mg/70kg *2–3 sessions*	CBT	NR

Author Year *N*	Psychedelic Medication *Follow-up*	Participant Characteristics	Dose *Sessions*	Co-intervention	Medication Tapered Prior to Intervention?
*Other Mental Health Diagnoses*b					
Davis 2020 [42] N=51	Ibogaine, 5-MeO-DMT *1 month–2 years*	Mean age: 40 % female: 4 % non-Hispanic White: 92%	Ibogaine: 10mg/kg MeO-DMT: 50mg *2 sessions (1 ibogaine, 1 MeO-DMT), 3 days of treatment*	Group therapy, psychological support	Yes

Notes.

[a] Lyons 2018 and Stroud 2018 included comparison groups to "healthy, non-treated controls."

[b] Other Mental Health Diagnoses contains 1 study of patients whose primary diagnosis was PTSD, SUD, depression, anxiety, cognitive problems, or suicidal thoughts and behaviors.

Abbreviations. 5-MeO-DMT=5-methoxy-N,N-dimethyltryptamine, a psychedelic of the tryptamine class; CBCT=cognitive-behavioral conjoint therapy; CBT=cognitive behavioral therapy; DMT=5-methoxy-N,N-dimethyltryptamine; hr=hour; MDMA=3,4-methylenedioxy-methamphetamine; NR=not reported; OUD=opioid use disorder; pts=patients.

Setting Characteristics of Included Primary Studies

Author Year	Treatment Setting	Treatment Administrators	Patient Instructions
Alcohol Use Disorder			
Bogenschutz 2022 [1]	Living room like setting, on a couch wearing eyeshades and headphones (providing a standardized program of music)	2 study therapists	NR
Major Depressive Disorder			

Author Year	Treatment Setting	Treatment Administrators	Patient Instructions
Carhart-Harris 2021 [2]	Clinical	2 mental health professions; 1 of the pair was a clinical psychologist, psychotherapist, or psychiatrist, and the other could be an equivalent grade clinician or trainee	Visit 2: 1st treatment dose. Patients also instructed to take daily placebo capsules until next dose Visit 5: Psychological integration session, instruction to take placebo or escitalopram daily
Davis 2021 [3] & Gukasyan 2022 [4]	Living-room like setting, on a couch wearing eyeshades and headphones (providing a standardized program of music)	2 facilitators with varying educational levels (*ie*, bachelor's, master's, doctorate, and medical degrees) and professional disciplines (*eg*, social work, psychology, and psychiatry)	Focus their attention inward and stay with any experience that arose.
Palhano-Fontes 2019 [5] & Zeifman 2019 [6]	Quiet, comfortable living room-like environment	2 investigators remained in room next door offering help when needed	Asked to remain quiet with their eyes closed while focusing on their body, thoughts, and emotions.
Opioid Use Disorder			
Glue 2016 [7]	NR	NR	Patients were given controlled release morphine and then immediate release morphine the week before ibogaine treatment. They were instructed to fast for 10 hours prior to ibogaine administration.
Posttraumatic Stress Disorder			

Author Year	Treatment Setting	Treatment Administrators	Patient Instructions
Bouso 2008 [8] [a]	Clinical	2 therapists	After drug administration: Lay in bed with eyes closed, relaxation techniques Hours 1–2: Confront traumatic event Hours 3–6: Share experience, talk therapy Hours 6–8: Session conclusion, shared meal
Mitchell 2021 [9]	NR	2-person therapy team; therapists had a master's degree or higher	Therapists helped participants work through memories of traumatic events, arrive at emotional resolution, and find new perspectives.
Mithoefer 2011 [10] & Mithoefer 2013 [11]	Comfortable, aesthetically pleasing outpatient office, patients reclining, listening to relaxing and then emotional evocative music	Male and female co-therapy team, 1 a psychiatrist and the other a psychiatric nurse	Equal balance between quiet introspection and therapeutic conversation
Mithoefer 2018 [12]	NR	Male and female co-therapy team	NR
Mithoefer 2019 [13] [b]	Designated are with futon or sofa with artwork or other objects to make the space esthetically pleasing	Male and female co-therapy team	Option to wear eye shades and listen to instrumental music and focus inward
Oehen 2013 [14]	Group psychotherapy room at the primary investigator's clinic	1 male and 1 female therapist	NR
Ot'alora 2018 [15]	Outpatient clinic furnished to look like a comfortable living room	Male and female co-therapy team	NR

Author Year	Treatment Setting	Treatment Administrators	Patient Instructions
NCT01958593	NR	Male and female co-therapy team	NR
NCT01689740	NR	Male and female co-therapy team	NR
Social Anxiety Disorder			
Dos Santos 2021 [16]	NR	NR	Researchers used a nondirective, supportive approach during drug sessions. Participants instructed to "remain as quiet and introspective as possible, with your eyes open or closed, while focusing on your body, thoughts, and emotions."

Notes.
[a] Bouso 2008 study terminated early due to "political pressure."
[b] Mithoefer 2019 is a pooled analysis of Mithoefer 2011, Mithoefer 2018, Oehen 2013, Otalora 2018, NCT0195893, and NCT01689740.
Abbreviations. MRI=magnetic resonance imaging; NR=not reported.

Observational Studies

Author Year	Treatment Setting	Treatment Administrators	Patient Instructions
Alcohol Use Disorder			
Bogenschutz 2015 [17]	Living-room like setting, on a couch wearing eyeshades and headphones (providing a standardized program of music)	2 study therapists	Direct attention toward their internal experience

Author Year	Treatment Setting	Treatment Administrators	Patient Instructions
Sessa 2021 [18]	NR	2 clinicians trained in delivering MDMA-assisted psychotherapy	NR
Major Depressive Disorder			
Carhart-Harris 2016 [19] & 2018 [20]	Pre-decorated dosing room with low lighting	2 psychiatrists	Patients were invited to relax on a ward bed while music played through speakers/earphones.
Lyons 2018 [21] [a]	Lyons 201821 a Same as Carhart-Harris 2016	Same as Carhart-Harris 2016	Same as Carhart-Harris 2016
Osorio 2015 [22]	Inpatient psychiatric ward, during treatment patients were seated in a comfortable recliner in a dimly lit room	NR	NR
Sanches 2016 [23] & Zeifman 2021 [24]	Quiet, dimly lit room	NR	NR
Stroud 2018 [25] [a]	Pre-decorated room with low light, fabric drapes, flowers at side of bed	2 psychiatrists	NR
Obsessive Compulsive Disorder			
Moreno 2006 [26]	Comfortable outpatient clinic setting	Principal investigator and trained sitter	Wear eye shades and listen to predetermined music
Opioid Use Disorder			
Brown 2018 [27]	NR	NR	Subjects were stabilized on shortacting opioids for 2–3 days prior to treatment. Test dose was administered in morning when subjects began feeling withdrawal symptoms.

Author Year	Treatment Setting	Treatment Administrators	Patient Instructions
Davis 2017 [28]	Residential care facility for adults with SUD and MH problems	Clinical	None
Knuijver 2022 [29]	Inpatient clinic	Clinical	None
Malcolm 2018 [30]	Medically supervised inpatient setting	Clinical	Prior to treatment, patients were converted to short-acting opioids. They received a medical eval upon arrival at the clinic. Ibogaine was administered 4 hours after last morphine dose.
Noller 2018 [31]	NR	2 ibogaine providers offering treatment on a fee-for-service basis, each associated with a physician. 1 was a registered addictions counselor.	NR
Posttraumatic Stress Disorder			
Jardim 2021 [32]	NR	Clinical	NR
Monson 2020 [33]	Combination of in person and video CBT sessions (MDMA sessions were in person)	Expert therapists in MDMA and CBCT	NR
Wang 2021 [34]	NR	Clinical	Introspection of trauma-related memories and feelings
Substance Use Disorder			
Thomas 201335	3-day spiritual retreat according to customs of Peruvian Shipibo people, during Ayahuasca	Master Ayahuasquero	NR

Author Year	Treatment Setting	Treatment Administrators	Patient Instructions
	sessions participants laid quietly on beds		
Mash 2000 [36]	Opiate detoxification facility	Clinical	NR
Mash 2018 [37]	Opiate detoxification facility	Clinical	NR
Mash 2018 [38]	Opiate detoxification facility	Clinical	NR
Schenberg 2014 [39]	Private hospital room	Physician administering Tx stayed onsite the entire time, checking in on pt. every ~30 min	Encouraged patients to be quiet, calm, and confident. Patients were advised to stay away from others or social activity for 7 days after treatment.
Tobacco Addiction			
Johnson 2014 [40] & 2017 [41]	NR	Clinical	NR
Other Mental Health Diagnoses[b]			
Davis 2020 [42]	Clinical/residential	Clinical	Patients were in a group setting, instructed to lie on a bed in a supine position. Integration session - Independent work, group discussion, psychological support.

Notes.

[a] Lyons 2018 and Stroud 2018 included comparison groups to "healthy, non-treated controls."

[b] Other Mental Health Diagnoses contains 1 study of patients whose primary diagnosis was PTSD, SUD, depression, anxiety, cognitive problems, or suicidal thoughts and behaviors.

Abbreviations. 5-MeO-DMT=5-methoxy-N,N-dimethyltryptamine; CBCT=cognitive-behavioral conjoint therapy; CBT=cognitive behavioral therapy; MDMA=3,4- methylenedioxy-methamphetamine; MH=mental health; MRI=magnetic resonance imaging; NR=not reported; pt.=patient; SUD=substance use disorder.

Outcome Data of Included Primary Studies

Disorder-specific Outcomes

Author Year *N*	Study Design	Intervention *Comparator*	Disorder-specific Outcomes
Alcohol Use Disorder			
Bogenschutz 2015 [17] *N=10*	Pre-post	Psilocybin none	% heavy drinking days weeks 5–12 relative to baseline: [mean difference (SD) = 26.0 (22.4), 95% CI 8.7–43.2, $p = 0.008$] and relative weeks 1–4: [mean difference (SD) = 18.2 (20.0), 95% CI 2.8–33.5, $p = 0.026$] % drinking days weeks 5–12 relative to baseline: [mean difference (SD) = 27.2 (23.7), 95% CI 9.0–45.4, $p = 0.009$] and relative weeks 1–4: [mean difference (SD) = 21.9 (21.8), 95% CI 5.1–38.6, $p = 0.017$]
Bogenschutz 2022 [1] *N=95*	RCT *Diphenhydramine*	Psilocybin	Mean (SD) % heavy drinking days at baseline and 32 weeks: 56.48 (31.77) and 9.71 (26.21) in the psilocybin group compared to 48.57 (28.73) and 23.57 (26.67) in the diphenhydramine group; between-group mean difference: 13.86 (95% CI 3.00, 24.72), $p = .01$ Mean (SD) % drinking days at baseline and 32 weeks: 78.03 (27.02) and 29.39 (32.86) in the psilocybin group compared to 71.68 (28.98) and 42.83 (33.43) in the diphenhydramine group; between-group mean difference: 13.44 (95% CI –0.18, 27.05), $p = .05$ Mean (SD) drinks per day at baseline and 32 weeks: 5.2 (2.81) and 1.17 (1.99) in the psilocybin group compared to 4.38 (2.39) and 2.26 (2.02) in the diphenhydramine group; between-group mean difference: 1.09 (95% CI 0.27, 1.92), $p = .01$
Sessa 2021 [43] N=14	Pre-post None	MDMA	9 participants were abstinent from alcohol and 2 reduced use to < 14 units of alcohol per week at 9 months follow-up
Major Depressive Disorder			
Carhart-Harris 201619 & 2018 [20] N=20	Pre-post	Psilocybin-assisted psychotherapy None	Mean change in QIDS-SR-16 from baseline to 6 months: − 14.9 (12.0), Cohen's d 1.4, $p < 0.001$ Mean reduction in suicidality scores on QIDS-SR-16 from baseline to 5 weeks: − 0.7, 95% CI = − 0.22 to − 1.2, $p = 0.01$ Relapse rate (QIDS score of 6+ or above) at 6 months among responders: 3/9 (33%)

Author Year *N*	Study Design	Intervention *Comparator*	Disorder-specific Outcomes
Carhart-Harris 2021 [2] N=59	RCT	Psilocybin-assisted psychotherapy Low-dose psilocybin & escitalopram	Mean (±SE) change in QIDS-SR-16 from baseline to week 6: −8.0±1.0 in the psilocybin group and −6.0±1.0 in the escitalopram group (difference, −2.0; 95% CI, −5.0 to 0.9; $p = 0.17$)
Davis 20213 & Gukasyan 2022 [4] N=27	RCT	Psilocybin-assisted psychotherapy Delayed treatment	Mean (±1 SD) GRID-HAMD at baseline 22.9 (3.6) and at 8 weeks 8.5 (5.7) for the immediate treatment group and 22.5 (4.4) at baseline and 23.5 (6.0) at 8 weeks for the delayed treatment group, Cohen's d = 2.6; 95% CI, 1.5-3.7; $p < .001$ For all participants: Mean (±1 SD) GRID-HAMD at baseline 22.8 (3.9) and at 12 months 7.7 (7.9); Cohen's d (95% CI) 2.4 (1.6–3.2) at 12 months
Lyons 2018 [21] [a] N=30	Open-label mixed design	Psilocybin-assisted psychotherapy Healthy untreated patients	Mean BDI at baseline (M = 34.33, SD = 7.44) and 1 week after psilocybin sessions (M = 12.13, SD = 9.80); $t(14) = 7.900$, 95% CI (16.17, 28.23) $p < 0.001$ No significant difference found in baseline vs follow-up BDI scores among the healthy comparison group.
Osorio 2015 [22] N=6	Pre-post None	Ayahuasca None	Reduction in mean HAM-D by 62% on day 1 ($p = 0.01$), 72% on day 7 ($p = 0.001$), and 45% on day 14 ($p = 0.11$). Scores significantly decreased at day 21 but % NR.
Palhano-Fontes 2019 [5] N=29	RCT	Ayahuasca 0mg placebo	Mean (SD) HAM-D at baseline and 1 week after dosing in the ayahuasca group: 24.07 (5.34) and 9.72 (7.39) compared to the placebo group: 19.73 (4.59) and 16.92 (7.36), within group Cohen's d = 2.22 (95% CI 1.28, 3.17) in the ayahuasca group compared to Cohen's d = 0.46 (95% CI -0.27, 1.18)
Sanches 201623 & Zeifman 2021 [24] N=17	Pre-post	Ayahuasca None	Administration of ayahuasca was associated with significant HAM-D and MADRS score decreases from 80 to 180 minutes ($p < 0.01$) and day 1 to day 21 ($p = 0.000$). Acute changes in suicidality (N=15): significant effect for time ($F(4,13.85) = 7.17$; $p = 0.002$). Within-subject t tests found the largest effect size at 180 min after administration (Hedges' g = 0.89). Post-acute changes in

Author Year *N*	Study Design	Intervention *Comparator*	Disorder-specific Outcomes
			suicidality (N=15): significant effect for time($F(4,10.69) = 15.65$; $p < 0.001$). Within-subject t tests found significant decreases in suicidality between baseline and 1, 7, 14, and 21 days after administration with the largest effect at 21 days ($g = 1.75$).
Stroud 2018[25] [a] N=32	Pre-post	Psilocybin-assisted psychotherapy Healthy untreated patients	Mean QIDS-16 at baseline ($M = 18.88$, $SD = 2.23$) and 1 week after psilocybin sessions ($M= 7.65$, $SD = 5.34$) ($p < .001$) No significant difference found in baseline vs follow-up QIDS-16 scores among the healthy comparison group.
Opioid Use			
Brown 2018 [27] N=30	Pre-post	Ibogaine None	Mean reduction in SOWS at mean time interval between first and second SOWS 76.5 ± 30 hrs: 17.0 ± 12.5 points ($t = 7.07$, $df = 26$, $p < .001$) ASI for drug use at baseline: 0.40 ± 0.08; at 12 months: 0.17 ± 0.10 Participants with opioid-free days in the previous 30 days at 12 months (missing values set to pretreatment baseline): 8.8 ± 12.7.
Davis 2017 [28] N=88	Pre-post	Ibogaine and participation in detoxification program None	% participants with reduction in cravings: 50% at 1 week; 35% at 3 or more months Opioid use post-treatment: 30% abstinent (variable duration); 48% returned to use; 17% no change; 6% use increased
Glue 2016 [7] N=27	RCT	Noribogaine 0mg placebo	Mean time to opioid substitution treatment: 8.6 hours in 60mg group, 22.5 hours in 120mg group, and 11.4 hours in 180mg group, and 13.9 hours in placebo group
Knuijver 2022 [29] N=14	Pre-post	Ibogaine None	Return to morphine use within 24 hours: 11/14 (79%); Median COWS among 5 not on morphine after 24 hours: 0
Malcolm 2018 [30] N=50	Pre-post	Ibogaine and participation in	Pre-ibogaine mean COWS: 8.2 ± 5.21 at 48 hours and 7.64 ± 5.27 at 24 hours; post-ibogaine mean COWS: 5.26 ± 4.31 at 24 hours and 3.30 ± 3.13) at 48 hours Pre-ibogaine mean SOWS: 20.51 ± 13.66 at 48 hours and 17.09 ± 12.95 at 24

Author Year *N*	Study Design	Intervention *Comparator*	Disorder-specific Outcomes
		detoxification program	hours; post-ibogaine mean SOWS: 12.63 ± 11.95 at 24 hours and 10.04 ± 11.65 at 48 hours Pre-ibogaine mean BSCS: 6.58 ± 3.08 at 48 hours and 5.98 ± 2.98 at 24 hours; post-ibogaine mean BSCS: 2.69 ± 2.68 at 24 hours and 1.92 ± 2.83 at 48 hours
Noller 2018 [31] N=14	Pre-post	Ibogaine and concomitant Diazepam and zopiclone	Mean SOWS (N=14) at baseline 25.21 (SD 12.57) and 12-24 hours 14.21 (SD 14.08), $p = 0.015$ Mean SOWS (N=6) at baseline 24 (SD 16.84) and 42-84 hours 8.5 (SD 3.72), $p = 0.070$ ASI for drug use (N=8) 0.32 (SD 0.07) at baseline compared to 0.06 (SD 0.08) $p < 0.01$ at 12-month follow-up Negative urine drug screen at 12 months (N=8): 6/8, 75%
Posttraumatic Stress Disorder			
Bouso 2008 [8] N=6	RCT	MDMA-assisted psychotherapy 0mg placebo	Mean SSSPTSD at baseline and post-treatment for the 50mg group: 37.3 vs 28.3 compared to the placebo group: 44.5 vs 40 Mean SSSPTSD at baseline and post-treatment for 1 participant who received 75mg: 48 vs 32
Jardim 202132 N=3	Pre-post	MDMA-assisted psychotherapy None	CAPS-5 at baseline per participant: 90, 78, and 72; 2 months post-treatment: 61, 27, and 8 respectively PCL-C at baseline per participant: 69, 59, 55; 2 months post-treatment: 57, 49, 20 respectively PTGI at baseline per participant: 9, 34, and 11; 2 months post-treatment: 66, 86, and 60 respectively
Mitchell 2021[9] [a] N=90	RCT	MDMA-assisted psychotherapy 0mg placebo	Participants no longer meeting PTSD diagnostic criteria: 14/42 (33%) MDMA group vs 2/37 (5%) placebo group
Mithoefer 2011[10] [b] & Mithoefer 2013 [11] N=20	RCT	MDMA-assisted psychotherapy 0mg placebo	Participants no longer meeting PTSD diagnostic criteria: 10/12 (83%) in MDMA group vs 2/8 (25%) in placebo group Participants with >30% reduction from baseline in CAPS total severity score: 10/12 (83%) in MDMA group vs 2/8 (25%) in placebo group
Mithoefer 201812 [b] N=26	RCT	MDMA-assisted psychotherapy Active control	Participants no longer meeting PTSD diagnostic criteria at 1 month follow-up: 6/7 (86%) of 75mg group, 7/12 (58%) of 125mg group, and 2/7 (29%) of control group Participants with >30% decrease in CAPS-4 total score at 1 month follow-up: 7/7 (100%) of 75mg group, 8/12 (67%) of 125mg group, and 2/7 (29%) of control group

Author Year *N*	Study Design	Intervention *Comparator*	Disorder-specific Outcomes
Mithoefer 2019 [13] N=105	RCT	MDMA-assisted psychotherapy 0mg placebo or active control	Pooled data from 6 RCTs: the active MDMA group had significantly greater reductions in CAPS-IV total scores from baseline than the control group [MMRM estimated mean difference (SE) between groups - 22.0 (5.17), $p < 0.001$].
Monson 2020 [33] N=12	Pre-post	MDMA and cognitive-behavioral conjoint therapy None	Mean (SD) CAPS-5 at baseline: 41.42 (5.76) and at 6 months: 15.52 (15.22) Patient PTSD Checklist-5: 62.64 (6.35) at baseline and 17.20 (16.76) at 6 months Partner-rated PTSD Checklist at baseline: 49.58 (8.52) at baseline and 16.64 (14.84) at 6 months
Oehen 2013 [14] [b] N=12	RCT	MDMA-assisted psychotherapy Active control	Participants with >30% decrease in CAPS-4 total score at 12-month follow-up after all had received full-dose MDMA: 9/12 (75%)
Ot'alora 2018 [15] [b] N=28	RCT	MDMA-assisted psychotherapy Active control	Participants no longer meeting PTSD diagnostic criteria at 12-month follow-up: 4/9 (44%) of 100mg group, 5/12 (42%) of 125mg group, and 2/6 (33%) of control group Participants with >30% decrease in CAPS-4 total score at 12-month follow-up: 5/9 (56%) of 100mg group, 6/12 (50%) of 125mg group, and 1/6 (17%) of control group
NCT0168974044 b N=8	RCT	MDMA-assisted psychotherapy Active control	See pooled analysis table
NCT01958593 [45] [b] N=6	RCT	MDMA-assisted psychotherapy 0mg placebo	See pooled analysis table
Wang 2021 [34] N=37	Pre-post	MDMA-assisted psychotherapy	Mean (SD) change CAPS-5: −29.89 (13.45)
Substance Use Disorder			
Thomas 2013 [35] N=12	Pre-post None	Ayahuasca None	No change was observed for opiate or cannabis use, and no serious adverse events were reported.

Author Year *N*	Study Design	Intervention *Comparator*	Disorder-specific Outcomes
Mash 2000 [36] N=27	Pre-post	Ibogaine and participation in detoxification program None	Ibogaine significantly decreased craving for cocaine and heroin during inpatient detoxification.
Mash 2001 [37] N=32	Pre-post	Ibogaine and participation in detoxification program None	Mean OOWS: 5.75 at 12 hours from last opiate dose (pre-ibogaine); mean OOWS 1.25 at 24 hours and 2 at 36 hours from last opiate dose (post-ibogaine)* Pre-ibogaine mean OP-SCL: 22 at 24 hours; post-ibogaine OP-SCL: 13 within 72 hours and 7 at 6-9 days*
Mash 201838 N=191	Pre-post	Ibogaine and participation in detoxification program None	Self-reported cravings as measured by the Heroin (HCQ-29) and Cocaine (CCQ-45) Craving Questionnaires were lower at the time of discharge compared to before treatment and remained lower among 37 participants with opioid dependence and 32 with cocaine dependence who completed follow-up at 1 month.
Schenberg 201439 N=75	Pre-post	Ibogaine None	The duration of reported abstinence was longer for participants who underwent multiple ibogaine dosing sessions compared to 1 dosing session (median 8.4 months compared to median 5.5 months).
Tobacco Addiction			
Johnson 201440 & 2017 [41] N=15	Pre-post	Psilocybin None	10/15 (67%) participants showed 7-day point prevalence abstinence as measured by smoking timeline follow-back assessments and verified by exhaled carbon monoxide and urinary cotinine levels. 9/12 (60%) smoking abstinent at mean 30 months post-TQD; range = 16–57 months
Other Mental Health Diagnoses[b]			
Davis 202042 N=51	Pre-post	Ibogaine None	Significant reductions in PTSD symptoms (SMD PTSD Checklist-5 = –3.6, p < 0.001), depression (SMD Patient Health Questionnaire-2 = -3.7, p < 0.001), anxiety (SMD Generalized Anxiety Disorder 2-Item = -3.1, p < 0.001), and suicidal ideation (SMD Depressive Symptom Index Suicidality Subscale = -1.9, p < 0.001) 30-days post-treatment
Social Anxiety Disorder			

Author Year *N*	Study Design	Intervention *Comparator*	Disorder-specific Outcomes
Dos Santos 202116 N=17	RCT	Ayahuasca Placebo	Compared with placebo, ayahuasca was associated with significant increases in self-perception during the public speaking test (F1,12 = 7.740, p = 0.017, .2 = 0.392).

Notes.

[a] Intervention group also formed part of the sample in Carhart-Harris 2016 and Carhart-Harris 2018.

[b] Mean change scores abstracted for pooled analysis.

Abbreviations. ASI=Addiction Severity Index; BDI=Beck Depression Inventory; BSCS=Brief Substance Craving Scale; CAPS-4/5=Clinician Administered PTSD Scale for Diagnostic and Statistical Manual of Mental Disorders 4th/5th Edition; CI=confidence interval; COWS=Clinical Opioid Withdrawal Scale; GRID-HAM- D=GRID-Hamilton Depression Rating Scale; HAM-D=Hamilton Depression Rating Scale; MADRS=Montgomery-Asberg Depression Rating Scale; MDMA=3,4- methylenedioxy-methamphetamine; NR=not reported; OOWS=Objective Opiate Withdrawal Scale; OP-SCL=Opiate Symptom Checklist; PCL-C=PTSD Checklist Civilian Version; PTGI=Posttraumatic Growth Inventory; PTSD=posttraumatic stress disorder; QIDS-SR-16=16-item Quick Inventory of Depressive Symptomatology; RCT=randomized controlled trial; SD=standard deviation; SE=standard error; SOWS=Subjective Opioid Withdrawal Scale; SSSPTSD=Severity of Symptoms Scale for Posttraumatic Stress Disorder.

Studies Used in Pooled Analysis (MDMA for PTSD)

Author Year	Comparator	MDMA Dose	N Overall	N MDMA	N Comparator	Outcome Timing	MDMA Mean (SD)	Comparator Mean (SD)
Mitchell 2021[9]	Placebo	80-120 mg +	N=79	N=42	N=37	18 weeks after	-24.4 (11.6)	-13.9 (11.5)
	(0mg)	supplemental				baseline (T4)		
		dose of 40–						
		60mg						
Mithoefer 2011[10]	Placebo (0mg)	125mg + supplemental	N=20	N=12	N=8	2 months after 2nd MDMA session	-55.2 (33.54)	-20.5 (20.47)
		dose of 62.5mg				(T4)		
Mithoefer 2018[12]	Active control (30mg)	125mg	N=19	N=12	N=7	1 month after 2nd MDMA session	-44.3 (28.7)	-11.4 (12.7)

Author Year	Comparator	MDMA Dose	N Overall	N MDMA	N Comparator	Outcome Timing	MDMA Mean (SD)	Comparator Mean (SD)
NCT01958593[4] 5	Placebo (0mg)	NR	N=6	N=4	N=2	1 month after 2nd MDMA session	-17.3 (13.05)	-21.5 (12.02)
NCT01689740[4] 4	Active control (25mg + 12.5mg)	125mg + 62.5mg supplemental dose	N=8	N=5	N=3	1 month after 2nd MDMA session	-34.6 (16.29)	-9 (15.62)
Oehen 2013[14]	Active control	125mg + 62.5mg	N=12	N=8	N=4	3 weeks after 3rd	-15.6 (18.1)	3.1 (15.3)
	(25mg +	supplemental				MDMA session		
	12.5mg)	dose				(T2)		
Ot'alora 2018[15]	Active control	125mg	N=18	N=12	N=6	1 month after 2nd	-29.2 (29.62)	-11.5 (21.21)
	(40mg)					MDMA session		

Abbreviations. MDMA=3,4-methylenedioxy-methamphetamine; NR=not reported; SD=standard deviation; T2/4=Timepoint 2/4.

Harms

Ayahuasca

Author, Year Diagnosis N	Headache	Nausea	Diarrhea	Vomiting	Anxiety	Restless-ness	Drowsiness	Confu-sion	Fear	Distress	Dissocia-tion/ Deperson-alization
Dos Santos, 2021[16]	2 (11.8%)	4 (23.5%)[a]	1 (5.9%)	3 (17.6%)	—	—	2 (11.8%)	2 (11.8%)	1 (5.9%)	1 (5.9%)	1 (5.9%)
Social Anxiety Disorder N=17											

Author, Year Diagnosis N	Headache	Nausea	Diarrhea	Vomiting	Anxiety	Restless-ness	Drowsiness	Confu-sion	Fear	Distress	Dissocia-tion/ Deperson-alization
Osorio, 2015 [22] MDD N=6	—	—	—	3 (50%)	—	—	—	—	—	—	—
Palhano-Fontes, 2019 [5] MDD N=29 (14 vs 15) [b]	6 (42%) vs 8 (53%)	10 (71%) vs 4 (26%)	—	8 (57%) vs 0 (0%)	7 (50%) vs 11 (73%)	7 (50%) vs 3 (20%)	—	—	—	—	—
Sanches, 2016 [23] MDD N=17	—	—	—	8 (47%)	—	—	—	—	—	—	—
Zeifman, 2021 [24] MDD N=17	—	—	—	—	—	—	—	—	—	—	—

Notes.
[a] Item is reported as "gastrointestinal discomfort and nausea."
[b] Data are reported as "treatment group vs control group," respectively.
Abbreviations. MDD=major depressive disorder.

Ibogaine

Author, Year Diagnosis N	Headache	Nausea	Vomiting	QTc > 500ms Event	Bradycardia	Death	Visual Impairment
Glue, 2016 [7]	60mg: 4	60mg: 0	—	—	—	—	60mg: 2
OUD	(66.7%)	120mg: 2 (33.3%)					(33.3%) 120mg: 5
(33.3%) 180mg: 2	120mg: 2	180mg: 2 (33.3%)					(83.3%) 180mg: 4
27	(33.3%)	Placebo: 1					(66.7%)
(60mg: 6	Placebo: 5	(11.1%)					Placebo: 2
120mg: 6	(55.6%)						(22.2%)
180mg: 6 Placebo: 9)							
Knuijver, 2022 [29]	—	—	2 (14.3%)	7 (50%)	7 (50%)	—	—
OUD							
N=14							
Noller, 2018 [31]	—	—	—	—	—	1 (7.1%)	—
OUD							
N=14							

Abbreviations. OUD=opioid use disorder.

MDMA

Author, Year Diagnosis N Follow-up	Psychiatric	Sleep/ Fatigue	Neurologic/ Sensory	Cardiac	ENT/ Respiratory	GI	Musculo-skeletal	Other
During Session								
Jardim, 2021[32] [a]	Irritability: 1 Anguish: 2	Insomnia: 1 Fatigue: 1	Dizziness: 1	—	Cough: 3	—	Pain: 1	Somatic pains: 4

Author, Year Diagnosis N Follow-up	Psychiatric	Sleep/ Fatigue	Neurologic/ Sensory	Cardiac	ENT/ Respiratory	GI	Musculo-skeletal	Other
PTSD N=3	Colic: 2 Despair: 1 Rage: 1 Sadness: 1				Nasal congestion: 1			

Author, Year Diagnosis N Follow-up	Psychiatric	Sleep/ Fatigue	Neurologic/ Sensory	Cardiac	ENT/ Respiratory	GI	Musculo-skeletal	Other
Mithoefer, 2011[10] PTSD N=20 (12 vs 8)	Anxiety: 14 (58%) vs 13 (81%) Restlessness: 5 (21%) vs 2 (13%) Low mood: 4 (17%) vs 2 (13%) Irritability: 2 (8%) vs 3 (19%) Rumination/ increased private worries: 1 (4%) vs 1 (6%) Difficulty concentrating: 3 (13%) vs 1 (6%)	Insomnia: 13 (54%) vs 10 (63%) Drowsiness: 2 (8%) vs 3 (19%) Need more sleep: 0 vs 1 (6%) Fatigue: 11 (46%) vs 8 (50%) Weakness: 1 (4%) vs 1 (6%)	Dizziness: 9 (38%) vs 2 (13%) Impaired balance/gait: 6 (25%) vs 0 Visual impairment/ disturbance: 1 (4%) vs 0 Nystagmus: 1 (4%) vs 0 Paresthesia/ tingling Sensation: 2 (8%) vs 0	—	—	Nausea: 12 (50%) vs 2 (13%) Upper GI burning: 1 (4%) vs 0 Reduced/ lack of appetite: 8 (33%) vs 1 (6%)	Headache: 14 (58%) vs 9 (56%) Pain: 1 (4%) vs 4 (25%) Jaw clenching/ tight jaw: 19 (79%) vs 3 (19%) Muscle tension: 4 (17%) vs 2 (13%)	Heavy legs: 2 (8%) vs 0 Somatic sensations: 1 (4%) vs 0 Sensitivity to cold/feeling cold: 10 (42%) vs 8 (50%) Dry mouth: 4 (17%) vs 1 (6%) Thirst: 2 (8%) vs 1 (6%)

Author, Year Diagnosis N Follow-up	Psychiatric	Sleep/ Fatigue	Neurologic/ Sensory	Cardiac	ENT/ Respiratory	GI	Musculo-skeletal	Other
								Perspiration: 4 (17%) vs 1 (6%) General infection: 1 (4%) vs 0
Mithoefer, 2018[12] PTSD N=26 30mg: 7 75mg: 7 125mg: 12	Anxiety: 4 (57%) vs 6 (86%) vs 11 (92%) Restlessness: 4 (57%) vs 5 (71%) vs 3 (25%) Suicidal ideation: 1 (3.8%) Depression: 1 (3.8%)	Fatigue: 5 (71%) vs 4 (57%) vs 7 (58%)	—	Premature ventricular contraction: 1 (3.8%)	—	Reduced/ lack of Appetite: 3 (43%) vs 4 (57%) vs 8 (67%) Appendicitis: 1 (3.8%)	Headache: 5 (71%) vs 5 (71%) vs 8 (67%) Jaw clenching/ tight jaw: 0 vs 4 (57%) vs 9 (75%) Muscle tension: 4 (57%) vs 3 (43%) vs 9 (75%)	Sensitivity to cold/feeling cold: 4 (57%) vs 4 (57%) vs 6 (50%) Perspiration: 2 (29%) vs 2 (29%) vs 5 (42%)
Monson, 2020[33] PTSD N=12	Anxiety: 1 (16.7%) vs 1 (16.7%) Difficulty con-centrating: 1 (16.7%) vs 1 (16.7%)	Insomnia: 0 vs 1 (16.7%) Fatigue: 2 (33.3%) vs 0	Tremor: 1 (16.7%) vs 0 Tic: 1 (16.7%) vs 0	—	Upper respiratory infection: 2 (33.3%) vs 1 (16.7%)	Nausea: 2 (33.3%) vs 0 Vomiting: 0 vs 1 (16.7%)	Oropharyn-geal pain: 0 vs 1 (16.7%) Painful urination: 1 (16.7%) vs 0	Skin irritation [b]: 1 (16.7%) vs 2 (33.3%)[b] Arthoropod bite: 0 vs 1 (16.7%)

Author, Year Diagnosis N Follow-up	Psychiatric	Sleep/ Fatigue	Neurologic/ Sensory	Cardiac	ENT/ Respiratory	GI	Musculo-skeletal	Other
		Weakness: 1 (16.7%) vs 0	Dizziness: 0 vs 1 (16.7%) Visual impairment/ disturbance: 0 vs 1 (16.7%) Paresthesia/ tingling sensation: 0 vs 1 (16.7%)		Sinusitis: 1 (16.7%) vs 0 Nasopharyn-gitis: 1 (16.7%) vs 0 Runny nose: 0 vs 1 (16.7%) Nasal congestion: 0 vs 1 (16.7%) Shortness of breath: 0 vs 1 (16.7%) Tinnitus: 1 (16.7%) vs 0	Reduced/ lack of appetite: 2 (33.3%) vs 0		
Oehen, 2013[14 c] PTSD N=12 (8 vs 4)	Anxiety: 10 (25%) / 1 (16%) vs 2 (15%) Restlessness: 15 (41%) / 2 (33%) vs NA Low mood: 4 (11%) / 0 vs 1 (8%)	Insomnia: 16 (43%) / 2 (50%) vs 4 (31%) Drowsiness: 2 (5%) / 0 vs 0	Dizziness: 8 (22%) / 3 (60%) vs 4 (31%) Impaired balance/gait: 12 (32%) / 4	—	—	Nausea: 6 (16%) / 2 (33%) vs 2 (15%) Reduced/ lack of appetite: 15	Headache: 11 (30%) / 2 (33%) vs 5 (38%) Jaw clenching/ tight jaw: 14	Heavy legs: 1 (3%) / 1 (16%) vs 0 Sensitivity to cold/feeling cold: 11 (30%) / 0 vs 1 (8%)

Author, Year Diagnosis N Follow-up	Psychiatric	Sleep/ Fatigue	Neurologic/ Sensory	Cardiac	ENT/ Respiratory	GI	Musculo-skeletal	Other
	Rumination/ Increased private worries: 2 (5%) / 0 vs 0 Difficulty concentrating: 6 (16%) / 0 vs 0	Need more sleep: 1 (3%) / 0 vs 0 Fatigue: 12 (35%) / 1 (16%) vs 2 (15%) Weakness: 3 (8%) / 1 (16%) vs 0	(66%) vs 3 (23%) Nystagmus: 3 (8%) / 1 (16%) vs 0 Paresthesia/ tingling sensation: 2 (5%) / 1 (16%) vs 0			(41%) / 2 (33%) vs 4 (31%)	(38%) / 4 (66%) vs 1 (8%)	Dry mouth: 7 (19%) / 2 (33%) vs 0 Thirst: 13 (35%) / 2 (33%) vs 0 Perspiration: 6 (16%) / 2 (33%) vs 0
Ot'alora, 2018[15] PTSD N=28 40mg: 6 100mg: 9 125mg: 13	Anxiety: • 40mg: 2 (33.3%) • 100mg: 6 (66.7%) • 125mg:7 (53.8%) • Total: 17 (60.7%) Low mood: 40mg: 0 • 100mg: 5 (55.6%) • 125mg: 2 (15.4%) • Total: 7 (25%)	Fatigue: • 40mg: 2 (33.3%) • 100mg: 4 (44.4%) • 125mg: 4 (30.8%) • Total: 11 (39.3%)	Dizziness: • 40mg: 1 (16.7%) • 100mg: 2 (22.2%) • 125mg: 7 (53.8%) • Total: 12 (42.9%)	—	—	—	Headache: • 40mg: 4 (66.7%) • 100mg: 4 (44.4%) • 125mg: 3 (23.1%) • Total: 13 (46.4%) Jaw clenching/ tight jaw: • 40mg: 2 (33.3%)	

Author, Year **Diagnosis** **N** **Follow-up**	**Psychiatric**	**Sleep/ Fatigue**	**Neurologic/ Sensory**	**Cardiac**	**ENT/ Respiratory**	**GI**	**Musculo-skeletal**	**Other**
							• 100mg: 5 (55.6%) • 125mg: 8 (61.5%) • Total: 18 (64.3%) Muscle tension: • 40mg: 2 (33.3%) • 100mg: 4 (44.4%) • 125mg: 7 (53.8%) • Total: 13 (46.4%)	
Sessa, 2021[43] AUD N=14	—	—	—	Rise in blood pressure: 1 (7.1%)	—	—	—	—
Wang, 2021[34] PTSD	Anxiety: 7 (19%) Suicidal ideation: 1 (3%)	Insomnia: 18 (49%) Fatigue: 5 (14%)	Dizziness: 9 (24%) Nystagmus: 11 (30%)	Palpita-tions/ Tachycar-dia: 3 (8%)	—	Nausea: 10 (27%)	Headache: 23 (62%) Pain in jaw: 3 (8%)	Perspiration: 4 (11%)

Author, Year Diagnosis N Follow-up	Psychiatric	Sleep/ Fatigue	Neurologic/ Sensory	Cardiac	ENT/ Respiratory	GI	Musculo-skeletal	Other
N=37			Vision blurred: 2 (5%) Paresthesia/ Tingling sensation: 3 (8%)			Reduced/lack of appetite: 7 (19%) Abdominal discomfort: 2 (5%)	Muscle tension: 27 (73%)	
Post-session								
Mithoefer, 2018[12] PTSD N=26 30mg: 7 75mg: 7 125mg: 12 Follow-up: 7 days	Anxiety: • 30mg: 4 (57%) • 75mg: 5 (71%) • 125mg: 10 (83%) • Total: 19 (73%) Low mood: • 30mg: 3 (43%) • 75mg: 0 • 125mg: 3 (25%) • Total: 6 (23%) Irritability: • 30mg: 4 (57%) • 75mg: 2 (29%) • 125mg: 6 (50%) • Total: 12 (46%)	Insomnia: • 30mg: 5 (71%) • 75mg: 3 (43%) • 125mg: 10 (83%) • Total: 18 (69%) Fatigue: • 30mg: 6 (86%) • 75mg: 7 (100%) • 125mg: 10 (83%) • Total: 23 (88%)	—	—	—	Reduced/ lack of appetite: • 30mg: 2 (29%) • 75mg: 1 (14%) • 125mg: 6 (50%) • Total: 9 (35%)	Headache: • 30mg: 2 (29%) • 75mg: 3 (43%) • 125mg: 7 (57%) • Total: 12 (46%) Muscle tension: • 30mg: 2 (29%) • 75mg: 3 (43%) • 125mg: 7 (58%)	—

Author, Year **Diagnosis** **N** **Follow-up**	Psychiatric	Sleep/ Fatigue	Neurologic/ Sensory	Cardiac	ENT/ Respiratory	GI	Musculo-skeletal	Other
	Difficulty concentrating: • 30mg: 2 (29%) • 75mg: 0 • 125mg: 5 (42%) • Total: 7 (27%)	Need more sleep: • 30mg: 6 (86%) • 75mg: 6 (86%) • 125mg: 9 (75%) • Total: 21 (81%)					• Total: 12 (46%)	
Mithoefer, 2011[10] PTSD N=20 (12 vs 8) Follow-up: 7 days	Anxiety: 13 (54%) vs 7 (44%) Restlessness: 1 (4%) vs 0 Distress/panic/ stress: 1 (4%) vs 1 (6%) Dissociation/ depersonalize-ation/dereal iz-ation/detachment: 1 (4%) vs 0 Low mood: 10 (42%) vs 8 (50%)	Insomnia: 9 (38%) vs 9 (56%) Drowsiness: 0 vs 2 (13%) Fatigue: 18 (75%) vs 12 (75%) Need more sleep: 5 (21%) vs 2 (13%) Weakness: 6 (25%) vs 0	Dizziness: 3 (13%) vs 1 (6%) Visual impairment/ Disturbance: 2 (8%) vs 0	—	Upper respiratory infection: 2 (8%) vs 2 (13%)	Nausea: 7 (29%) vs 4 (25%) Diarrhea: 3 (13%) vs 0 Reduced/ lack of appetite: 9 (38%) vs 0	Headache: 6 (25%) vs 4 (25%) Jaw clenching/ tight jaw: 6 (25%) vs 2 (13%) Muscle tension: 2 (8%) vs 1 (6%)	Perspiration: 0 vs 1 (6%) Sensitivity to cold/feeling cold: 18 (75%) vs 12 (75%) Dry mouth: 1 (4%) vs 0 General infection: 0 vs 2 (13%) Heavy legs: 1 (4%) vs 0

Author, Year Diagnosis N Follow-up	Psychiatric	Sleep/ Fatigue	Neurologic/ Sensory	Cardiac	ENT/ Respiratory	GI	Musculo-skeletal	Other
	Irritability: 8 (33%) vs 3 (19%) Difficulty concentrating: 6 (25%) vs 0 Rumination/ increased private worries: 3 (13%) vs 2 (13%)							Pain: 1 (4%) vs 1 (6%) Somatic sensations: 1 (4%) vs 0
Oehen, 2013[14 d] PTSD N=12 (8 vs 4) Follow up: 7	Anxiety: 11 (26%) vs 2 (15%) Restlessness: 6 (14%) vs 0 Distress/panic/ Stress: 1 Low mood: 20 (47%) vs 6 (46%) Irritability: 9 (21%) vs 1 (8%)	Insomnia: 20 (47%) vs 6 (46%) Drowsiness: 2 (5%) vs 1 (8%) Fatigue: 24 (56%) vs 5 (38%) Need more sleep: 6 (14%) vs 3 (23%)	Dizziness: 8 (18%) vs 3 (23%) Nystagmus: 1 (2%) vs 0 Impaired balance/gait: 3 (7%) vs 0	—	—	Nausea: 5 (12%) vs 2 (15%) Reduced/ lack of appetite: 7 (16%) vs 5 (38%)	Headache: 10 (23%) vs 4 (31%) Jaw clenching/ tight jaw: 7 (16%) vs 0	Perspiration: 1 (2%) vs 0 Sensitivity to cold/feeling cold: 6 (14%) vs 1 (8%) Dry mouth: 5 (12%) vs 0 Heavy legs: 0 vs 1 (8%) Thirst: 1 (2%) vs 0

Author, Year **Diagnosis** **N** **Follow-up**	Psychiatric	Sleep/ Fatigue	Neurologic/ Sensory	Cardiac	ENT/ Respiratory	GI	Musculo-skeletal	Other
	Difficulty concentrating: 10 (23%) vs 0 Rumination/ increased private worries: 9 (21%) vs 3 (23%)	Weakness: 5 (12%) vs 0						
Monson, 2020[33] PTSD N=12 Follow-up: 6 months	—	—	—	—	—	—	—	Urithritis/UTI: 1 (16.7%) vs 0 Hypothyroid-ism: 1 (16.7%) vs 0 Tooth infection: 1 (16.7%) vs 0 Abortion: 0 vs 1 (16.7%)
Ot'alora, 2018[15] PTSD N=28 40mg: 6	Anxiety: • 40mg: 2 (33.3%) • 100mg: 8 (88.9%) • 125mg: 10 (76.9%) • Total: 20 (71.4) Low mood:	Insomnia: • 40mg: 3 (50%) • 100mg: 7 (77.8%) • 125mg: 6 (46.2%)	—	—	—	Nausea: • 40mg: 1 (16.7%) • 100mg: 3 (33.3%) • 125mg: 8 (61.5%)	Headache: • 40mg: 4 (66.7%) • 100mg: 3 (33.3%) • 125mg: 5 (38.5%)	—

Author, Year **Diagnosis** **N** **Follow-up**	Psychiatric	Sleep/ Fatigue	Neurologic/ Sensory	Cardiac	ENT/ Respiratory	GI	Musculo-skeletal	Other
100mg: 9 125mg: 13 Follow-up: 7 days	• 40mg: 2 (33.3%) • 100mg: 6 (66.7%) • 125mg: 9 (69.2%) • Total: 17 (60.7%) Irritability: • 40mg: 2 (33.3%) • 100mg: 5 (55.6%) • 125mg: 6 (46.2%) • Total: 13 (46.4%) Difficulty concentrating: • 40mg: 2 (33.3%) • 100mg: 5 (55.6%) • 125mg: 2 (15.4%) • Total: 9 (32.1%) Rumination/ increased private worries: • 40mg: 1 (16.7%) • 100mg: 5 (55.6%) • 125mg: 6 (46.2%) • Total: 12 (42.9%)	• Total: 16 (57.1%) Fatigue: • 40mg: 2 (33.3%) • 100mg: 7 (77.8%) • 125mg: 9 (69.2%) • Total: 18 (64.3%) Need more sleep: • 40mg: 2 (33.3%) • 100mg: 5 (55.6%) • 125mg: 8 (61.5%) • Total: 15 (53.6%)				• Total: 12 (42.9%) Reduced/ lack of appetite: • 40mg: 1 (16.7%) • 100mg: 1 (11.1%) • 125mg: 8 (61.5%) • Total: 10 (35.7%)	• Total: 12 (42.9%) Muscle tension: • 40mg: 2 (33.3%) • 100mg: 1 (11.1%) • 125mg: 6 (46.2%) • Total: 9 (32.1%)	

Author, Year Diagnosis N Follow-up	Psychiatric	Sleep/ Fatigue	Neurologic/ Sensory	Cardiac	ENT/ Respiratory	GI	Musculo-skeletal	Other
Jardim, 2021[32] PTSD N=3 Follow-up: 7 days	Fear: 1 Anguish: 10	Fatigue: 3 Nightmares: 1 Sleepless-ness: 1	—	—	Cough: 2	—	Headache: 3 Muscle tension: 1	Pain: 1 Somatic pains: 3
Bouso, 2008[8] PTSD N=6 Follow-up: 24 hours	Depression: 1 Difficulty concentrating: 1 Failing memory: 1 Tension/inner unrest: 2 Emotional indifference: 1	Sleepiness: 2 Fatigue: 2	Visual impairment/ Disturbance: 1	Palpita-tions/ tachycard-ia: 1	—	Diarrhea: 1	Tension headache/ migraine: 2	Lack of libido: 1
Wang, 2021[34] PTSD N=37	Anxiety: • 1 day: 1 (3%) • 2 days: 2 (5%) Suicidal ideation: • 1 Day: 2 (5%)	Insomnia: • 1 day: 2 (5%) • 2 days: 3 (8%) Fatigue:	Dizziness: • 1 day: 3 (8%) • 2 days: 0	Palpita-tions/ Tachycard-ia: • 1 day: 1 (3%) • 2 days: 0	—	Nausea: • 1 day: 3 (8) • 2 days: 0 Reduced/lack of appetite:	Headache: • 1 day: 13 (35%) • 2 days: 1 (3%)	—

Author, Year **Diagnosis** **N** **Follow-up**	**Psychiatric**	**Sleep/ Fatigue**	**Neurologic/ Sensory**	**Cardiac**	**ENT/ Respiratory**	**GI**	**Musculo-skeletal**	**Other**
Follow-up: 1-2 days	• 2 days: 1 (3%)	• 1 day: 3 (8%) • 2 days: 2 (5%)				• 1 day: 1 (3%) • 2 days: 0 Abdominal discomfort: • 1 day: 1 (3%) • 2 days: 0	Jaw clenching/ tight jaw: • 1 day: 1 (3%) • 2 days: 1 (3%)	
Total/Timing Unspecified								
Sessa, 2021[43] AUD N=14				Rise in blood pressure: 1				
Mithoefer, 2018[12] PTSD N=26 30mg: 7 75mg: 7 125mg: 12	Suicidal ideation: 1 Depression: 1	—	—	Premature ventricular contraction: 1	—	—	—	—

Author, Year Diagnosis N Follow-up	Psychiatric	Sleep/ Fatigue	Neurologic/ Sensory	Cardiac	ENT/ Respiratory	GI	Musculo-skeletal	Other
Mitchell, 2021[9] PTSD N=90 (46 vs 44)	Anxiety: 3 (6.5%) vs 0 Restlessness: 7 (15.2%) vs 0 Distress/panic/ stress: 4 (8.7%) vs 0 Suicidal ideation: 3 (6.5%) vs 5 (10.9%) Substance use: 3 (6.5%) vs 0 Feeling jittery: 5 (10.9%) vs 0 Intrusive thoughts: 4 (8.7%) vs 0	Drowsiness: 3 (6.5%) vs 0	Visual impairment/ disturbance: 4 (8.7%) vs 1 (2.3%) Dizziness: 6 (13%) vs 2 (4.5%) Nystagmus: 6 (13%) vs 0 Mydriasis/ dilated pupils: 7 (15.2%) vs 0	Rise in blood pressure: 5 (10.9%) vs 0	—	Nausea: 14 (30.4%) vs 5 (11.4%) Vomiting: 4 (8.7%) vs 0 Reduced/ lack of appetite: 24 (52.2%) vs 5 (11.4%)	Muscle twitching: 3 (6.5%) vs 0 Jaw clenching/ tight jaw: 6 (13%) vs 1 (2.3%) Muscle tension: 29 (63%) vs 5 (11.4%) Pain: 4 (8.7%) vs 0 Non-cardiac chest pain: 5 (10.9%) vs 1 (2.3%)	Perspiration: 9 (19.6%) vs 1 (2.3%) Sensitivity to cold/feeling cold: 9 (19.6%) vs 3 (6.8%) Dry mouth: 5 (10.9%) vs 2 (4.5%) Pollakiuria/ frequent urination: 4 (8.7%) vs 1 (2.3%) Fever: 3 (6.5%) vs 1 (2.3%) Chills: 3 (6.5%) vs 0

Author, Year Diagnosis N Follow-up	Psychiatric	Sleep/ Fatigue	Neurologic/ Sensory	Cardiac	ENT/ Respiratory	GI	Musculo-skeletal	Other
								Urinary urgency: 3 (6.5%) vs 0
Ot'alora, 2018[15] PTSD N=28 40mg: 6 100mg: 9 125mg: 13	Anxiety: • 40mg: 0 • 100mg: 3 (33.3%) • 125mg: 4 (30.8%) • Total: 7 (25%) Restlessness: • 40mg: 0 • 100mg: 1 (11.1%) • 125mg: 0 • Total: 1 (3.6%) Distress/panic/ stress: • 40mg: 0 • 100mg: 0 • 125mg: 1 (7.7%) • Total: 1 (3.6%) Depression (TEAE): • 40mg: 0 • 100mg: 2 (22.2%) • 125mg: 2 (15.4%)	—	—	—	—	—	—	—

Author, Year **Diagnosis** **N** **Follow-up**	**Psychiatric**	**Sleep/ Fatigue**	**Neurologic/ Sensory**	**Cardiac**	**ENT/ Respiratory**	**GI**	**Musculo-skeletal**	**Other**
	• Total: 4 (14.3%) Irritability (TEAE): • 40mg: 0 • 100mg: 2 (22.2%) • 125mg: 1 (7.7%) • Total: 3 (10.7%) Rumination/ increased private worries (TEAE): • 40mg: 0 • 100mg: 1 (11.1%) • 125mg: 1 (7.7%) • Total: 2 (7.1%)							
Jardim, 2021[32] PTSD N=3	Anxiety: 7 Fear: 7 Distress/panic/ stress: 3 Depression: 2 Irritability: 2 Anguish: 21	Insomnia: 1 Drowsiness: 2 Fatigue: 9 Nightmares: 3 Sleeplessness: 1	Dizziness: 2	—	Nasal congestion: 1 Shortness of breath: 1 Cough: 11	Nausea: 2 Diarrhea: 1	Headache: 6 Jaw clenching/ tight jaw: 1 Muscle tension: 1 Pain: 6	—

Author, Year **Diagnosis** **N** **Follow-up**	Psychiatric	Sleep/ Fatigue	Neurologic/ Sensory	Cardiac	ENT/ Respiratory	GI	Musculo-skeletal	Other
	Colic: 7 Rage: 3 Sadness: 6 Stress: 1 Rumination/ increasing private worries: 1 Despair: 2 Frustration: 1 Crying: 1						Non-cardiac chest pain: 1 Somatic pains: 22 Impotence: 2 Lack of libido: 1 Lack of trust: 1 Loneliness: 2 Vulnerability: 3	
Wang, 2021[34] PTSD N=37	Anxiety: 12 (32%) Suicidal ideation: 10 (27%)	Insomnia: 13 (35%) Fatigue: 10 (27%)	Visual impairment/ disturbance: 4 (11%) Dizziness: 7 (19%)	Palpita-tions/ tachycardia: 5 (14%)	—	Nausea: 11 (30%) Reduced/ lack of appetite: 5 (14%)	Headache: 25 (68%) Pain in jaw: 4 (11%) Muscle tension: 18 (49%)	Hyperhidrosis: 4 (11%)

Author, Year Diagnosis N Follow-up	Psychiatric	Sleep/ Fatigue	Neurologic/ Sensory	Cardiac	ENT/ Respiratory	GI	Musculo-skeletal	Other
			Nystagmus: 8 (22%) Vision blurred: 4 (11%) Paresthesia/ tingling sensation: 4 (11%)			Abdominal discomfort: 5 (14%)		
NCT01689740[44] PTSD N=10	Anxiety: • Lead in: 1/2 (50%) • Active placebo: 0/3 • Full dose 1: 4/7 (57.14%) • Full dose 2: 0/2 Suicidal ideation: • Lead in: 0/2 • Active placebo: 0/3 • Full dose 1: 1/7 (14.29%) • Full dose 2: 0/2 Depression: • Lead in: 0/2 • Active placebo: 0/3	Insomnia: • Lead in: 1/2 (50%) • Active placebo: 0/3 • Full dose 1: 0/7 • Full dose 2: 0/2	Tremor: • Lead in: 0/2 • Active placebo: 0/3 • Full dose 1: 0/7 • Full dose 2: 1/2 (50%) Dizziness: • Lead in: 0/2 • Active placebo: 0/3 • Full dose 1: 2/7 (28.57%) • Full dose 2: 0/2	—	Upper respiratory infection: • Lead in: 1/2 (50%) • Active placebo: 0/3 • Full dose 1: 1/7 (14.29%) • Full dose 2: 0/2 Shortness of breath (asthma): • Lead in: 1/2 (50%)	Nausea: Lead in: 0/2 Active placebo: 0/3 Full dose stage 1: 1/7 (14.29%) Full dose stage 2: 0/2 Intestinal obstruction: Lead in: 0/2 Active placebo: 0/3 Full dose stage 1: 1/7 (14.29%)	Headache: Lead in: 0/2 Active placebo: 0/3 Full dose 1: 1/7 (14.29%) Full dose 2: 0/2	Fever: Lead In: 1/2 Active placebo: 0/3 Full dose 1: 1/7 (14.29%) Full dose 2: 0/2 Skin hypersensitivity: Lead in: 0/2 Active placebo: 0/3 Full dose 1: 0/7 Full dose 2: 1/2 (50%)

Author, Year Diagnosis N Follow-up	Psychiatric	Sleep/ Fatigue	Neurologic/ Sensory	Cardiac	ENT/ Respiratory	GI	Musculo-skeletal	Other
	• Full dose 1: 1/7 (14.29%) • Full dose 2: 0/2 Anger: • Lead in: 0/2 • Active placebo: 0/3 • Full dose 1: 0/7 • Full dose 2: 1/2 (50%) PTSD: • Lead in: 0/2 • Active placebo: 0/3 • Full dose 1: 0/7 • Full dose 2: 1/2 (50%) Major depression: • Lead lin: 0/2 • Active placebo: 0/3 • Full dose 1: 1/7 (14.29%) • Full dose 2: 0/2				• Active placebo: 0/3 • Full dose 1: 0/7 • Full dose 2: 0/2 Oropharynge-al pain: • Lead in: 1/2 (50%) • Active placebo: 0/3 • Full dose 1: 0/7 • Full dose 2: 0/2 Influenza: • Lead in: 0/2 • Active placebo: 1/3 (33.33%)	Full dose stage 2: 0/2		Exposure to violent event: Lead in: 0/2 Active placebo: 0/3 Full dose 1: 0/7 Full dose 2: 1/2 (50%)

Author, Year Diagnosis N Follow-up	Psychiatric	Sleep/ Fatigue	Neurologic/ Sensory	Cardiac	ENT/ Respiratory	GI	Musculo-skeletal	Other
					• Full dose 1: 1/7 (14.29%) • Full dose 2: 0/2			
NCT01958593[45] PTSD N=6	Anxiety: • Placebo: 0/2 • MDMA 1: 2/4 (50%) • MDMA 2: 0/2 Restlessness: • Placebo: 0/2 • MDMA 1: 1/4 (25%) • MDMA 2: 0/2 Distress/panic/stress: • Placebo: 1/2 (50%) • MDMA 1: 1/4 (25%) • MDMA 2: 0/2 Dissociation/ depersonalization/ derealization/detach-ment: • Placebo: 1/2 (50%) • MDMA 1: 0/4	Insomnia: • Placebo: 0/2 • MDMA 1: 1/4 (25%) • MDMA 2: 0/2 Fatigue: • Placebo: 0/2 • MDMA 1: 1/4 (25%) • MDMA 2: 0/2	Paresthesia/ tingling sensation: • Placebo: 0/2 • MDMA 1: 1/4 (25%) • MDMA 2: 0/2	—	—	Nausea: • Placebo: 0/2 • MDMA 1: 1/4 (25%) • MDMA 2: 0/2	Headache: • Placebo: 0/2 • MDMA 1: 1/4 (25%) • MDMA 2: 0/2 Jaw clenching/ tight jaw: • Placebo: 0/2 • MDMA 1: 1/4 (25%) • MDMA 2: 0/2 Muscle tension: • Placebo: 0/2	—

Author, Year Diagnosis N Follow-up	Psychiatric	Sleep/ Fatigue	Neurologic/ Sensory	Cardiac	ENT/ Respiratory	GI	Musculo-skeletal	Other
	• MDMA 2: 0/2 Low mood: • Placebo: 0/2 • MDMA 1: 2/4 (50%) • MDMA 2: 0/2 Intentional self-injury: • Placebo: 1/2 (50%) • MDMA 1: 0/4 • MDMA 2: 1/2 (50%)						• MDMA 1: 1/4 (25%) • MDMA 2: 0/2 Pain: • Placebo: 0/2 • MDMA 1: 1/4 (25%) • MDMA 2: 0/2 Concussion: • Placebo: 0/2 • MDMA 1: 0/4 • MDMA: 1/2 (50%)	

Note: An analytic dataset of effect sizes used in reported meta-analyses is available upon request to esp.cc@va.gov.

[a] Percentages not calculated because count/denominator are unclear.

[b] "Erythema," "Pruritis," and "Rash" were combined as "skin irritation."

[c] Data are presented as "125mg session/150mg session vs placebo."

[d] Thirty-seven sessions had a full dose of 125 mg. Six sessions had a full dose of 150mg.

Abbreviations. AUD=alcohol use disorder; ENT=ear, nose, and throat; GI=gastrointestinal; MDMA=3,4-methylenedioxy-methamphetamine; PTSD=posttraumatic stress disorder; TEAE=treatment emergent adverse event; UTI=urinary tract infection.

Psilocybin

Author, Year Diagnosis	Psychiatric	Sleep/ Fatigue	Neurologic/ Sensory	Cardiac	ENT/ Respiratory	GI	Musculo- skeletal	Other
N								
Follow-up								
Pre-session								
Carhart-Harris, 2016 [19] MDD N=12	Anxiety: 6 (50%)	—	—	—	—	—	—	—
Carhart-Harris, 2021 [2] MDD N=59 (30 psilocybin vs 29 escitalopram) 6-week trial period	Anxiety: 0 vs 4 (14%) Feeling jittery: 2 (7%) vs 1 (3%) Feeling abnormal: 0 vs 3 (10%)	Sleep disorder: 1 (3%) vs 3 (10%) Fatigue: 2 (7%) vs 7 (24%)	—	Palpitations/ Tachycardia: 1 (3%) vs 3 (10%)	—	Nausea: 8 (27%) vs 9 (31%) Diarrhea: 1 (3%) vs 2 (7%) Vomiting: 2 (7%) vs 1 (3%)	Headache: 20 (67%) vs 15 (52%) Migraine: 3 (10%) vs 1 (3%)	Dry mouth: 0 vs 4 (14%)
During Session								

Author, Year Diagnosis	Psychiatric	Sleep/ Fatigue	Neurologic/ Sensory	Cardiac	ENT/ Respiratory	GI	Musculo- skeletal	Other
N								
Follow-up								
Bogenschutz, 2015 [1] AUD N=10	—	—	—	—	—	Nausea: 1 (10%) Diarrhea: 1 (10%)	Headache: 5 (50%)	—
Davis, 2021 [3] MDD N=27 (15 in treatment group)	Anxiety: 27 (56%) Fear: 26 (54%)	—	Tremor: 32 (67%)	Blood pressure event: 1 (2%) Heart rate	—	—	Headache: 16 (33%) Pressure in chest/	Isolation/ loneliness: 28 (58%) Feeling of
	"I felt			event: 4 (8%)			abdomen: 32 (67%)	isolation from people/
	frightened": 21 (44%)							things: 26 (54%)
	Distress/ panic/stress: 19 (40%) Emotional/							"I felt isolated from everything/ everyone": 22 (46%)
	physical suffering: 37 (77%)							
	Despair: 28 (58%)							
	Feelings of despair: 23 (48%)							

Author, Year Diagnosis	Psychiatric	Sleep/ Fatigue	Neurologic/ Sensory	Cardiac	ENT/ Respiratory	GI	Musculo- skeletal	Other
N								
Follow-up								
	Sadness: 38 (79%)							
	Feel shaky inside: 30 (63%)							
	Grief: 29							
	(60%)							
Carhart- Harris, 2021 [2]	—	—	—	—	—	Nausea: 4 (13%) vs 0	Headache: 13 (43%) vs5 (17%)	—
MDD								
N=59 (30								
psilocybin vs								
29								
escitalopram)								
Carhart-	Anxiety: 6	—	—	—	—	Nausea: 3	Headache: 4	—
Harris, 2016 [19]	(50%)					(25%)	(33.3%)	
	Confusion: 9							
MDD	(75%)							
N=12	Paranoia: 2							
	(16.7%)							
Johnson, 2014 [40]	Fear, fear of insanity,	—	—	—	—	—	—	—
	feeling							
Tobacco	trapped: 5							

Author, Year Diagnosis	Psychiatric	Sleep/ Fatigue	Neurologic/ Sensory	Cardiac	ENT/ Respiratory	GI	Musculo- skeletal	Other
N								
Follow-up								
addiction	(33.3%)							
N=15								
Post-session								
Bogenschutz, 2015 [17]	—	Insomnia: 1 (10%)	—	—	—	—	—	—
AUD								
N=10								
Follow-up: 1								
day								
Davis, 2021 [3]	—	Nightmares	Visual	—	—	—	Headache	Somatic
		(post-	impairment/				(post-session	sensations:
MDD		session 2): 1	Disturbance				1): 7 (29%)	(post-
		(4%)	(post-session					session 2): 1
N=27 (15 in			1): 1 (4%)				Headache	(4%)
treatment							(post-session	
group)			Visual				2): 7 (29%)	
			impairment/					
Follow-up: 2			Disturbance				Physical	
weeks			(post-session				discomfort	
			2): 2 (8%)				(post-session1): 1 (4%)	
							Muscle tension	
							(post-session2): 2 (8%)	

Author, Year Diagnosis	Psychiatric	Sleep/ Fatigue	Neurologic/ Sensory	Cardiac	ENT/ Respiratory	GI	Musculo- skeletal	Other
N								
Follow-up								
							Non-cardiac chest pain (post-session2): 1 (4%)	
							Muscle twitching: (post-session 1): 1 (4%)	
Gukasyan, 2022 [4] MDD N=24 Follow up: 3 months	—	—	1-min episode of visual distortions: 1 (4.2%)	—	—	—	—	—
Johnson, 2014 [40] Tobacco Addiction N=15 Follow up: NR	—	—	—	—	—	—	Headache: 8/10 (80%) a	—
Total/timing Unspecified								
Carhart- Harris, 2018 [20] MDD N=20	Anxiety: 15 (75%) Paranoia: 3 (15%)	—	Autobio - graphical visions: 14 (70%)	—	—	Nausea: 5 (25%)	Headache: 8 (40%)	—

Author, Year Diagnosis	Psychiatric	Sleep/ Fatigue	Neurologic/ Sensory	Cardiac	ENT/ Respiratory	GI	Musculo- skeletal	Other
N								
Follow-up								
Moreno, 2006 [26] OCD N=9	—	—	—	Transient hypertension: 1 (11.1%)	—	—	—	—

Abbreviations. ENT=ear, nose, and throat; GI=gastrointestinal; MDD=major depressive disorder; NR=not reported; OCD=obsessive compulsive disorder.
Notes. a Mean onset was 6.2 hours.

Quality Assessment of Included Primary Studies

RCTs – RoB 2 Tool

Author	Risk of Bias	Risk of Bias	Risk of Bias	Risk of Bias	Risk of Bias in	Risk of Bias in	Overall Bias
Year	from	from Deviation	from Deviation	from Missing	Measurement	Selection of	(High, Low,
	Randomizatio	from Intended	from Intended	Outcome Data	of Outcome	Reported	Some
	n Process	Interventions	Interventions			Result	Concerns)
		(Assignment)	(Adherence)				
Bouso 2008[8]	Unclear	Unclear	High	Unclear	Unclear	Low	High
	Limited	Participants and	Only 6 (of 29)	Unclear level or	Unclear if	Appear to have	
	information	investigators	participants	handling of	outcome	reported all	
	about	blinded, but no	completed	missing data.	assessors were	prespecified	

	randomization process or	information about deviations	intervention prior to study		blinded.	findings.	
	allocation	or experiment	termination.				
	concealment.	flow.					
Bogenschutz	Low	Low	Low	Low	Low	Low	Low
2022 [1]	Randomization	Participants and	98% received	Analyzed 98% of	Outcome	Appear to have	
	through	investigators	first medication	randomized	assessors	reported all	
	independent	blinded, although	session, 82%	participants.	blinded, but	prespecified	
	pharmacist	90%+ guessed assignment	received second medication	Missing values imputed with	90%+ guessed assignment	findings	
		correctly. No deviation from assignments.	session.	multivariate imputation.	correctly.		
Mitchell	Low	Low	Low	Unclear	Low	Low	Some concerns
2021 [9]	Randomization	Participants and	87–98% of	Omitted	Outcome	Appear to have	
	blinded through	investigators	participants	withdrawals from	assessors	reported all	
	centralized	blinded. No	completed 1st,	data set for 2nd	blinded	prespecified	
	web-based system	deviation from assignments.	2nd, and 3rd sessions.	(93% complete) and 3rd session		findings	
			Patients required	(88% complete)			
			to discontinue				
			medications prior				
			to study.				
Carhart-	Low	Unclear	Unclear	Unclear	Unclear	Low	Some concerns
Harris 2021 [2]	Randomization	Participants and	86% of	Unclear level of	Unclear if	Appear to have	
	by independent	investigators	participants	missing data. No	outcome	reported all	
	staff members.	blinded. Unclear	adhered to	imputation for	assessors were	prespecified	
	Baseline characteristics	if there were deviations from	intervention. 39%	missing data.	blinded.	findings	

	balanced except alcohol	assignment, no participant flow	discontinued medications and				
	use.	diagram.	7% discontinued				
			psychotherapy.				
Davis 2021 [3]	Low	Unclear	Low	Low	Low	Low	Low
& Gukasyan	Randomization	Participants and	88% received	No primary	Outcome raters	Appear to have	
2022 [4]	described,	investigators	adhered to	outcome data	blinded to	reported all	
	performed by	unblinded	intervention. All	were missing.	treatment status.	prespecified	
	investigator not involved in	because of delayed	patients required to discontinue			findings	
	enrollment and screening. No baseline	treatment. No deviations from assignment.	medications prior to study.				
	differences						
	between						
	groups.						
Dos Santos	Unclear	Unclear	Low	Unclear	Unclear	Low	Some concerns
2021 [16]	"simple"	Participants and	100% adhered to	82% had	Outcomes were	Appear to have	
	randomization	investigators	intervention.	complete data	self-reported and	reported all	
	performed by	blinded. Unclear	Patients	for analysis	100% guessed	prespecified	
	independent researcher. Unclear	if deviations from assignment.	discontinued medications prior to study.		group assignment.	findings	
	balance of						
	baseline						
	characteristics.						
Glue 2016 [7]	Unclear	Unclear	Unclear	Unclear	Low	Low	Some concerns
	Randomization	Participants and	No description of	Unclear level	Participants	Appear to have	
	described.	investigators	adherence, but	and handling of	blinded for self-	reported all	

	Allocation concealment not described.	blinded. Unclear if deviations from assignment.	single-dose so likely high. All patients	missing data.	reported outcomes.	prespecified findings	
	Baseline characteristics		switched to morphine prior to				
	not presented.		study.				
Mithoefer	Low	Low	Low	Unclear	Low	Low	Low
2019 [13]	Randomization	Participants and	7.6% dropout	Missing data not	Outcome raters	Appear to have	
	described and	investigators	rate, 6/105	imputed. From	were masked to	reported all	
	similar across	blinded. No	terminated early	individual	intervention	prespecified	
	studies. No significant differences in baseline	deviation from assignments.	but completed at least 1 session and follow-up assessment.	studies, 15% and lower	assignment.	findings	
	characteristics.		91% took				
			supplemental				
			dose.				
Mithoefer	Unclear	Low	Unclear	Unclear	Low	Low	Some concerns
2011 [10] &	Randomization	Participants and	87% received	All patients who	Outcome raters	Appear to have	
2013 [11]	described.	investigators	allocated	completed	were masked to	reported all	
	Allocation	blinded. No	intervention.	treatment had	records of	prespecified	
	concealment not described. Most baseline characteristics	deviation from assignment in initial phase.	27% in the intervention group got an additional dose	outcome data (87%).	treatment sessions.	findings	
	similar except # months of prior		as a protocol amendment. All				
	therapy.		patients received				
			non-drug therapy				
			and discontinued				

			medications prior				
			to study.				
Mithoefer	Low	Low	Low	Low	Low	Low	Low
2018 [12]	Randomization	Investigators,	2/26 patients	All patients	Outcome raters	Appear to have	
	and allocation	participants, and	discontinued	completed	were masked to	reported all	
	concealment	outcome raters	treatment. All	primary	dosage for	prespecified	
	described. Some differences in baseline characteristics,	masked until primary endpoint. Blind broken after primary	patients received psychotherapy and discontinued other medications prior	assessment and 24/26 completed 12-month follow-up	primary assessment.	findings	
	likely due to small sample	endpoint.	to study.				
	size.						
Oehen	Unclear	Low	Low	Unclear	Low	Low	Some concerns
2013 [14]	No description	Double blind	Few participants	Excluded data	Outcomes were	Results appear	
	of allocation	study until open	continued on to	from 2/14 (15%)	assessed by	to follow pre-	
	process. No significant differences	label arm. No reported deviations from	the open label phase (T3 and beyond), but	of sample.	blinded study staff. Investigators	specified analysis plan.	
	between groups	assignment.	results are only		provided		
	at baseline.		provided for T1 and T2,		guesses on condition		
			representing the		assessments		
			full sample. 2 participants		with an accuracy rate of 59%,		
			withdrew after first dose due to		indicating that blinding was		
			AEs.		effective.		
Ot'alora	Low	Low	Unclear	Low	Low	Low	Some concerns
2018 [15]	Allocation was	Participants and	5/28 (18%) did	Data from 1	Outcomes were	Appear to have	

	completed	all study staff	not complete	participant who	measured by	reported all	
	through a web-	were blinded to	intervention	withdrew was	blinded	prespecified	
	based system and was blinded to study	assignment until open label phase		excluded.	independent raters.	findings	
	staff						
Palhano-	Unclear	Low	Unclear	Low	Unclear	Low	Some concerns
Fontes 2019 [5]	Allocation via	All investigators	17% didn't	Several patients	Psychiatrists'	Results appear	
& Zeifman	permuted	and patients	receive	did not meet	blindness was	to follow pre-	
2019 [6]	blocks of size	were blind to	intervention.	criteria after	not assessed,	specified	
	10. Zeifman 2019 describes low suicidality in placebo group despite randomization. Intervention assignment was stored in database and only known to pharmacy administrators.	intervention. Each patient was assigned a different blinded psychiatrist for each dosing session.	Investigators and participants blinded with placebo participants were given a substance that resembled ayahuasca and produced GI distress. Participants with past ayahuasca	washout and were excluded from analysis. 1 patient dropped out of study. Missing data imputed.	but they were randomly assigned to each patient each dosage session. Zeifman 2019 does not clarify if clinicians administering MADRS were blinded to assignment.	analysis plan.	
			use were				
			excluded to				
			enhance				
			intervention				
			blindness.				

Abbreviations. AE=adverse event; GI=gastrointestinal; MADRS=Montgomery-Asberg Depression Rating Scale; T1/2/3=timepoint 1/2/3.

Observational Studies – ROBINS-I Tool for Cohort Studies

Author Year	Selection Bias	Bias in Classification of Interventions	Bias Due to Departures from Intended Intervention	Bias Due to Measurement of Outcomes	Bias Due to Confounding	Bias Due to Missing Data	Bias in the Selection of Reported Results	Overall Bias (High, Low, Unclear)
Lyons 2018 [21]	Unclear Control group matched on age, gender, and education, and was assessed over a similar timeframe, but minimal information about how patients were selected into study.	Unclear Intervention clearly defined. Unclear what (if anything) controls received - says "untreated."	Unclear No information on patient adherence or if controls received any type of intervention during the period.	Unclear Self-reported depression measures may have been influenced by knowledge of intervention.	High Control group differed significantly from intervention group in baseline depression. Matched on other factors, but for outcome of depression there is high risk of confounding.	Unclear Unclear level and handling of missing data	Unclear No protocol identified.	High
Stroud 2018 [25]	High Minimal information about control group. Controls had no psychiatric illness and likely differed	Unclear Intervention clearly defined. Unclear what (if anything) controls received.	Unclear No information on patient adherence or if controls received any type of	Unclear Self-reported depression measures may have been influenced by knowledge of intervention.	High Minimal information about control group and likely that they differed from	High Missing data handled with likewise deletion. Unclear level of missing data.	Unclear No protocol identified.	High

Author Year	Selection Bias	Bias in Classification of Interventions	Bias Due to Departures from Intended Intervention	Bias Due to Measurement of Outcomes	Bias Due to Confounding	Bias Due to Missing Data	Bias in the Selection of Reported Results	Overall Bias (High, Low, Unclear)
	from those in the trial which comprised the intervention group.		intervention during the period.		intervention group. No adjustment for confounding.			
Bogenschutz Low 2015 [17]	Same groups of patients followed for pre-post assessments	Low Time points for pre- and post-assessments clearly defined.	Unclear 3/10 patients didn't complete 2nd psilocybin session	Unclear Outcome assessment similar pre and post intervention. Outcome self-reported may be influenced by study participation.	High Single pre-treatment measurement. No analysis of potential confounders.	Low Omitted missing data, but low level	Unclear No protocol identified	High
Brown 2018 [27]	Low Same groups of patients followed for pre-post assessments	Low Time points for pre- and post-assessments clearly defined.	Unclear No information on adherence, but likely high since it was a single administration.	Unclear Outcome assessment similar pre and post intervention. Outcome self-reported may be influenced by study participation.	High Single pre-treatment measurement. No analysis of potential confounders.	Unclear Did analyses either omitting missing data or setting it to baseline values. Unclear level of missing data.	Unclear No protocol identified	High

Author Year	Selection Bias	Bias in Classification of Interventions	Bias Due to Departures from Intended Intervention	Bias Due to Measurement of Outcomes	Bias Due to Confounding	Bias Due to Missing Data	Bias in the Selection of Reported Results	Overall Bias (High, Low, Unclear)
Carhart-Harris 2016 [19], 2018 [20]	Low Same groups of patients followed for pre-post assessments	Low Time points for pre- and post-assessments clearly defined	Unclear No information on adherence. Intensive preparatory visit prior to psychedelic visit.	Unclear Outcome assessment similar pre and post intervention. Outcome self-reported may be influenced by study participation.	High Single pre-treatment measurement. No analysis of potential confounders.	Low All patients completed measures	Unclear No protocol identified	High
Davis 2017 [28]	Low Same groups of patients followed for pre-post assessments	High Pre- and post-assessment were done at the same time through a survey.	Unclear No information on intervention adherence, only that they had received treatment during a certain time period.	High Measures self-reported and collected pre- and post-measure both post-intervention in a single survey.	High Single pre-treatment measurement. No analysis of potential confounders.	Low Table 1 indicates that they had data for all but 1 participant.	Unclear No protocol identified	High
Davis 2020 [42]	Low Same groups of patients followed for pre-post assessments	High Pre- and post-assessment were done at the same time through a	Unclear No information on intervention adherence, only that they had received	High Measures self-reported and collected pre- and post-measure both	High Single pre-treatment measurement. No analysis of potential	Unclear Unclear level and handling of missing data.	Unclear No protocol identified	High

Author Year	Selection Bias	Bias in Classification of Interventions	Bias Due to Departures from Intended Intervention	Bias Due to Measurement of Outcomes	Bias Due to Confounding	Bias Due to Missing Data	Bias in the Selection of Reported Results	Overall Bias (High, Low, Unclear)
		survey.	treatment during a certain time period.	post-intervention in a single survey.	confounders.			
Jardim 2021 [32]	Low Same groups of patients followed for pre-post assessments	Low Time points for pre- and post-assessments clearly defined	Unclear 3 patients, all completed program. Several pre-intervention sessions.	Unclear Outcome assessment similar pre and post intervention. Outcome self-reported may be influenced by study participation.	High Single pre-treatment measurement. No analysis of potential confounders.	Low Appears data were available for all patients.	Unclear No protocol identified	High
Johnson 2014 [40] & 2017 [41]	Low Same groups of patients followed for pre-post assessments	Low Time points for pre- and post-assessments clearly defined	Unclear 12/15 completed all 3 sessions. Program also involved CBT.	Unclear Outcome assessment similar pre and post intervention. Outcome self-reported may be influenced by study participation.	High Single pre-treatment measurement. No analysis of potential confounders.	Low Appears data were available for all patients.	Unclear No protocol identified	High
Knuijver	Low	Low	Low	Low	High	Low	Unclear	High

Author Year	Selection Bias	Bias in Classification of Interventions	Bias Due to Departures from Intended Intervention	Bias Due to Measurement of Outcomes	Bias Due to Confounding	Bias Due to Missing Data	Bias in the Selection of Reported Results	Overall Bias (High, Low, Unclear)
2022 [29]	Same groups of patients followed for pre-post assessments	Time points for pre- and post-assessments clearly defined	All patients completed study	Outcome assessment similar pre and post intervention. Outcomes were clinician assessed.	Single pre-treatment measurement. No analysis of potential confounders.	Appears data were available for all patients.	No protocol identified	
Malcolm 2018 [30]	Low Same groups of patients followed for pre-post assessments	Low Time points for pre- and post-assessments clearly defined	Unclear No information on intervention adherence.	Low Outcome assessment similar pre and post intervention. Outcomes were clinician assessed.	Unclear Two pre-treatment measures and multiple post-treatment measures. No assessment of confounders.	Unclear Omitted missing data from 10/50 patients on baseline demographics.	Unclear No protocol identified	Unclear
Mash 2001 [37]	Low Same groups of patients followed for pre-post assessments	Low Time points for pre- and post-assessments clearly defined	Unclear No information on intervention adherence.	Unclear Outcome assessment similar pre and post intervention. Outcome self-reported may be influenced by study	High Single pre-treatment measurement. No analysis of potential confounders.	Unclear Unclear level and handling of missing data.	Unclear No protocol identified	High

Author Year	Selection Bias	Bias in Classification of Interventions	Bias Due to Departures from Intended Intervention	Bias Due to Measurement of Outcomes	Bias Due to Confounding	Bias Due to Missing Data	Bias in the Selection of Reported Results	Overall Bias (High, Low, Unclear)
				participation.				
Mash 2000 [36]	Low Same groups of patients followed for pre-post assessments	Low Time points for pre- and post-assessments clearly defined	Unclear No information on intervention adherence.	Unclear Outcome assessment similar pre and post intervention. Outcome self-reported may be influenced by study participation.	High Single pre-treatment measurement. No analysis of potential confounders.	Unclear Unclear level and handling of missing data.	Unclear No protocol identified	High
Mash 2018 [38]	Low Same groups of patients followed for pre-post assessments	Low Time points for pre- and post-assessments clearly defined	Unclear No information on intervention adherence.	Unclear Outcome assessment similar pre and post intervention. Outcome self-reported may be influenced by study participation.	High Single pre-treatment measurement. No analysis of potential confounders.	Unclear Unclear level and handling of missing data.	Unclear No protocol identified	High
Monson 202033	Low Same groups of patients followed for	Low Time points for pre- and	Low All couples completed the protocol.	Low Outcome assessment similar pre and post	High Single pretreatment measurement. No analysis of	Low No missing data for clinicianassesse	Unclear No protocol identified	High

Author Year	Selection Bias	Bias in Classification of Interventions	Bias Due to Departures from Intended Intervention	Bias Due to Measurement of Outcomes	Bias Due to Confounding	Bias Due to Missing Data	Bias in the Selection of Reported Results	Overall Bias (High, Low, Unclear)
	pre-post assessments	postassessments clearly defined	Intervention included CBCT therapy	intervention. Outcomes clinician assessed.	potential confounders.	d PTSD data. Overall assessment completion 86%.		
Moreno 2006 [26]	Low Same groups of patients followed for pre-post assessments	Low Time points for pre- and postassessments clearly defined	Unclear 2/9 did not complete study. 6/9 received all doses.	Unclear Outcome assessment similar pre and post intervention. Outcome selfreported may be influenced by study participation.	High Single pretreatment measurement. No analysis of potential confounders.	Unclear Unclear level and handling of missing data.	Unclear No protocol identified	High
Noller 2018 [31]	Low Same groups of patients followed for pre-post assessments	Low Time points for pre- and postassessments clearly defined	Low 14/15 completed treatment.	Unclear Outcome assessment changed over time (inperson, over the phone, mailed surveys).	High Single pretreatment measurement. No analysis of potential confounders.	High (urine screen)/unclear (other outcomes) High levels of missing urine screen data. Level of missing data unclear for	Unclear No protocol identified	High

Author Year	Selection Bias	Bias in Classification of Interventions	Bias Due to Departures from Intended Intervention	Bias Due to Measurement of Outcomes	Bias Due to Confounding	Bias Due to Missing Data	Bias in the Selection of Reported Results	Overall Bias (High, Low, Unclear)
						other outcomes, but states 14/14 were analyzed.		
Osorio 2015 [22]	Low Same groups of patients followed for pre-post assessments	Low Time points for pre- and postassessments clearly defined	Unclear No information on intervention adherence.	Low Outcome assessment similar pre and post intervention. Outcomes clinician assessed.	High Single pretreatment measurement. No analysis of potential confounders.	Unclear Data missing for 1 patient on blood pressure measures. Unclear if there were missing data for other outcomes.	Unclear No protocol identified	High
Sanches 2016 [23] & Zeifman 2021 [24]	Low Same groups of patients followed for pre-post assessments	Low Time points for pre- and postassessments clearly defined	Unclear No information on intervention adherence.	Low Outcome assessment similar pre and post intervention. Outcomes clinician assessed.	High Single pretreatment measurement. No analysis of potential confounders.	Unclear No information on level and handling of missing data.	Unclear No protocol identified	High
Schenberg 2014 [39]	Low Same groups of patients followed for pre-post assessments	Unclear Unclear how long since intervention the interviews were conducted.	Unclear Unclear if patients adhered to planned intervention.	High Measures assessed after intervention. Non-patients were interviewed in	High Appears that pre-treatment use was assessed in post-treatment interview.	Unclear No information on level and handling of missing data.	Unclear No protocol identified	High

Author Year	Selection Bias	Bias in Classification of Interventions	Bias Due to Departures from Intended Intervention	Bias Due to Measurement of Outcomes	Bias Due to Confounding	Bias Due to Missing Data	Bias in the Selection of Reported Results	Overall Bias (High, Low, Unclear)
				almost 20% of cases.				
Sessa 2021 [43]	Low Same groups of patients followed for pre-post assessments	Low Time points for pre- and postassessments clearly defined	Low 12/14 received both sessions.	Low Outcome assessment similar pre and post intervention. Outcomes clinician assessed.	High Single pretreatment measurement. No analysis of potential confounders.	Unclear Mean data used for missing data. 4/14 had missing data for 1 question on SADQ.	Unclear No protocol identified	High
Thomas 2013 [35]	Unclear Data came from 2 different retreats.	Low Time points for pre- and postassessments clearly defined	Unclear 3/18 did not complete retreat. Unclear adherence to all aspects of retreat.	Unclear Outcome assessment similar pre and post intervention. Outcome selfreported may be influenced by study participation.	High Single pretreatment measurement. No analysis of potential confounders.	Unclear 3/18 with missing data excluded from analysis.	Unclear No protocol identified	High
Wang 2021 [34]	Low Same groups of patients followed for	Low Time points for pre- and postassessments clearly defined.	Unclear Describes mean # of sessions, but unclear	Low Outcome assessment similar pre and post intervention.	High Single pretreatment measurement. No analysis of	Low 1/37 did not complete primary endpoint assessment.	Unclear No protocol identified	High

Author Year	Selection Bias	Bias in Classification of Interventions	Bias Due to Departures from Intended Intervention	Bias Due to Measurement of Outcomes	Bias Due to Confounding	Bias Due to Missing Data	Bias in the Selection of Reported Results	Overall Bias (High, Low, Unclear)
	pre-post assessments		adherence to all sessions.	Outcomes clinician assessed.	potential confounders.			

Abbreviations. CBCT=cognitive-behavioral conjoint therapy; CBT=cognitive behavioral therapy; PTSD=posttraumatic stress disorder; SADQ=Severity of Alcohol Dependence Questionnaire; SUD=substance use disorder.

Strength of Evidence for Included Studies

Outcome	Psychedelic	Studies	Study Limitations	Directness	Consistency	Precision	Reporting Bias	Rating and Summary of Evidence
Alcohol Use Disorder								
Drinking behavior	Psilocybin	Bogenschutz 2022, [1] Bogenschutz 201517	Low to high	Direct	Consistent	Imprecise	Unknown	Low Psilocybin may decrease drinking behavior based on an RCT and pre-post study.
Drinking	MDMA	Sessa 2021 [43]	High	Direct	Unknown	Unknown	Unknown	Insufficient
behavior								It is unclear whether MDMA
								decreases drinking behavior
								based on a single pre-post
Major Depressive Disorder								study.
Depressive symptoms	Psilocybin	Carhart- Harris 2016 [19], Carhart- Harris 2018 [20], Davis 20213,	Low to high	Direct	Consistent	Imprecise	Unknown	Low Psilocybin with psychotherapy may reduce depressive symptoms compared to no treatment, based on a single

Outcome	Psychedelic	Studies	Study Limitations	Directness	Consistency	Precision	Reporting Bias	Rating and Summary of Evidence
		Gukasyan 2022 [4], Lyons 2018 [21], Stroud 2018 [25]						RCT and 3 pre-post studies with small sample sizes.
Depressive symptoms	Psilocybin	Carhart- Harris 20212	Moderate	Direct	Unknown	Imprecise	Unknown	Low Psilocybin-assisted psychotherapy may not reduce depressive symptoms compared to psychotherapy and daily escitalopram.
Depressive symptoms	Ayahuasca	Palhano- Fontes 2019, [5] Osorio 2015 [22], Sanches 2016 [23], Zeifman 2021 [24]	Moderate to high	Direct	Consistent	Unknown	Unknown	Low Ayahuasca may reduce depressive symptoms based on a single RCT and 2 pre-post study with small sample sizes.
Suicidal ideation	Psilocybin	Carhart- Harris 2021 [2]	Moderate	Direct	Unknown	Imprecise	Unknown	Insufficient It is unclear whether psilocybin improves suicidal ideation compared to escitalopram based on a single RCT.
Suicidal ideation	Psilocybin	Psilocybin Davis 2021 [3], Gukasyan 2022 [4]	Low	Direct	Unknown	Unknown Imprecise	Unknown	Insufficient It is unclear whether psilocybin improves suicidal ideation based on a single RCT compared to delayed treatment.
Suicidal ideation	Ayahuasca	Palhano- Fontes 2019, [5] Zeifman 2019, [6] Sanches 2016, [23]	Moderate to high	Direct	Consistent	Imprecise	Unknown	Insufficient Ayahuasca may improve suicidal ideation over time, but it is unclear whether it differs from placebo based on a

Outcome	Psychedelic	Studies	Study Limitations	Directness	Consistency	Precision	Reporting Bias	Rating and Summary of Evidence
		Zeifman 2021 [24]						single RCT and a single pre-post study with small sample sizes.
Opioid Use Disorder								
Opioid use	Ibogaine	Davis 2017 [28], Brown 2018 [27], Noller 2018 [31], Glue 20167	High	Direct	Consistent	Unknown	Unknown	Low Ibogaine may reduce opioid use immediately after treatment, but limited by prepost studies with high RoB. Single RCT showed similar time to resumption of opioid substitution therapy among participants on methadone.
Withdrawal	Ibogaine	Davis 2017 [28], Brown 2018 [27], Knuijver 2022 [29], Malcom 2018 [30], Noller 2018 [31], Glue 2016 [7]	High	Direct	Consistent	Unknown	Unknown	Low Ibogaine may reduce opioid withdrawal symptoms immediately after treatment, but limited by pre-post studies with mostly high RoB. Single RCT showed increases in withdrawal symptoms within 10 hours of last morphine dose among participants on methadone.
Posttraumatic Stress Disorder								
Remission	MDMA	Mitchell 2021 [9], Mithoefer 2011 [10], Mitheofer 2018 [12], Ot'alora 201815	Low - some concerns	Direct	Consistent	Unknown	Unknown	Low: MDMA-assisted psychotherapy may result in PTSD remission compared to placebo based on 4 RCTs.

Outcome	Psychedelic	Studies	Study Limitations	Directness	Consistency	Precision	Reporting Bias	Rating and Summary of Evidence
Clinically meaningful improvement	MDMA	Mitheofer 201110, Mithoefer 201812, Ot'alora 201815, Oehen 201314	Low - some concerns	Direct	Consistent	Unknown	Unknown	Low: MDMA-assisted psychotherapy may result in a clinically meaningful reduction in symptom burden (defined as a >30% improvement on CAPS total severity scores) compared to placebo based on 4 RCTs.
Change in mean symptom scores	MDMA	Mitchell 2021 [9], Mithoefer 2011 [10], Mitheofer 2018 [12], Ot'alora 2018 [15], Oehen 2013 [14], Bouso 2008 [8], Jardim 2021 [32], Monson 2020 [33], Wang 2021 [34], NCT0195859 3 [45], NCT0168974 0 [44]	Low to high	Direct	Consistent	Imprecise	Unknown	*Low SOE:* MDMA-assisted psychotherapy may reduce PTSD symptoms (in 7 trials, the pooled mean difference in PTSD symptom change for intervention dose MDMA compared with 0mg or low-dose placebo is -18.0 (95% CI [-30.0, -6.0]).
Tobacco Use								
Tobacco Use	Psilocybin	Johnson 2014 [40], Johnson 2017 [41]	High	Direct	Unknown	Unknown	Unknown	Insufficient It is unclear whether psilocybin influences tobacco use based on a single pre-post study.

Outcome	Psychedelic	Studies	Study Limitations	Directness	Consistency	Precision	Reporting Bias	Rating and Summary of Evidence
Mixed Substance Use								
Substance use	Ayahuasca	Thomas 2013 [35]	High	Direct	Unknown	Unknown	Unknown	Insufficient It is unclear whether ayahuasca reduces substance use in participants of a substance use program based on a single study.
Opiate and cocaine craving	Ibogaine	Mash 2000, [36] Mash 2001, [37] Mash 2018 [38]	High	Direct	Unknown	Unknown	Unknown	Insufficient It is unclear whether ibogaine reduces opiate and cocaine craving in participants of a substance use program based on a single study.
Substance use	Ibogaine	Schenberg 2014 [39]	High	Direct	Unknown	Unknown	Unknown	Insufficient It is unclear whether ibogaine reduces substance use in participants of a substance use program based on a single study.
Other Conditions								
Mood and anxiety symptoms	Ibogaine	Davis 2020 [42]	High	Indirect	Unknown	Unknown	Unknown	Insufficient It is unclear whether ibogaine reduces mood and anxiety symptoms in US special operations forces based on a single study.
Social anxiety symptoms	Ayahuasca	Dos Santos 2021 [16]	Some concerns	Indirect	Unknown	Unknown	Unknown	Insufficient It is unclear whether ayahuasca improves social anxiety symptoms based on a single pre-post study.
OCD Symptoms	Psilocybin	Moreno 2006 [26]	High	Direct	Unknown	Unknown	Unknown	Insufficient It is unclear whether psilocybin impacts OCD symptoms based on a single pre-post study.

Abbreviations. MDMA=3,4-methylenedioxy-methamphetamine; OCD=obsessive compulsive disorder; PTSD=posttraumatic stress disorder; RCT=randomized controlled trial; RoB=risk of bias; US=United States.

Appendix D: Peer Review Disposition

Comment #	Reviewer #	Comment	Author Response
Are the objectives, scope, and methods for this review clearly described?			
1	1	Yes	*None*
2	3	Yes	*None*
3	4	Yes	*None*
4	5	Yes	*None*
5	6	Yes	*None*
6	7	Yes	*None*
7	8	Yes	*None*
Is there any indication of bias in our synthesis of the evidence?			
8	1	No	*None*
9	2	No	*None*
10	3	Yes - Pg22, 5 & Pg32, 21: "but whether effects are primarily due to psilocybin exposure or intensive psychotherapy remains unclear", can you expand on the inclusion of this statement? This doesn't seem to address a key question of this evidence review. This statement perhaps presents a false dichotomy unnecessarily, I suggest more framing or removing.	*Thank you for this comment. We agree that this wording is problematic without additional context and have removed it. In the section pertaining to PTSD, we now discuss in more detail our assessment of what the evidence can and cannot tell us about the relative contribution of the intervention components.*
11	4	No	*None*
12	5	No	*None*
13	6	No	*None*

Comment #	Reviewer #	Comment	Author Response
14	7	No	*None*
15	8	No	*None*
Are there any published or unpublished studies that we may have overlooked?			
16	1	No	
17	2	No	
18	3	Yes - Anderson BT, et al. (2020). Psilocybin-assisted group therapy for demoralized older long-term AIDS survivor men: an open-label safety and feasibility pilot study. EClinicalMedicine. 100538.	*Thank you for identifying this study, which we did not find in our search. This study does not meet our inclusion criteria as we excluded studies of adults with serious medical illness (eg terminal cancer, end-stage renal disease, and in this case HIV/AIDS) experiencing secondary mental health symptoms.*
19	4	No	*None*
20	5	No	*None*
21	6	No	*None*
22	7	No	*None*
23	8	No	*None*
Additional suggestions or comments can be provided below. If applicable, please indicate the page and line numbers from the draft report.			
24	1	Overall I think this is a good draft. I found it helpful to see the data summarized this way. My overarching concern is the lack of attention to the adequacy of placebo control in this research. It is a known challenge because it is difficult to plausibly mimic the effects of psychedelic drugs, e.g., https://doi.org/10.1038/s41591- 021-01524-1. The limited use of active placebos and reduced adequacy of blinding tempers the evidence of effectiveness. I am commenting on the MDMA-assisted psychotherapy studies for PTSD but the issue is broadly relevant.	*Thank you for your comments regarding the use of different placebos. In the Results section pertaining to MDMA-assisted psychotherapy, we have expanded our discussion on the use of inactive (0mg) and low-dose placebos. We comment that low-dose placebos are meant to produce some of the sensations of having ingested a psychedelic but are thought to have a subtherapeutic effect that is distinct from psychedelic doses used in intervention groups. We revised Figure 3 (forest plot) to separate the studies using inactive and low-dose placebos and now provide pooled estimates for the study sub-groups. We comment that use of inactive placebos with inadequate blinding is a potential source of bias in the Results section and in the Limitations sections.*
25	1	In MDMA-assisted psychotherapy for PTSD, 2 of the 5 published studies used inactive placebo	*As stated above, we now explicitly discuss the use of 2 placebo types – 0mg placebo and low-dose placebo.*

Comment #	Reviewer #	Comment	Author Response
		(Mithoefer et al., 2011; Mitchell et al., 2021), whereas the other studies used lose-dose MDMA: 25 mg (Oehen et al., 2013), 30 mg (Mithoefer et al., 2018), and 40 mg (Ot'alora, 2018). This is a particular problem for interventions like psychedelics, for which there is a lot of hype and public-facing "evidence" on the efficacy of these interventions.	
26	1	Blinding was inadequate in the studies that used inactive placebo. In the Mithoefer et al. (2011) study, 95% of participants correctly guessed their assigned condition, and in the Mitchell study, 84%/96% guessed correctly in the inactive/MDMA groups, respectively. Guessing was less accurate in studies that used active placebo, but still incomplete: 46% overall in Mithoefer (2018); 46% vs. 66% in 25mg vs. 125 mg in Oehen (2013); and 73% vs. 58% in 40mg vs. 100/125 mg in Ot'alora (2018). Even if the effect sizes in the ESP report do not vary as a function of blinding—and for MDMA I think they probably do not due to the Mitchell study having a relatively small effect and the Mithoefer 2018 study having a large effect—this is a key issue that should be addressed in the report to caution readers.	*Thank you for your comments regarding the potential for ineffective blinding. As stated above, we comment that use of inactive placebos with inadequate blinding is a potential source of bias in the Results section and in the Limitations sections. We also recommend use of lowdose placebo in the Future Research section and recommend that studies report data on blinding effectiveness.*
27	1	Another concern is the limited number of total as well as Veteran participants that have been studied in MDMA-assisted psychotherapy for	*Thank you for this comment. We added a sentence to the Key Findings in the Executive Summary to highlight the low inclusion rates of Veterans. In the Discussion and Limitations section, we*

Comment #	Reviewer #	Comment	Author Response
		PTSD. Looking at the 5 published studies, these trials have included a total of only 176 participants in the ITT samples.* All except one study (Mitchell et al., 2021, N = 90) included fewer than 30 participants. Almost 2 out of 3 participants (64%) have been female and almost no participants have experienced combat trauma or were military veterans, with the exception of the study by Mithoefer et al. (2018), which enrolled 22 Veterans. The existing data therefore have limited generalizability to VA patients. The ongoing MAPS study (https://clinicaltrials.gov/ct2/show/NCT04077437) may mitigate this limitation, but it is unlikely that many Veterans will be enrolled given that the protocol does not focus specifically on Veterans. Effect sizes in PTSD medication and psychotherapy studies are smaller in Veteran and active duty samples relative to non-military samples, so the lack of Veteran data is likely to cause the effects on Veterans to be overestimated.	*comment on concerns related to generalizing study findings to VHA populations. We have also recommended inclusion of Veteran populations as a priority in the Future Research section.*
28	1	*I was surprised to see the sample sizes listed for these trials because they are smaller than those reported in the studies. I looked at one trial, Mitchell, in which the sample size is 90 overall and 89 in the primary MMRM analysis, even though data are missing for some participants in later assessments. Figure 3 in the ESP	*Thank you for this comment. In this particular study, the outcome of change from baseline in PTSD symptoms was only reported for participants who completed the intervention, which was 79. We reviewed the report Tables and Figures for consistency and clarified when we were referencing the "analytic N" rather than the study's total N.*

Comment #	Reviewer #	Comment	Author Response
		report lists the N as 79; however, the authors say the N for T4, the final endpoint, was 82. So even if the ESP report is using the T4 N, it is difficult to understand how the total was 79. I assume that the language on the calculation of effect sizes is standard, but in this and future reports, it would be helpful to clarify how the Ns were determined.	
29	1	Pg 1 Line 11-12: It is extremely important to present the effect sizes for the active and placebo controlled studies separately. Also, one of the major issues in this literature is the problem of unblinding in placebo control. IT is a key issue that undermines the interpretation of findings. Having just reviewed this literature carefully, I don't think this interpretation is valid given the serious limitations in the literature.	As stated above, we now explicitly discuss the use of 2 placebo types – 0mg placebo and low-dose placebo. We revised Figure 3 (forest plot) to separate the studies using inactive and low-dose placebos and now provide pooled estimates for the study sub-groups.
30	1	Pg 1 Line 33: What about the challenges of placebo blinding--finding credible active placebo is challenging, especially for long-acting medications like MDMA and psilocybin	*Please see responses to Comments #24-26.*
31	1	Pg 2 Line 18-19: Please see prior comments about the importance of presenting effect sizes for active and placebo control separately. This is analagous to presenting separate effect sizes for in psychotherapy studies for active and waitlist, for example. And placebo control is inadequate, so interpretation needs to be tempered.	*Please see responses to Comments #24-26.*
32	1	Pg 31 Line 48-49: This section [Discussion] needs to address the issue of placebo plinding and the need for adequate control. The possibility of	*Please see responses to Comments #24-26.*

Comment #	Reviewer #	Comment	Author Response
		plcebo effects is especially concerning for threatments like MDMA that have been promoted in the popular press	
33	1	Pg 31 Line 48-49: please see: Caution at psychiatry's psychedelic frontier. Matthew J. Burke1,2,3,4 ☐ and Daniel M. Blumberger1,5 arising from J. M. Mitchell et. al. Nature Medicine https://doi.org/10.1038/s41591- 021-01336-3 (2021)	*Thank you for highlighting this commentary. In the Results section pertaining to MDMA-assisted psychotherapy for PTSD, we discuss the use of different placebo types and specifically highlight that Mitchell 2021 used an inactive placebo.* *As above, we recommend use of low-dose placebo in the Future Research section and recommend that studies report data on blinding effectiveness.*
34	1	Pg 31 Line 57: Two of the 5 published MDMA studies used inactive placebo (Mithoefer et al., 2011; Mitchell et al., 2021), whereas the other studies used lose-dose MDMA: 25 mg (Oehen et al., 2013), 30 mg (Mithoefer et al., 2018), and 40 mg (Ot'alora, 2018). Blinding was inadequate in the studies that used inactive placebo. In the Mithoefer et al. (2011) study, 95% of participants correctly guessed their assigned condition, and in the Mitchell study, 84%/96% guessed correctly in the inactive/MDMA groups, respectively. Guessing was less accurate in studies that used active placebo: 46% overall in Mithoefer (2018); 46% vs. 66% in 25mg vs. 125 mg in Oehen (2013); and 73% vs. 58% in 40mg vs. 100/125 mg in Ot'alora (2018). **The data indicate that active placebo is needed in order to achieve adequate blinding, which is especially important given the novelty of MDMA and the media's portrayal of its efficacy.**	*Please see responses to Comments #24-26.*

Comment #	Reviewer #	Comment	Author Response
35	1	Pg. 32 Line 16-17: Limitations of findings: These trials have included a total of only 176 participants. All except one study (Mitchell et al., 2021, N = 90) included fewer than 30 participants. Almost 2 out of 3 participants (64%) have been female and almost no participants have experienced combat trauma or were military veterans, with the exception of the study by Mithoefer et al. (2018), which enrolled 22 Veterans. The existing data therefore have limited generalizability to VA patients. The ongoing MAPS study (https://clinicaltrials.gov/ct2/show/NCT04077437) may mitigate this limitation, but it is unlikely that many Veterans will be enrolled given that the protocol does not focus specifically on Veterans.	*Please see response to Comment #27.*
36	1	Pg 33 Line 39-40: active placebo-controlled studies	*Please see responses to Comments #24-26.*
37	1	Pg 33 Line 44-45: include veterans	*Please see response to Comment #27.*
38	2	This review is thorough and comprehensive and provides a detailed overview of the full landscape of psychedelic use in MH and SUD conditions, which is much needed and appreciated. However, I am concerned that the summary of findings for MDMA for PTSD is overstating the strength of the evidence. The limitations of studies were not as fully explored in this section as I think is warranted. For example, there was little mention of the problematic nature of the 2 studies that are	*Thank you for these comments. Please see our responses to Comments #24-27 above, which address similar concerns raised by Reviewer 1. We reassessed our Strength of Evidence (SOE) rating for MDMAassisted psychotherapy for PTSD (now rated as low SOE) accounting for the limitations that you and other reviewers highlighted.*

Comment #	Reviewer #	Comment	Author Response
		placebo controlled, especially given in those studies the participants had very high rates of identifying whether they received treatment or placebo (hence very high risk of being unblinded). Lumping these studies together with the active comparator studies is problematic. Also, the total N across all MDMA studies is only 176, with all but the 2021 Mitchell study having N<30. Also - there is little note of the study population of greatest interest to VA - Veterans. Most of these psychedelic studies are lacking in veteran participants, especially combat veterans (of particularly important note for PTSD studies). This is something that should be added to the discussion as well as an area needed to expand upon findings with future research.	
39	3	Pg2, Ln58: long-term, cite long-term MDMA studies clearly	*We have removed this sentence from the Executive Summary to improve clarity. In our discussion of evidence gaps and areas for future research, we include the durability of treatment effects as a gap.*
40	3	Pg6, 41: "expectations" should maybe be changed to "intentions"? (a tenet of this intervention is "intention without expectation", i.e., expectation/expectancy is a component of 'set' that is mitigated)	*Change made.*
41	3	P6,58: comma after "feasibility"	*Change made.*
42	3	Pg11, 29: Mitchell used CAPS-5, which has a different score range	*We have corrected the text regarding CAPS-5 scoring.*

Comment #	Reviewer #	Comment	Author Response
43	3	Pg13, 53: consider making it clear that participants were able to continue psychotherapy with outside provider(s) during study participation	*Thank you for this comment. In the Results section, we now provide more detail (when reported by individual studies) on how many study participants continued or restarted other treatments during the study period or follow-up period.*
44	3	Pg24, 51: "3-4 integration sessions"; the protocol from Mitchell (2021) included 9 integration sessions total and many Phase 2 MDMA studies included 6-9 integration sessions	*We had originally counted only the sessions that were not aligned with the experimental sessions. We have revised the wording to reflect the total number of sessions.*
45	3	Pg32, 27: edit "estimate draw conclusions"	*Removed "estimate"*
46	4	Thank you for the opportunity to review this ESP. I found the summary to be thorough in highlighting the limitations of current psychedelic research (which includes small size of trials, inconsistency in intervention and co-intervention, risk of bias, limitations in blinding, and lack of data on long-term durability). The recommendations for future research are prudent, as preliminary data is positive. The clinical implication of discontinuing current treatment is certainly relevant as more people seek these compounds worldwide and standard treatments are lacking.	*Thank you for your comments*
47	5	The authors conducted a systematic review of studies examining the effects of psychedelic medications for mental health and substance use disorders. They included 38 studies. They found moderate strength evidence indicating that MDMA likely improves PTSD symptoms. The strength of evidence for the remaining effects were deemed either low or insufficient.	*None*

Comment #	Reviewer #	Comment	Author Response
48	5	This is a very well written and comprehensive review of the literature. In my view, the authors provided a balanced portrayal and contextualized their findings as applied to the veteran population nicely. I have a few suggestions they might consider addressing.	*Thank you for your comments. Suggestions are addressed below.*
49	5	I wonder if it would be helpful to spend a bit more time discussing the content of the psychotherapy component of the psychedelic-assisted psychotherapies. A brief description of this treatment component is included in Table 2 but was discussed only briefly in the text. A better understanding of what this psychotherapy component entails may be helpful for stakeholders, particularly given issues related to accessibility and scalability which were highlighted. For example, how equipped might VA mental health providers / systems be to deliver the interventions that are being tested in these trials?	*We agree and have expanded our discussion of the psychotherapy component of the interventions for PTSD and depression in particular.*
50	5	I may have missed this, but I was curious what sample size cutoff was used to evaluate whether a trial was small or not for the purposes of grading the strength of evidence. In particular, I was curious why the Carhart- Harris et al. (2021) psilocybin for depression trial (n = 59) provided insufficient evidence. In comparison, the authors graded evidence from the Davis et al. (2020) trial (n = 27) when combined with 4 pre-post studies	*Thank you for this comment. We reassessed our Strength of Evidence (SOE) ratings for the outcomes related to depression to be consistent with the algorithm we presented in the Methods section ("low strength evidence consisted of a single trial or multiple small trials and/or multiple observational studies, with unclear to high risk of bias, consistent findings, and clinically relevant outcomes"). In this case, we rated the SOE as low for the outcomes informed by the Carhart-Harris 2021 trial and the Davis 2020 trial.*

Comment #	Reviewer #	Comment	Author Response
		as providing low strength of evidence (i.e., not insufficient).	
51	5	I realize this may not be typically done for VA ESP reviews, but I wondered whether it would be helpful to calculate standardized effect sizes for those studies that reported mean differences (e.g., MDMA for PTSD, Carhart-Harris et al., 2020). From my perspectives, effect sizes provide another helpful metric of potential magnitude of effects beyond the grading of the strength of evidence.	*Thank you for this comment. Given this and other reviewers' feedback, we have calculated SMDs for CAPS outcomes of MDMA for PTSD studies.*
52	5	I wondered about the authors' choice to combine MDMA trials that included placebo and active controls. In general, I think it is much preferred to avoid combining across control condition types. At the very least, the authors might discuss why this is appropriate (e.g., active control MDMA dose was too low to be considered therapeutic and/or unlikely to produce a perceptible effect). Might it be possible to examine whether control condition type moderated treatment effects?	*Thank you for these comments. Please see our responses to Comments #24-25 above, which address similar concerns raised by Reviewer 1. We revised Figure 3 (forest plot) to separate the studies using 0mg and low-dose placebos and now provide pooled estimates for the study sub-groups.*
53	5	Two potential typos to correct: p. 2, line 60 ("PTSDassisted psychotherapy -> "psychedelic-assisted psychotherapy"), p. 11, line 35 ("PI" -> "CI").	*"PTSD-assisted" has been changed to "psychedelicassisted". "PI" is correct as it is referring to the prediction interval, not the confidence interval.*
54	6	None	None
55	7	This is a concisely written report summarizing the evidence to date on the use of psychedelic pharmacotherapy for the treatment of mental health and substance use disorder. The overall	*Thank you for your comments. Suggestions are addressed below*

Comment #	Reviewer #	Comment	Author Response
		report was informative, accurate and portrayed a non-biased review of classic and non-classic psychedelics, with their evolution, history, structure, and proposed mechanism of action. A comprehensive review of the evidence to date on efficacy, risks and benefits was well summarized. As stated in the review, the evidence on psychedelics for the treatment of mental health and substance use disorders is insufficient or low strength in evidence for most of the psychedelics. The one caveat to this is the evidence for MDMA-assisted therapy for PTSD where research according to this report is moderately strong in favor of the benefits of MDMA for improving PSTD. While the evidence does in fact support a strong signal for the efficacy of MDMA for treating PTSD with associated serious risks being rare, there are several practical, methodological and generalizability concerns with these studies that should be made more explicit - as they potentially mitigate this favorable rating. These concerns are summarized below.	
56	7	The "psychotherapy" component across all the MDMAassisted therapy studies for PTSD is vague and varies significantly in session number and likely content, except Monson et al., 2020. It is unclear if any of the strides made in PTSD psychotherapy research over the past 2 decades have been integrated into the "therapy" component of the MAPS MDMA-assisted therapy	*Thank you for this comment. We added a paragraph to the Limitations section to discuss the lack of clarify on to what extent, if any, protocols such as those used by MAPS overlap with recommended VA/DoD psychotherapy approaches.*

Comment #	Reviewer #	Comment	Author Response
		protocol for PTSD. Current MAPS protocol for preparation and integration is loosely structured and not in line with current best practice for PTSD therapy. This has significant implications for replication and implementation in settings such as VHA. Future studies examining MDMA-assisted evidence-based psychotherapy for PTSD are needed.	
57	7	A significant methodological concern across the MDMA studies is the placebo comparator. Given the subjective experience of MDMA there is a clear placebo problem with many of these studies and this should temper enthusiasm of findings. Although this is highlighted in the review, this point should be made more explicit.	*Thank you for these comments. Please see our responses to Comments #24-25 above, which address similar concerns raised by Reviewer 1.*
58	7	Most of the published MDMA studies are small. The largest study to date is Mitchell and colleagues (2021) which was only an N=90. This is a relatively small sample size for a phase III trial and raises concern with replication in a larger more diverse samples and settings, as noted. The moderate rating would be more compelling if there were larger more diverse samples.	*Thank you for this comment. We reassessed our Strength of Evidence (SOE) rating for MDMA-assisted psychotherapy for PTSD (now rated as low SOE) accounting for the limitations that you and other reviewers highlighted.*
59	7	All MDMA studies were funded/sponsored by MAPS raising concern re bias.	*In the Result section, we state that all studies were funded or sponsored by MAPS.*
60	7	The lack of current MDMA evidence with military veterans' seeking mental health treatment in a VA setting is perhaps the largest concern. Given the medical and psychiatric complexity of the veteran mental health treatment seeking	*Thank you for these comments. Please see our responses to Comment #27 above, which address similar concerns raised by Reviewer 1.*

Comment #	Reviewer #	Comment	Author Response
		population, this is a significant gap. This current evidence cannot be generalized to this important population.	
61	7	Given these important concerns I believe a strong cautionary statement should be included regarding the moderate favorable evidence for MDMA-assisted therapy for PTSD.	*Thank you for this comment. As stated above, we reassessed our Strength of Evidence (SOE) rating for MDMA-assisted psychotherapy for PTSD (now rated as low SOE) accounting for the limitations that you and other reviewers highlighted. We also provide more context regarding generalizability and emphasize that findings are preliminary.*
62	8	Minor edit needed on page 2 - I believe that "PTSDassisted psychotherapy" should be changed to "MDMAassisted psychotherapy for PTSD"	*Change made.*

Appendix E: Research in Progress

Status	Study Title	Study Design	Information Resources
Clinical Trials			
Substance Use Disorder			
Not yet recruiting	Safety and Feasibility of Psilocybin in Methamphetamine Use Disorder in a Community- Based Sample	Pre-post study	ClinicalTrials.gov Identifier: NCT05322954
Not yet recruiting	A Randomized, Double-Blind Study of Psilocybin for Opioid Use Disorder in Patients on Methadone Maintenance with Ongoing Opioid Use	Crossover RCT	ClinicalTrials.gov Identifier: NCT05242029
Not yet recruiting	Psilocybin-Enhanced Psychotherapy for Methamphetamine Use Disorder	RCT	ClinicalTrials.gov Identifier: NCT04982796
Not yet recruiting	Psilocybin for Treatment of Alcohol Use Disorder: a Feasibility Study	Pre-post study	ClinicalTrials.gov Identifier: NCT04718792
Active, not recruiting	Pilot Trial of Visual Healing®, a Nature-themed Virtual Immersive Experience, to Optimize Set and Setting in Psilocybin-assisted Therapy for Alcohol Use Disorder	RCT	ClinicalTrials.gov Identifier: NCT04410913
Recruiting	Phase I Study of the Safety and Adjunctive Effects of Psilocybin in Adults with Opioid Use Disorder Maintained on Buprenorphine/ Naloxone	Pre-post study	ClinicalTrials.gov Identifier: NCT04161066
Unknown	Open-Label Proof of Concept Feasibility Study to Explore the Safety, Tolerability and Potential Role of MDMA-Assisted Psychotherapy for the Treatment of Detoxified Patients with Alcohol Use Disorder	Pre-post study	ClinicalTrials.gov Identifier: NCT04158778
Recruiting	Phase II, Randomized, Double Blind, Placebo Controlled, Parallel Group, Single Center Study of Psilocybin Efficacy and Mechanism in Alcohol Use Disorder	RCT	ClinicalTrials.gov Identifier: NCT04141501
Recruiting	Preliminary Efficacy and Safety of Ibogaine in the Treatment of Methadone	RCT	ClinicalTrials.gov Identifier: NCT04003948
Not yet recruiting	Tolerability and Efficacy of Ibogaine in the Treatment of Alcoholism: The First Randomized, Double-blind, Placebo-controlled, Escalating-dose, Phase 2 Trial	RCT	ClinicalTrials.gov Identifier: NCT03380728
Recruiting	Psilocybin-facilitated Treatment for Cocaine Use: A Pilot Study	RCT	ClinicalTrials.gov Identifier: NCT02037126
Recruiting	Psilocybin-facilitated Smoking Cessation Treatment: A Pilot Study	RCT	ClinicalTrials.gov Identifier: NCT01943994

Status	Study Title	Study Design	Information Resources
Unknown	Effects and Therapeutic Potential of Psilocybin in Alcohol Dependence	Pre-post study	ClinicalTrials.gov Identifier: NCT01534494
Recruiting	Ibogaine to Determine Maximum Tolerated Dose (MTD) or Treat-to-Target Dose (TTD) for the Evaluation of Efficacy and Safety	RCT	ClinicalTrials.gov Identifier: NCT05029401
Anxiety Disorders			
Not yet recruiting	Effects of Repeated Dosing of Psilocybin on Obsessive-Compulsive Disorder: A Randomized, Waitlist-Controlled Study	RCT	ClinicalTrials.gov Identifier: NCT05370911
Recruiting	Social Anxiety MDMA-Assisted Therapy Investigation (SAMATI): A Randomized, Delayed Treatment Control Phase 2 Study of the Safety and Effectiveness of Manualized MDMA-Assisted Therapy for the Treatment of Social Anxiety Disorder	RCT	ClinicalTrials.gov Identifier: NCT05138068
Not yet recruiting	Open Label, Phase 1 Study for Evaluating the Feasibility, Safety and Efficacy of Psychotherapy Assisted Psilocybin for Treatment of Severe OCD	Pre-post study	ClinicalTrials.gov Identifier: NCT04882839
Recruiting	Psilocybin Treatment in Obsessive-Compulsive Disorder: a Preliminary Efficacy Study and Exploratory Investigation of Neural Correlates.	RCT	ClinicalTrials.gov Identifier: NCT03356483
Completed	LSD Treatment in Persons Suffering from Anxiety Symptoms in Severe Somatic Diseases or in Psychiatric Anxiety Disorders: a Randomized, Double-blind, Placebo-controlled Phase II Study	Crossover RCT	ClinicalTrials.gov Identifier: NCT03153579
Mood Disorders			
Not yet recruiting	An Open Label Study of Single-Dose Psilocybin for Major Depressive Disorder with Co-occurring Borderline Personality Disorder	Pre-post study	ClinicalTrials.gov Identifier: NCT05399498
Not yet recruiting	A Phase I/IIa, Randomized, Double Blind, Placebo-Controlled Study to Assess Safety, Tolerability, Pharmacokinetics and Pharmacodynamics of Multiple Ascending Oral Doses of CYB003 in Participants with Major Depressive Disorder	RCT	ClinicalTrials.gov Identifier: NCT05385783
Recruiting	Psilocybin Versus Ketamine - Fast Acting Antidepressant Strategies in Treatment-resistant Depression	RCT	ClinicalTrials.gov Identifier: NCT05383313
Not yet recruiting	The Effects of Psilocybin on Self-Focus and Self-Related Processing in Treatment Resistant MDD	Pre-post study	ClinicalTrials.gov Identifier: NCT05381974
Not yet recruiting	Microdosing Psychedelics to Improve Mood	Crossover RCT	ClinicalTrials.gov Identifier: NCT05259943
Not yet recruiting	Psilocybin-assisted Cognitive Behavioral Therapy for Depression	Pre-post study	ClinicalTrials.gov Identifier: NCT05227612

Appendix E. (Continued)

Recruiting	An Open-Label Pilot Study Examining the Feasibility, Safety, and Effectiveness of Psilocybin Therapy for Depression in Bipolar II Disorder	Pre-post study	ClinicalTrials.gov Identifier: NCT05065294
Active, not recruiting	The Efficacy and Tolerability of Psilocybin in Participants With Treatment-Resistant Depression: a Phase 2, Randomized Feasibility Study	RCT	ClinicalTrials.gov Identifier: NCT05029466
Not yet recruiting	Randomized Double Blind Placebo Controlled Assessing the Efficacy of Micro-dosed Psilocybin in Reducing Anxiety and or Depression Levels in Adults	RCT	ClinicalTrials.gov Identifier: NCT04989972
Completed	The Safety and Efficacy Of Psilocybin as an Adjunctive Therapy in Participants With Treatment Resistant Depression	Pre-post study	ClinicalTrials.gov Identifier: NCT04739865
Active, not recruiting	Fixed Order, Open-Label, Dose-Escalation Study of DMT in Humans	Non-randomized crossover trial	ClinicalTrials.gov Identifier: NCT04711915
Completed	A Phase 1/2 Study of GH001 in Patients With Treatment-Resistant Depression	Non-randomized sequential trial	ClinicalTrials.gov Identifier: NCT04698603
Recruiting	A Double-blind, Randomised, Placebo-controlled Study of Intravenous Doses of SPL026 (DMT Fumarate), a Serotonergic Psychedelic, in Healthy Subjects (Part A) and Patients With Major Depressive Disorder (Part B)	RCT	ClinicalTrials.gov Identifier: NCT04673383
Recruiting	A Phase II Randomized, Double-blind, Active Placebo-controlled Parallel Group Trial to Examine the Efficacy and Safety of Psilocybin in Treatment-resistant Major Depression	RCT	ClinicalTrials.gov Identifier: NCT04670081
Recruiting	The Effect of Psilocybin on MDD Symptom Severity and Synaptic Density - A Single Dose Randomized, Double Blind, Placebo- Controlled Phase 2 Positron Emission Tomography Study	RCT	ClinicalTrials.gov Identifier: NCT04630964
Recruiting	Psilocybin Treatment of Major Depressive Disorder With Co-occurring Alcohol Use Disorder	RCT	ClinicalTrials.gov Identifier: NCT04620759
Recruiting	Multicentre Study To Assess Safety And Efficacy Of Psilocybin In Patients With Treatment-Resistant Depression Following Completion Of COMP 001 And COMP 003 Trials (P-TRD LTFU)	Prospective cohort	ClinicalTrials.gov Identifier: NCT04519957

Status	Study Title	Study Design	Information Resources
Recruiting	An Open Label Study of the Safety and Efficacy of Psilocybin in Participants With Treatment-Resistant Depression (P-TRD)	Pre-post study	ClinicalTrials.gov Identifier: NCT04433858
Recruiting	The Safety and Efficacy of Psilocybin in Participants With Type 2 Bipolar Disorder (BP-II) Depression	Pre-post study	ClinicalTrials.gov Identifier: NCT04433845
Enrolling by invitation	A Two-Year Observational Follow-up Study of Subjects With Major Depressive Disorder Following a Randomized, Double-Blind Single-Dose of Psilocybin or Niacin-Control	Cohort (long-term follow-up)	ClinicalTrials.gov Identifier: NCT04353921
Active, not recruiting	LSD Therapy for Persons Suffering From Major Depression: A Randomised, Double-blind, Active-placebo Controlled Phase II Study	RCT	ClinicalTrials.gov Identifier: NCT03866252
Completed	The Safety and Efficacy of Psilocybin in Participants With Treatment Resistant Depression	RCT	ClinicalTrials.gov Identifier: NCT03775200
Completed	Phase II, Randomized, Double Blind, Placebo Controlled, Parallel Group, Single Center Study of Psilocybin Efficacy in Major Depression	RCT	ClinicalTrials.gov Identifier: NCT03715127
Active, not recruiting	Psilocybin - Induced Neuroplasticity in the Treatment of Major Depressive Disorder	Crossover RCT	ClinicalTrials.gov Identifier: NCT03554174
Unknown	Psilocybin and Depression - Assessing the Long-term Effects of a Single Administration of Psilocybin on the Psychiatric Symptoms and Brain Activity of Patients With Severe Depression	RCT	ClinicalTrials.gov Identifier: NCT03380442
PTSD			
Recruiting	The Safety and Tolerability of COMP360 in Participants With Post-traumatic Stress Disorder	Pre-post study	ClinicalTrials.gov Identifier: NCT05312151
Recruiting	Sustaining Remission From Posttraumatic Stress Disorder (PTSD) Using Tuned Vibroacoustic Stimulation (TVS) Following MDMA-Assisted Psychotherapy	Pre-post study	ClinicalTrials.gov Identifier: NCT05274230
Not yet recruiting	Investigating the Therapeutic Effects of Psilocybin in Treatment-Resistant Post-Traumatic	Pre-post study	ClinicalTrials.gov Identifier: NCT05243329
Not yet recruiting	MDMA-Assisted Therapy for Postpartum People With Opioid Use Disorder and Coexisting Post Traumatic Stress Disorder	Pre-post study	ClinicalTrials.gov Identifier: NCT05219175
Not yet recruiting	An Open-Label Feasibility and Safety Study of MDMA-Assisted Group Therapy for the Treatment of Posttraumatic Stress Disorder in Veterans	Pre-post study	ClinicalTrials.gov Identifier: NCT05173831
Suspended	A Phase 2 Open-Label Treatment Development Study of MDMA-Assisted Cognitive Processing Therapy (CPT) for Posttraumatic Stress Disorder (PTSD)	Pre-post study	ClinicalTrials.gov Identifier: NCT05067244

Appendix E. (Continued)

Enrolling by Invitation *Withdrawn*	Long-Term Safety and Persistence of Effectiveness of Manualized MDMA-Assisted Therapy for the Treatment of Posttraumatic Stress Disorder A Phase 2, Open Label Study of the Safety and Effectiveness of MDMA-assisted Therapy for Participants With Posttraumatic Stress Disorder	Retrospective Cohort Pre-post study	ClinicalTrials.gov Identifier: NCT05066282 ClinicalTrials.gov Identifier: NCT04968938
Recruiting	A Phase 2, Open-Label, Randomized Comparative Effectiveness Study for MDMA-Assisted Psychotherapy in U.S. Veterans With Chronic PTSD	RCT	ClinicalTrials.gov Identifier: NCT04784143
Enrolling by invitation	A Multi-Site Open-Label Safety Extension Study of Manualized MDMA-Assisted Psychotherapy for the Treatment of Participants With Posttraumatic Stress Disorder	Pre-post study	ClinicalTrials.gov Identifier: NCT04714359
Available	A Multi-site Expanded Access Program for MDMA-assisted Psychotherapy for Patients With Treatment-resistant PTSD	Expanded access protocol	ClinicalTrials.gov Identifier: NCT04438512
Recruiting	Open-label Phase 2 Study of MDMA-Assisted Psychotherapy in Veterans With Combat-Related, Refractory PTSD	Pre-post study	ClinicalTrials.gov Identifier: NCT04264026
Active, not recruiting	A Randomized, Double-Blind, Placebo-Controlled, Multi-Site Phase 3 Study of the Efficacy and Safety of Manualized MDMA-Assisted Psychotherapy for the Treatment of Posttraumatic Stress Disorder of Moderate or Greater Severity	RCT	ClinicalTrials.gov Identifier: NCT04077437
Recruiting	An Open-Label, Phase 2, Multicenter Feasibility Study of Manualized MDMA-Assisted Psychotherapy With an Optional fMRI Sub-Study Assessing Changes in Brain Activity in Subjects With Posttraumatic Stress Disorder	Pre-post study	ClinicalTrials.gov Identifier: NCT04030169
Completed	An Open-Label, Multi-Site Phase 2 Study of the Safety and Effect of Manualized MDMA-Assisted Psychotherapy for the Treatment of Severe Posttraumatic Stress Disorder (Canada)	Pre-post study	ClinicalTrials.gov Identifier: NCT03485287
Completed	An Open-Label, Multi-Site Phase 2 Study of the Safety and Effect of Manualized MDMA-Assisted Therapy for the Treatment of Severe Posttraumatic Stress Disorder	Pre-post study	ClinicalTrials.gov Identifier: NCT03282123
Completed	A Phase 1/2 Open-Label Treatment Development Study of Methylenedioxymethamphetamine (MDMA)-Assisted Cognitive-Behavioral Conjoint Therapy (CBCT) in Dyads in Which 1 Member	Pre-post study	ClinicalTrials.gov Identifier: NCT02876172

Status	Study Title	Study Design	Information Resources
	Has Chronic Posttraumatic Stress Disorder (PTSD)		
Completed	An Open-Label Proof-of-Principle Study Testing the Use of an Additional MDMA-Assisted Therapy Session in People Who Relapsed After Participating in a Phase 2 Clinical Trial of MDMA-Assisted Therapy to Treat Chronic, Treatment-Resistant Posttraumatic Stress Disorder (PTSD)	Pre-post study	ClinicalTrials.gov Identifier: NCT01458327
Terminated	MDMA-assisted Therapy in Twelve People With War and Terrorism-related Posttraumatic Stress Disorder (PTSD)	RCT	ClinicalTrials.gov Identifier: NCT00402298
Eating Disorders Recruiting	A Phase 2a Safety and Feasibility Study Evaluating Psilocybin (TRP-8802) Administration in Concert With Psychotherapy in the Treatment of Binge Eating Disorder	Pre-post study	ClinicalTrials.gov Identifier: NCT05035927
Active, not recruiting	Evaluation of Psilocybin in Anorexia Nervosa: Safety and Efficacy	Pre-post study	ClinicalTrials.gov Identifier: NCT04661514
Active, not recruiting	Safety and Efficacy of Psilocybin for Body Dysmorphic Disorder	Pre-post study	ClinicalTrials.gov Identifier: NCT04656301
Not yet recruiting	An Open-Label, Multi-Site Phase 2 Study of the Safety and Feasibility of MDMA-Assisted Psychotherapy for Eating Disorders	Non-randomized controlled trial	ClinicalTrials.gov Identifier: NCT04454684
Recruiting	Effects of Psilocybin in Anorexia Nervosa	Pre-post study	ClinicalTrials.gov Identifier: NCT04052568
Other			
Recruiting	Safety and Efficacy of Repeated Low Dose MM-120 as Treatment for Attention Deficit Disorder (ADHD) in Adults: a Multi-center, Randomized, Double-blind, Placebo-controlled Phase 2a Proof of Concept Trial	RCT	ClinicalTrials.gov Identifier: NCT05200936
Recruiting	The Safety and Efficacy of Psilocybin in Patients With Treatment-resistant Depression and Chronic Suicidal Ideation	Pre-post study	ClinicalTrials.gov Identifier: NCT05220410

Notes. MM-120 is a form of LSD. SPL026 is also known as DMT Fumarate.

Abbreviations. ADHD=attention-deficit/hyperactivity disorder; BP-II=bipolar disorder II; CPT=cognitive processing therapy; DMT=5-methoxy-N,N-dimethyltryptamine; fMRI=functional magnetic resonance imaging; GH001=5 methoxy N,N dimethyltryptamine; LSD=lysergic acid diethylamide; LTFU=long-term follow up; MDD=major depressive disorder; MDMA=3,4-methylenedioxy-methamphetamine; MTD=maximum tolerated dose; OCD=obsessive compulsive disorder; RCT=randomized controlled trial; SAMATI=social anxiety MDMA-assisted therapy investigation; TRD=treatment resistant depression; TTD=treat-to-target dose; TVS=tuned vibroacoustic stimulation.

References

[1] Bogenschutz M P, Ross S, Bhatt S, et al. Percentage of Heavy Drinking Days Following Psilocybin-Assisted Psychotherapy vs Placebo in the Treatment of Adult Patients With Alcohol Use Disorder: A Randomized Clinical Trial. *JAMA Psychiatry.* 2022.

[2] Carhart-Harris R, Giribaldi B, Watts R, et al. Trial of Psilocybin versus Escitalopram for Depression. *New England Journal of Medicine.* 2021;384(15):1402-1411.

[3] Davis A K, Barrett F S, May D G, et al. Effects of Psilocybin-Assisted Therapy on Major Depressive Disorder: A Randomized Clinical Trial. *JAMA Psychiatry.* 2021;78(5):481- 489.

[4] Gukasyan N, Davis A K, Barrett F S, et al. Efficacy and safety of psilocybin-assisted treatment for major depressive disorder: Prospective 12-month follow-up. *Journal of Psychopharmacology.* 2022;36(2):151-158.

[5] Palhano-Fontes F, Barreto D, Onias H, et al. Rapid antidepressant effects of the psychedelic ayahuasca in treatment-resistant depression: a randomized placebo-controlled trial. *Psychological Medicine.* 2019;49(4):655-663.

[6] Zeifman R J, Palhano-Fontes F, Hallak J, Arcoverde E, Maia-Oliveira JP, Araujo DB. The Impact of Ayahuasca on Suicidality: Results From a Randomized Controlled Trial. *Frontiers in Pharmacology.* 2019;10.

[7] Glue P, Cape G, Tunnicliff D, et al. Ascending Single-Dose, Double-Blind, Placebo-Controlled Safety Study of Noribogaine in Opioid-Dependent Patients. *Clinical Pharmacology in Drug Development.* 2016;5(6):460-468.

[8] Bouso J C, Doblin R, Farre M, Alcazar MA, Gomez-Jarabo G. MDMA-assisted psychotherapy using low doses in a small sample of women with chronic posttraumatic stress disorder. *Journal of Psychoactive Drugs.* 2008;40(3):225-236.

[9] Mitchell J M, Bogenschutz M, Lilienstein A, et al. MDMA-assisted therapy for severe PTSD: a randomized, double-blind, placebo-controlled phase 3 study. *Nature Medicine.* 2021;27(6):1025-1033.

[10] Mithoefer M C, Wagner M T, Mithoefer A T, Jerome L, Doblin R. The safety and efficacy of {+/-}3,4-methylenedioxymethamphetamine-assisted psychotherapy in subjects with chronic, treatment-resistant posttraumatic stress disorder: the first randomized controlled pilot study. *Journal of Psychopharmacology.* 2011;25(4):439-452.

[11] Mithoefer M C, Wagner M T, Mithoefer A T, et al. Durability of improvement in post- traumatic stress disorder symptoms and absence of harmful effects or drug dependency after 3,4-methylenedioxymethamphetamine-assisted psychotherapy: a prospective long- term follow-up study. *Journal of Psychopharmacology.* 2013;27(1):28-39.

[12] Mithoefer M C, Mithoefer A T, Feduccia A A, et al. 3,4-methylenedioxy methamphetamine (MDMA)-assisted psychotherapy for post-traumatic stress disorder in military veterans, firefighters, and police officers: a randomised, double-blind, dose-response, phase 2 clinical trial. *The Lancet Psychiatry.* 2018;5(6):486-497.

[13] Mithoefer M C, Feduccia A A, Jerome L, et al. MDMA-assisted psychotherapy for treatment of PTSD: study design and rationale for phase 3 trials based on pooled analysis of six phase 2 randomized controlled trials. *Psychopharmacology.* 2019;236(9):2735- 2745.

[14] Oehen P, Traber R, Widmer V, Schnyder U. A randomized, controlled pilot study of MDMA (+/- 3,4-Methylenedioxymethamphetamine)-assisted psychotherapy for treatment of resistant, chronic Post-Traumatic Stress Disorder (PTSD). *Journal of Psychopharmacology.* 2013;27(1):40-52.

[15] Ot'alora G M, Grigsby J, Poulter B, et al. 3,4-Methylenedioxymethamphetamine-assisted psychotherapy for treatment of chronic posttraumatic stress disorder: A randomized phase 2 controlled trial. *Journal of Psychopharmacology.* 2018;32(12):1295-1307.

[16] Dos Santos R G, Osorio F L, Rocha J M, et al. Ayahuasca Improves Self-perception of Speech Performance in Subjects With Social Anxiety Disorder: A Pilot, Proof-of- Concept, Randomized, Placebo-Controlled Trial. *Journal of Clinical Psychopharmacology.* 2021;41(5):540-550.

[17] Bogenschutz M P, Forcehimes AA, Pommy JA, Wilcox CE, Barbosa PC, Strassman R J. Psilocybin-assisted treatment for alcohol dependence: a proof-of-concept study. *Journal of Psychopharmacology.* 2015;29(3):289-299.

[18] Sessa B, Aday J S, O'Brien S, et al. Debunking the myth of 'Blue Mondays': No evidence of affect drop after taking clinical MDMA. *Journal of Psychopharmacology.* 2022;36(3):360-367.

[19] Carhart-Harris R L, Bolstridge M, Rucker J, et al. Psilocybin with psychological support for treatment-resistant depression: an open-label feasibility study. *The Lancet Psychiatry.* 2016;3(7):619-627.

[20] Carhart-Harris R L, Bolstridge M, Day CMJ, et al. Psilocybin with psychological support for treatment-resistant depression: six-month follow-up. *Psycho pharmacology.* 2018;235(2):399-408.

[21] Lyons T, Carhart-Harris RL. More realistic forecasting of future life events after psilocybin for treatment-resistant depression. *Frontiers in Psychology.* 2018;9.

[22] Osorio L, Sanches RF, Macedo LR, et al. Antidepressant effects of a single dose of ayahuasca in patients with recurrent depression: a preliminary report. *Revista Brasileira de Psiquiatria.* 2015;37(1):13-20.

[23] Sanches R F, de Lima Osorio F, Dos Santos RG, et al. Antidepressant Effects of a Single Dose of Ayahuasca in Patients With Recurrent Depression: A SPECT Study. *Journal of Clinical Psychopharmacology.* 2016;36(1):77-81.

[24] Zeifman R J, Singhal N, Dos Santos RG, et al. Rapid and sustained decreases in suicidality following a single dose of ayahuasca among individuals with recurrent major depressive disorder: results from an open-label trial. *Psychopharmacology.* 2021;238(2):453-459.

[25] Stroud JB, Freeman TP, Leech R, et al. Psilocybin with psychological support improves emotional face recognition in treatment-resistant depression. *Psychopharmacology.* 2018;235(2):459-466.

[26] Moreno F A, Wiegand CB, Taitano EK, Delgado PL. Safety, tolerability, and efficacy of psilocybin in 9 patients with obsessive-compulsive disorder. *Journal of Clinical Psychiatry.* 2006;67(11):1735-1740.

[27] Brown T K, Alper K. Treatment of opioid use disorder with ibogaine: detoxification and drug use outcomes. *American Journal of Drug & Alcohol Abuse.* 2018;44(1):24-36.

[28] Davis A K, Barsuglia J P, Windham-Herman A-M, Lynch M, Polanco M. Subjective effectiveness of ibogaine treatment for problematic opioid consumption: Short- and long- term outcomes and current psychological functioning. *Journal of Psychedelic Studies.* 2017;1(2):65-73.

[29] Knuijver T, Schellekens A, Belgers M, et al. Safety of ibogaine administration in detoxification of opioid-dependent individuals: a descriptive open-label observational study. *Addiction.* 2022;117(1):118-128.

[30] Malcolm B J, Polanco M, Barsuglia JP. Changes in Withdrawal and Craving Scores in Participants Undergoing Opioid Detoxification Utilizing Ibogaine. *Journal of Psychoactive Drugs.* 2018;50(3):256-265.

[31] Noller G E, Frampton C M, Yazar-Klosinski B. Ibogaine treatment outcomes for opioid dependence from a twelve-month follow-up observational study. *American Journal of Drug & Alcohol Abuse.* 2018;44(1):37-46.

[32] Jardim A V, Jardim D V, Chaves B R, et al. 3,4-methylenedioxymethamphetamine (MDMA)-assisted psychotherapy for victims of sexual abuse with severe post-traumatic stress disorder: an open label pilot study in Brazil. *Revista Brasileira de Psiquiatria.* 2021;43(2):181-185.

[33] Monson C M, Wagner A C, Mithoefer A T, et al. MDMA-facilitated cognitive-behavioural conjoint therapy for posttraumatic stress disorder: An uncontrolled trial. *European Journal of Psychotraumatology.* 2020;11(1):1840123.

[34] Wang J B, Lin J, Bedrosian L, et al. Scaling Up: Multisite Open-Label Clinical Trials of MDMA-Assisted Therapy for Severe Posttraumatic Stress Disorder. *Journal of Humanistic Psychology.* 2021;0(0):00221678211023663.

[35] Thomas G, Lucas P, Capler NR, Tupper KW, Martin G. Ayahuasca-assisted therapy for addiction: results from a preliminary observational study in Canada. *Current Drug Abuse Reviews.* 2013;6(1):30-42.

[36] Mash D C, Kovera C A, Pablo J, et al. Ibogaine: complex pharmacokinetics, concerns for safety, and preliminary efficacy measures. *Annals of the New York Academy of Sciences.* 2000;914:394-401.

[37] Mash D C, Kovera C A, Pablo J, et al. Ibogaine in the treatment of heroin withdrawal. *The Alkaloids Chemistry & Biology.* 2001;56:155-171.

[38] Mash D C, Duque L, Page B, Allen-Ferdinand K. Ibogaine Detoxification Transitions Opioid and Cocaine Abusers Between Dependence and Abstinence: Clinical Observations and Treatment Outcomes. *Front Pharmacol.* 2018;9:529.

[39] Schenberg E E, de Castro Comis M A, Chaves B R, da Silveira D X. Treating drug dependence with the aid of ibogaine: a retrospective study. *Journal of Psychopharmacology.* 2014;28(11):993-1000.

[40] Johnson M W, Garcia-Romeu A, Cosimano MP, Griffiths RR. Pilot study of the 5-HT2AR agonist psilocybin in the treatment of tobacco addiction. *Journal of Psychopharmacology.* 2014;28(11):983-992.

[41] Johnson M W, Garcia-Romeu A, Griffiths RR. Long-term follow-up of psilocybin-facilitated smoking cessation. *The American Journal of Drug and Alcohol Abuse.* 2017;43(1):55-60.

[42] Davis A K, Averill L A, Sepeda ND, Barsuglia JP, Amoroso T. Psychedelic treatment for trauma-related psychological and cognitive impairment among US Special Operations Forces Veterans. *Chronic Stress.* 2020;4:2470547020939564.

[43] Sessa B, Higbed L, O'Brien S, et al. First study of safety and tolerability of 3,4-methylenedioxymethamphetamine-assisted psychotherapy in patients with alcohol use disorder. *Journal of Psychopharmacology.* 2021;35(4):375-383.

[44] Kotler M. A Randomized, Double-Blind, Active Placebo-Controlled Phase 2 Pilot Study of MDMA-assisted Psychotherapy in People With Chronic, Treatment-Resistant Posttraumatic Stress Disorder (PTSD). NCT01689740. Multidisplinary Association for Psychedelic Studies. https://clinicaltrials.gov/ct2/show/record/NCT01689740?term=NCT01689740&draw=2& rank=1. Published 2017. Accessed August 22, 2022.

[45] Pacey I. A Randomized, Double-Blind, Controlled Phase 2 Pilot Study of Manualized 3,4-methylenedioxymethamphetamine (MDMA)-Assisted Psychotherapy in 12 Subjects With Treatment-Resistant Posttraumatic Stress Disorder (PTSD) - Canada. NCT01958593. Multidisciplinary Association for Psychedelic Studies. https://clinicaltrials.gov/ct2/show/record/NCT01958593?term=NCT01958593&draw=2& rank=1. Published 2017. Accessed August 22, 2022.

Chapter 5

Protecting Public Health and Safety with Psychedelics Advancing Therapies (PATH)*

Jack Bergman

Tuesday, November 5, 2024

Mr. BERGMAN. Mr. Speaker, I rise today to include in the RECORD an updated open letter from myself and Congressman CORREA. the founders of the PATH Caucus, to ensure stakeholders have a voice in crafting the rules and regulations surrounding psychedelic assisted treatments. This is an updated version of the letter from my previous submission to the RECORD on August 9, 2024. It serves to extend our requested deadline for responses to February 28, 2025.

DEAR COMMENTER: In 2022, a new Congressional caucus was created to raise awareness among federal lawmakers about the therapeutic potential of psychedelic and entactogenic drugs to treat several mental health conditions that were refractory to contemporary evidence-based therapies. The Congressional Psychedelics Advancing Therapies (PATH) Caucus aimed to accelerate and support clinical research in the use of these novel substances, specifically psilocybin and 3,4- methylenedioxymethamphetamine (MDMA).

To better inform Congressional members, the bipartisan PATH Caucus is seeking input on how to implement programs and policies that address the range of complex issues with potential novel therapies that may use a psychedelic or entactogenic drug in medically supervised and interpersonally supportive settings.

---

* This is an edited, reformatted and augmented version of CREC, E1112, Congressional Record-Extensions of Remarks, dated November, 5, 2024.

In: The Psychedelic Landscape
Editor: James P. Macintosh
ISBN: 979-8-89530-991-9

To gain a more complete understanding of the issues associated with use of these substances, the PATH Caucus believes that taking an inclusive, intentional, and reasoned approach to gathering input from the public may engender valuable insights that can more accurately and comprehensively characterize how different modalities incorporate the use of these substances while also ensuring responsible, accountable, safe, and ethical use. We seek information from the general public, those who have received psychedelic-assisted therapies as an intervention, interested stakeholders, and those individuals and entities working within the bipsycho-social-spiritual behavioral health ecosystem (e.g., palliative care, addiction services), which stresses a holistic system of care comprised of clinical providers, counseling, and peer support (Courtney et al., 2023; D'Souza, 2007; Urutia et al., 2023).

It will be essential to receive input from people and organizations with specialized experience in implementing therapies where psychedelic or entactogenic drug substances are administered, such as in clinical research protocols (e.g., depression, palliative care, substance use disorders, post-traumatic stress disorder (PTSD)), or experience in training others for such therapies. As a part of the PATH Caucus information gathering effort, we acknowledge the significant anthropological role of certain psychedelic substances such as ayahuasca, peyote, and Psilocybe mushrooms. Some indigenous peoples of the Americas have extensive traditions dating back hundreds to thousands of years, where they incorporated these substances into spiritual ceremonial or ritual healing practices. The PATH Caucus believes that respectful, inclusive, cultural knowledge sharing from these communities may provide substantial insights, further informing our overall understanding, and we welcome their input.

In medications derived from psychedelic or entactogenic drug substances are ultimately approved for therapeutic indications by the FDA, it is important for States to understand the risk mitigations frameworks FDA has established and develop ways to make sure they are supported. Aspects of real-world risk reduction and mitigation frameworks may include, but are not limited to, providing comprehensive transparent public education, implementing substance misuse prevention programs, minimizing the potential for adverse reactions, and developing implementable risk mitigation, safety, and ethical monitoring strategies. Moreover, it will be vital to consider how Congress can best support states in developing and adopting scalable infrastructures and sustainable service delivery systems that ensure proper accountability and monitoring, as well as facilitate access and equity in utilization, with a particular focus on communities that may be at risk for experiencing inequities in care resulting in disparate health outcomes (e.g., veterans, the uninsured, those who are experiencing homelessness, people with lower incomes, and individuals living with mental illness and/or co-occurring substance use disorders; Ortiz et al., 2022). In addition, when federal agencies such as the Department of Veterans Affairs make these products available, we need to be sure there is sufficient infrastructure to ensure patient safety. All of these components, when collectively addressed, may contribute to more responsible, accountable, safe, and ethical use of psychedelic and entactogenic derived substances in medically supervised and interpersonally supportive settings.

The PATH Caucus seeks input that can inform Congress so any potential future appropriations will support states collectively addressing the relevant issues and support necessary federal initiatives such as research, implementation and FDA regulation. Congress believes that by listening and learning from the broader ecosystem, staying abreast of potential innovative evidence-based therapies that may treat individuals with behavioral health disorders refractory to current treatment modalities, and simultaneously undertaking proactive measures for developing real-world risk reduction and mitigation frameworks, will help protect public health and safety.

Current State of Psychedelic and Entactogenic Clinical Research

Clinical data continue to be collected regarding the safety profiles and potential benefits from therapies that use psychedelic or entactogenic drug substances across a variety of diagnoses such as major depressive disorder (MDD), treatment resistant depression (TRD), demoralization, PTSD, generalized anxiety disorder (GAD) and substance use disorders, in conjunction with appropriate supervision and support from qualified mental health professionals (Belouin et al., 2022; Carhart-Harris et al., 2021; Davis et al., 2021; Griffiths et al., 2016; Jerome et al., 2020; Mitchell et al., 2021; Ross et al., 2016; Siegel et al., 2021; Xi et al., 2023). Additionally, FDA has granted requests for Breakthrough Therapy designation to specific development programs involving MDMA for the treatment of PTSD (Multidisciplinary Association of Psychedelic Studies, 2017), psilocybin for TRD (COMPASS Pathways, 2018; Goodwin, G.M. et al., 2022) and MDD (Khan, 2019; Raison et al., 2023), CYB003 for MDD (Cybin, 2024), and MM120 (lysergide dtartrate) for GAD (MindMed, 2024). The Breakthrough Therapy designation process facilitates and expedites the development and review of certain new drugs that have the potential to address unmet medical needs. This designation is available for drugs that are intended to treat a serious or life-threatening disease or condition and where preliminary clinical evidence indicates that the drug may demonstrate substantial improvement over available treatments on clinically significant endpoint(s) (U.S. Food and Drug Administration, 2022). It should be noted that a Breakthrough Therapy designation does not mean that the FDA has made a safety or efficacy determination for a drug, and the Breakthrough Therapy designation is not a substitute for marketing approval. Currently, FDA has not approved any drug containing MDMA, psilocybin, psilocybin analogs, or LSD or other psychedelics or entactogens as being safe and effective for any therapeutic indication(s).

Acknowledging the Need to Address Complex Issues

Use of these substances is not without risk. A psychedelic (e.g, psilocybin) or entactogenic (e.g., MDMA) drug can temporarily alter a person's mood, thoughts, and perceptions, and lead to heightened suggestibility, anxiety/panic, and/or paranoia, among other outcomes. For psychedelics, a participant can experience vast changes in their perceptions of reality, including time and space. Moreover, an individual can become extremely sensitive to internal and external stimuli and altered in their cognitive functioning and visuoperceptual skills. Knowing these realities, any therapy that uses psilocybin or MDMA, for example, should involve thorough participant screening, education, and preparation, supportive settings, and close supervision by credentialed and qualified medical and mental health professionals to maximize safety and promote potential therapeutic outcomes (Davis et al., 2021; Johnson et al., 2008; Nichols, 2016; Phelps, 2017).

Furthermore, acknowledging that it has been suggested that some therapies could potentially lead to blurring of ethical boundaries between participants and provider(s) in some cases, as well as the potential for enhanced suggestibility, there might be increased risk for serious intimate ethical boundary violations by session facilitators/ monitors, including emotional, physical, and sexual abuse (Anderson, B., Danforth, A., Grob, C., 2020; Goldhill, 2020; Pilecki et al., 2021), though psychedelics and entactogens are by no means unique in this regard. Some populations might have a higher risk for adverse reactions from psychedelic or entactogenic drugs, such as people with a known history of serious cardiac conditions or serious mental conditions such as borderline personality disorder or bipolar disorder (Bender and Hellerstein, 2022; Bradberry et al., 2022; Leonard et al., 2018; Lim et al., 2012; Malcolm and Thomas, 2021).

Given the broad array of potential challenges with therapies that may use psychedelics (e.g., psilocybin) or entactogens (e.g., MDMA), compounded by an absence of consensus about how best to address these challenges, a proactive collaborative approach may be most effective, where a partnership of subject matter expertise can consolidate efforts and collectively work to address relevant issues (Belouin et al., 2022; Belouin and Henningfield, 2018; Xi et al., 2023). Best practices good, credentialling, et.

Information Being Requested

This letter seeks broad input to address five major landscape domains that may contribute to developing real-world risk reduction and mitigation frameworks that protect public health and safety when considering implementing potential therapies that use a psychedelic or entactogenic drug substance in medically supervised and interpersonally supportive settings. These include: (1) service delivery, (2) promoting participant protections, (3) engagement of communities, (4) safeguarding equitable access, and (5) best practices for data standards.

Service Delivery

What is the spectrum of interdisciplinary practitioners who will be held accountable as session facilitators/monitors for the potential use of these substances in medically supervised and interpersonally supportive settings?

Training Considerations

What are the minimal training standards for integrated care delivery?

What curriculum is needed that best addresses variations in psychotherapy (e.g., how best to address a participant's vulnerability and manage psychedelic-related challenging experiences)?

Credentialing Considerations

What are the relevant background education, qualifications, professional experiences, and potential examinations that might be considered for interdisciplinary credentialing?

Which disciplines may represent 'service providers' (e.g., clinical practitioners, counselors, peer support)?

What might be appropriate supervision and practice hour requirements?

What types of guidance documents may be necessary for those who provide close supervision/monitoring of participants using psychedelics or entactogens?

Promoting Participant Protections

Provide input on strategies that may be critical to protecting participants, including:

What strategies will be needed to ensure participant education, screening for medical or mental health conditions that may disqualify from participation, and informed consent prior to an individual participating in a therapy that may use a psychedelic or entactogenic drug substance?

What is needed to assess baseline pre-dose and adverse event monitoring post-dose (e.g., suicidal ideation or behavior, physiological reactions, psychological harm, substance misuse, and drug-drug interactions)?

What information is available or needed on how medically supervised and interpersonally supportive settings might incorporate substance misuse screening and prevention, risk mitigation, safety and ethical monitoring strategies that protect participants from potential ethical boundary violations from providers?

What components need to be developed to support ethical-vigilance reporting systems (e.g., state departments of consumer protection, professional societies, state licensing bodies, and law enforcement)?

What data might be collected that improves existing pharmacovigilance reporting systems?

How will these strategies complement existing patient protection regulations enforced by FDA that reduce risk for clinical trial participants as well as for users of approved and regulated products?

Engagement of Communities

The PATH Caucus invites input to help identify best mechanisms/approaches that achieve engagement with diverse communities, including:

How might some indigenous people's use of psychedelics (e.g., ayahuasca, peyote) as sacraments in spiritual ceremonial or ritual healing practices, improve our understanding to protect public health and safety? How might we ensure engagement with vulnerable populations disproportionately affected by mental health conditions, including people experiencing homelessness, racial/ ethnic minorities, sexual and gender minorities, older adults, people living with disabilities and chronic health conditions, and individuals in the criminal justice system (Ortiz et al., 2022)?

Are there examples of best practices that facilitate provider (e.g., clinical practitioners, counselors, and peer support) engagement with vulnerable populations?

How do we effectively navigate societal stigma associated with psychedelic or entactogenic use?

How do we effectively educate healthcare, local crisis response systems, and law enforcement?

How do we best engage in comprehensive transparent community educational outreach?

Safeguarding Equitable Access

What should be considered critical elements to the development of capabilities across the following domains or activities?

Reimbursements that ensure equitable access to services.

Healthcare economic impact analyses. Types of medically supervised and interpersonally supportive therapy settings. Collaboration on activities that may include input on prescribing, administering, and dispensing.

Manufacturing and distribution standards. Supporting oversight of the available supply of substances.

Diversion Control Monitoring

Information on how potential psychedelic and entactogenic medicinal use might fit within the medication use process and workflow of health care systems.

How should these activities be performed in a manner that complements and supports FDA's regulation of development, manufacturing, distribution, marketing and use of psychedelics?

Best Practices for Data Standards

What types of data standards and repositories (e.g., Coordinated Registry Networks) may be created to collect data that continually informs best practices and vice versa? How might current surveillance systems of regulated and unregulated settings be improved?

For example, Researched Abuse, Diversion and Addiction-Related Surveillance (RA- DARS®), Monitoring the Future, National Survey on Drug Use and Health, and the Drug Abuse Warning Network, collect actionable data on psychedelic and entactogenic use; associated adverse events; prevalence of medical and non-medical use; frequency, dose, and use settings; and participant comorbidities, health concerns, long- term effects, as well as demographic characteristics.

Please email your input and feedback to PATH@mail.house.gov by close of business on February 28, 2025. Your responses to these questions are crucial, as they will directly inform Congress on how best to contribute to protecting public health and safety, acknowledging the complex nature of issues associated with these novel therapies that use psychedelic or entactogenic substances in medically supervised and interpersonally supportive settings. We aim to ensure the path we walk is illuminated for all Congressional members where they can make informed decisions on the relevant issues.

Chapter 6

To Amend Title 38, United States Code, to Direct the Secretary of Veterans Affairs to Report on Whether the Secretary Will Include Certain Psychedelic Drugs in the Formulary of the Department of Veterans Affairs*

The Committee on Veterans' Affairs

Purpose and Summary

H.R. 7347, ''To amend Title 38, United States Code, to direct the Secretary of Veterans Affairs to report on whether the Secretary will include certain psychedelic drugs in the formulary of the Department of Veterans Affairs,'' was introduced by Representative Derrick Van Orden of Wisconsin on February 14, 2024. H.R. 7347 would require the U.S. Department of Veterans Affairs (VA) to submit a report to Congress no later than 180 days after the U.S. Food and Drug Administration (FDA) approval of a psychedelic drug, outlining whether or not VA is choosing to include the drug in the VA formulary, as well as justifications as to why or why not.

---

* This is an edited, reformatted and augmented version of the Report of The Committee on Veterans' Affairs [To accompany H.R. 7347] Committed to the Committee of the Whole House on the State of the Union and ordered to be printed, Publication No. 118–647, dated September 6, 2024.

In: The Psychedelic Landscape
Editor: James P. Macintosh
ISBN: 979-8-89530-991-9

Background and Need for Legislation

Section 1. Reporting of Determination of the Secretary of Veterans Affairs Whether to Include Newly Approved or Licensed Psychedelic Drugs in the Formulary of the Department of Veterans Affairs.

Under current law, psychedelic assisted therapy and the drugs associated with it are only authorized for use in clinical trials to study the effects of these drugs on patients with severe suicidality and Post Traumatic Stress Disorder (PTSD). This bill would require VA to send a report to the House and Senate Committees on Veterans' Affairs on whether VA has decided to include psychedelics in the VA formulary if the FDA approves the drug, as part of the list of approved drugs for prescription and clinical use for veterans struggling with PTSD, thoughts of suicide, or other conditions that may benefit from the use of the approved drug as determined by the veterans' primary care physician. The VA formulary is a list of approved drugs for prescription and clinical use approved by the Department. As the FDA continues to study and approve psychedelic drugs for clinical use, the Committee recognizes the potential benefits these treatments have in saving veteran lives and mitigating some of the symptoms of PTSD. VA's ongoing clinical trials are an important part of the research which can inform the benefits of the use of these drugs. According to VA's 2023 Annual Suicide Prevention Report, around 17 veterans per day die by suicide.[1] Some of VA's research at local medical facilities show that psychedelic assisted therapy has strong positive effects on the treatment of PTSD. This indicates that the use of psychedelics has the potential to significantly reduce suicides. However, if these drugs are not placed on the VA formulary, VA providers may not be able to consider the use of the drug in the veterans' treatment plan.

In 2023, the Committee conducted site visits to the Bronx VA Medical Center, New York University (NYU), and Johns Hopkins University (JHU) to meet with researchers at the forefront of ongoing clinical trials aimed at addressing severe suicidality and depression with psychedelic assisted therapy. Committee staff learned that NYU has conducted extensive trials with Methylenedioxymethamphetamine (MDMA). The results of one trial indicate that 88% of MDMA assisted therapy trial participants have significantly reduced PTSD symptoms after their third and final dosing session, with 67%

---

[1] 2023 National Veteran Suicide Prevention Annual Report, Department of Veterans Affairs, 2023, https://www.mentalhealth.va.gov/docs/data-sheets/2023/2023-National-Veteran-Suicide- Prevention-Annual-Report-FINAL-508.pdf.

achieving remission.[2] The duration of this treatment spans three months, with patients being monitored by their physician throughout the duration of the trial. Studies show that psychedelic assisted therapy may also have tremendous potential in addressing alcoholism and substance use disorders. Researchers at NYU have seen an 83% reduction in heavy drinking among patients undergoing psilocybin assisted therapy treatment, with 48% stopping drinking altogether.[3]

Based upon the results of those trials, the Committee believes that time is of the essence in getting these therapies approved for wide-scale use at VA upon FDA approval, which could happen as soon as the Fall of 2024. The Committee believes this bill would put pressure on VA to establish a timeline on the availability of these life saving drugs so that proper oversight can be conducted, as the Committee does not want VA to fall behind the private sector in the availability of these breakthrough treatments that could be available to veterans through VA.

Hearings

On March 21, 2024, the subcommittee on Health held a legislative hearing on H.R. 7347. The following witnesses testified:

> The Honorable Mike Bost, U.S. House of Representatives, Illinois 12th; The Honorable Chris Deluzio, U.S. House of Representatives, Pennsylvania 17th; The Honorable Jack Bergman, U.S. House of Representatives, Michigan 1st; The Honorable Greg Murphy, U.S. House of Representatives, North Carolina 3rd; The Honorable Derrick Van Orden, U.S. House of Representatives, Wisconsin 3rd; The Honorable Nick LaLota, U.S. House of Representatives, New York 1st; The Honorable Debbie Dingell, U.S. House of Representatives, Michigan 6th; The Honorable Lauren Underwood, U.S. House of Representatives, Illinois 14th; Dr. Ajit Pai, Executive Director, Office of Rehabilitation and Prosthetic Services, Veterans Health Administration, U.S. Department of Veterans Affairs; Dr. Michael Brennan, Executive

---

[2] MDMA Assisted Therapy for PTSD Completion of Phase 3 Study, Psychiatric Times, 2022, https://www.psychiatrictimes.com/view/mdma-assisted-therapy-for-ptsd-completion-of-phase-3-study.

[3] Psychedelic Drug Therapy May Help Treat Alcohol Addiction, NYU Langone Health, 2022, https://nyulangone.org/news/psychedelic-drug-therapy-may-help-treat-alcohol-addiction.

Director, Office of Construction and Facilities Management, U.S. Department of Veterans Affairs; Dr. Wendy Tenhula, Deputy Chief Research and Development Officer, Office of Research and Development, Veterans Health Administration, U.S. Department of Veterans Affairs; Dr. David Perry Chief Officer, Workforce Management and Consulting, Veterans Health Administration, U.S. Department of Veterans Affairs; Mr. Jon Retzer, Assistant National Legislative Director, Disabled American Veterans; Mr. Roscoe Butler, Senior Health Policy Advisor, Paralyzed Veterans of America; Ms. Brittany Elliot, Veteran (USMC), Advocate; Ms. Melissa Bryant, Chair, Board of Directors, Minority Veterans of America.

The following individuals and organizations submitted statements for the record:

Wounded Warrior Project, Treat Now, Superior Ambulance.

Subcommittee Consideration

On April 16, 2024, the Health Subcommittee met in an open markup session, a quorum being present, and ordered H.R. 7347 to be reported favorably to the Full Committee by voice vote.

Committee Consideration

On May 1, 2024, the full Committee met in open markup session, a quorum being present, and ordered H.R. 7347 be reported favorably to the House of Representatives by voice vote.

A motion by Ranking Member Takano of California to report H.R. 7347 favorably to the House of Representatives was agreed to by voice vote.

Committee Votes

In compliance with clause 3(b) of rule XIII of the Rules of the House of Representatives, no recorded votes were taken with ordering H.R. 7347 reported to the House.

Committee Oversight Findings

In compliance with clause 3(c)(1) of rule XIII and clause (2)(b)(1) of rule X of the Rules of the House of Representatives, the Committee's oversight findings and recommendations are reflected in the descriptive portions of this report.

Statement of General Performance Goals and Objectives

In accordance with clause 3(c)(4) of rule XIII of the Rules of the House of Representatives, the Committee's performance goals and objectives of H.R. 7347 are to provide a report to Congress on the plans of the Department of Veterans Affairs to include psychedelic drugs in the formulary.

Earmarks and Tax and Tariff Benefits

H.R. 7347 does not contain any Congressional earmarks, limited tax benefits, or limited tariff benefits as defined in clause 9 of rule XXI of the Rules of the House of Representatives.

Committee Cost Estimate

The Committee adopts as its own the cost estimate on H.R. 7347 prepared by the Director of the Congressional Budget Office.

H.R. 7347 would require the Department of Veterans Affairs (VA) to report to the Congress whenever a decision is made about whether to include on VA's prescription formulary, psychedelic drugs that have been approved by the Food and Drug Administration.

Under current law, VA publicizes its decisions about what to include in the department's formulary, and to date, no psychedelic drugs have been approved for medical use by the Food and Drug Administration. CBO estimates that satisfying the requirement to report to the Congress would cost less than $500,000 over the 2024–2034 period.

Budget Authority and Congressional Budget Office Cost Estimate

H.R. 7347, a bill to amend title 38, United States Code, to direct the Secretary of Veterans Affairs to report on whether the Secretary will include certain psychedelic drugs in the formulary of the Department of Veterans Affairs
As ordered reported by the House Committee on Veterans Affairs on May 1, 2024

By Fiscal Year, Millions of Dollars	2024	2024-2029	2024-2034
Direct Spending (Outlays)	0	0	0
Revenues	0	0	0
Increase or Decrease (-) in the Deficit	0	0	0
Spending Subject to Appropriation (Outlays)	*	*	*

Increases *net direct spending* in any of the four consecutive 10-year periods beginning in 2035?	No	Statutory pay-as-you-go procedures apply?	No
		Mandate Effects	
Increases *on-budget deficits* in any of the four consecutive 10-year periods beginning in 2035?	No	Contains intergovernmental mandate?	No
		Contains private-sector mandate?	No

* = between zero and $500,000.

The CBO staff contact for this estimate is Matt Schmit. The estimate was reviewed by Christina Hawley Anthony, Deputy Director of Budget Analysis.

Phillip L. Swagel,
Director, Congressional Budget Office.

Federal Mandates Statement

Section 423 of the Congressional Budget and Impoundment Control Act (as amended by Section 101(a)(2) of the Unfunded Mandate Reform Act, P.L. 104–4) is inapplicable to H.R. 7347.

Advisory Committee Statement

No advisory committees within the meaning of section 5(b) of the Federal Advisory Committee Act would be created by H.R. 7347.

Applicability to Legislative Branch

The Committee finds that H.R. 7347 does not relate to the terms and conditions of employment or access to public services or accommodation within the meaning of section 102(b)(3) of the Congressional Accountability Act.

Statement on Duplication of Federal Programs

Pursuant to clause 3(c)(5) of rule XIII of the Rules of the House of Representatives, the Committee finds that no provision of H.R. 7347 establishes or reauthorizes a program of the Federal Government known to be duplicative of another Federal program, a program that was included in any report from the Government Accountability Office to Congress pursuant to section 21 of Public Law 111–139, or a program related to a program identified in the most recent Catalog of Federal Domestic Assistance.

Section-by-Section Analysis of the Legislation

Section 1. Reporting of determination of the Secretary of Veterans Affairs whether to include newly approved or licensed psychedelic drugs in the formulary of the Department of Veterans Affairs.

This section would amend Chapter 81 of title 38, United States Code, by inserting, a new section § 8125A, which would require, no later than 180 days after a psychedelic drug is approved under section 505 of the Federal Food, Drug, and Cosmetic Act (21 U.S.C. 355) or licensed under section 351 of the Public Health Service Act (42 U.S.C. 262), the Secretary to submit to the House and Senate Committees on Veterans' Affairs a report regarding such drug, that includes the determination of the Secretary whether to include such drug in the formulary of the Department, and the justification of the Secretary for such determination.

Changes in Existing Law Made by the Bill, as Reported

In compliance with clause 3(e) of rule XIII of the Rules of the House of Representatives, changes in existing law made by the bill, as reported, are shown as follows (existing law proposed to be omitted is enclosed in black brackets, new matter is printed in italics, existing law in which no change is proposed is shown in roman):

Changes in Existing Law Made by the Bill, as Reported

In compliance with clause 3(e) of rule XIII of the Rules of the House of Representatives, changes in existing law made by the bill, as reported, are shown as follows (new matter is printed in italics and existing law in which no change is proposed is shown in roman):

TITLE 38, UNITED STATES CODE

* * * * * * *

PART VI—ACQUISITION AND DISPOSITION OF PROPERTY

* * * * * * *

Chapter 81—Acquisition and Operation of Hospital and Domiciliary Facilities; Procurement and Supply; Enhanced-Use Leases of Real Property

* * * * * * *

* * * * * * *

SUBCHAPTER II—PROCUREMENT AND SUPPLY

SEC. 8125A. Reporting of determination whether to include newly approved or licensed psychedelic drugs in the formulary of the Department.

Not later than 180 days after a psychedelic drug is approved under section 505 of the Federal Food, Drug, and Cosmetic Act (21 U.S.C. 355) or licensed under section 351 of the Public Health Service Act (42 U.S.C. 262), the

Secretary shall submit to the Committees on Veterans' Affairs of the Senate and House of Representatives a report regarding such drug, that includes—

1) the determination of the Secretary whether to include such drug in the formulary of the Department; and
2) the justification of the Secretary for such determination.

* * * * * * *

* * * * * * *

8125A. Reporting of determination whether to include newly approved or licensed psychedelic drugs in the formulary of the Department.

* * * * * * *

SUBCHAPTER II—PROCUREMENT AND SUPPLY

* * * * * * *

Chapter 7

Drug Control: DEA Should Improve its Religious Exemptions Petition Process for Psilocybin (Mushrooms) and Other Controlled Substances*

United States Government Accountability Office

Abbreviations

BIA	Bureau of Indian Affairs
CBP	U.S. Customs and Border Protections
DOJ	Department of Justice
DEA	Drug Enforcement Administration
DMT	Dimethyltryptamine
EOUSA	Executive Office for United States Attorneys
FBI	Federal Bureau of Investigation
FDA	Food and Drug Administration
IND	Investigational New Drug
LSD	lysergic acid diethylamide
MDMA	3,4-methylenedioxymethamphetamine
ONDCP	Office of National Drug Control Policy
USPIS	U.S. Postal Inspection Service

* This is an edited, reformatted and augmented version of the United States Government Accountability Office Report to Congressional Committees, Publication No. GAO-24-106630, dated May 2024.

In: The Psychedelic Landscape
Editor: James P. Macintosh
ISBN: 979-8-89530-991-9

Why GAO Did This Study

DEA is responsible for investigating and enforcing violations of the Controlled Substances Act; overseeing, and coordinating with the Food and Drug Administration (FDA), on the process to study controlled substances; and reviewing petitions for religious exemptions to the Controlled Substances Act. Historically, psilocybin has been used in Indigenous cultures for spiritual ceremonies. Some states have taken steps to legalize the adult use of psilocybin or establish programs to study psilocybin for therapeutic applications.

The Joint Explanatory Statement accompanying the Consolidated Appropriations Act, 2023, includes a provision for GAO to review the use of psilocybin. Among other objectives, this report addresses (1) what federal data show on psilocybin's enforcement; and (2) reported barriers to the legal access and use of psilocybin for religious practices under the Religious Freedom Restoration Act.

GAO analyzed data from DEA related to enforcement and religious exemption processes, and interviewed officials at professional associations, DEA, FDA, research institutions, selected attorney and associated advocacy groups; and officials from two states that legalized psilocybin use.

What GAO Recommends

GAO is making four recommendations to DEA, including that DEA should establish timeframes to make determinations on completed religious exemption petitions under the Religious Freedom Restoration Act. DEA concurred with each of the recommendations.

What GAO Found

Psilocybin is a naturally occurring hallucinogenic substance found in certain types of mushrooms. Generally, it is a federal crime for any person to possess, manufacture or distribute this controlled substance. However, numbers of investigations and seizures for psilocybin are small compared to other Schedule I controlled substances. During fiscal years 2018 through 2023, psilocybin cases (identified as the harshest or primary drug of concern) represented less than 1 percent of all cases the Drug Enforcement Administration (DEA) investigated and closed. Over the same period, psilocybin accounted for about 2 percent of all the U.S. Customs and Border Protection's drug seizures.

Depiction of Various Forms of Psilocybin (Mushrooms)

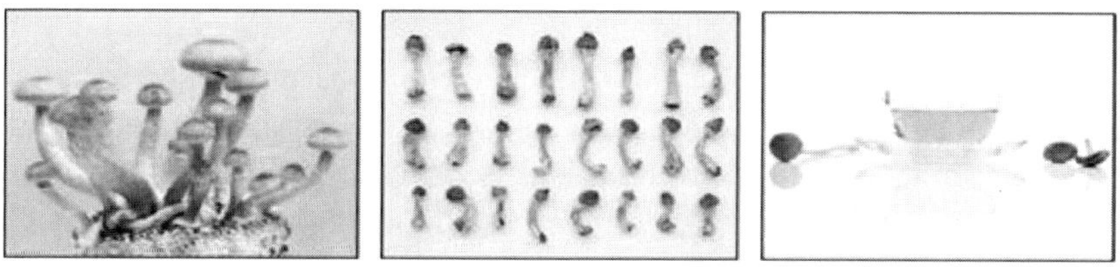

Source: mindhive/stock.adobe.com. Cannabis_Pic/stock.adobe.com. and Esymaks/ stock.adobe.com. | GAO-24-106630.

Selected stakeholders reported several barriers to the legal access and use of psilocybin for religious practices under the Religious Freedom Restoration Act. For example, DEA established a process for parties to petition for a religious exemption from the Controlled Substances Act to use controlled substances for religious purposes. However, DEA's guidance does not inform petitioners on its timeframes to make determinations on completed petitions. DEA officials stated the agency is aware of public concerns on the need to better understand its policies and processes that impact the petitions for religious exemptions. In 2019, DEA initiated a draft notice of proposed rulemaking related to its process for petitioning for religious exemptions. Four years later, in February 2023, the final draft notice was submitted to DEA's Office of the Administrator, according to DEA officials; but there is no timeframe for issuance of the notice or final regulations.

Over an 8-year period—from fiscal year 2016 through January 2024—DEA reported that 24 petitioners requested a religious exemption for various controlled substances. As of January 2024, DEA reported that none of these petitions had been granted an exemption and of the 6 for psilocybin, three were withdrawn and three were pending a DEA determination. The three pending religious exemption petitions related to psilocybin ranged from about 8 months to over 3 years from the date of receipt. DEA's information also showed instances where finalized actions regarding exemption petitions related to other controlled substances have been pending a determination for an extensive period—one almost 5 years and one almost 8 years.

Including timeframes to make determinations about religious exemption petitions in DEA's guidance will provide better transparency about the agency's process.

May 30, 2024

Congressional Committees

Psilocybin is a naturally occurring hallucinogenic substance found in certain types of mushrooms in South America, Mexico, and the United States. Psilocybin is a Schedule I controlled substance under the Controlled Substances Act, as amended,[1] meaning that it has a high potential for abuse, no currently accepted medical use in treatment in the United States, and there is a lack of accepted safety for use of the substance under medical supervision.[2] In addition, as a Schedule I controlled substance, generally it is a federal crime for any person to knowingly or intentionally possess, manufacture, distribute, or dispense psilocybin under federal law.[3]

However, some states and localities have taken steps to legalize, decriminalize or deprioritize the personal use or possession of psilocybin under state or local law.[4] Alternatively, other states have established initiatives supporting psilocybin-based research or pilot programs administering psilocybin services in a limited capacity. Some medical researchers are exploring how psilocybin may be used as an alternative psychedelic treatment to provide relief to individuals with certain conditions, such as depressive

---

[1] Pub. L. No. 91-513, 84 Stat. 1242. The Controlled Substances Act classifies all federally controlled substances into categories known as schedules depending upon, among other things, the drug's likelihood for abuse or dependence, and whether the drug has an accepted medical use. These schedules range from I through V – with Schedule I having the greatest restrictions. Schedule I substances are those that have been found by the federal government to have a high potential for abuse, no currently accepted medical use in treatment in the United States, and a lack of accepted safety for use under medical supervision.

[2] 21 U.S.C. § 812(c), Schedule I (c)(15) and 21 U.S.C. § 812(b)(1).

[3] 21 U.S.C. §§ 841, 844.

[4] We defined "deprioritize" generally as instances where states or localities have passed laws reducing the criminal penalties associated with the personal use or possession of psilocybin from a felony to a lesser crime or fine; stating that non-commercial planting, cultivating, transporting, or possession of psilocybin is among law enforcement's lowest enforcement priorities; or preventing public funds from being used to enforce criminal laws related to the personal use or possession of psilocybin. A state or local entity's alteration of its laws or priorities with respect to a particular substance has no effect on the legal status under federal law. Generally, possession or distribution of a Schedule I controlled substance continues to violate the Controlled Substances Act even if a state no longer imposes separate penalties for that conduct.

disorders and addictions. Reportedly, psilocybin has historically been used ritualistically as a psychedelic or hallucinogenic agent in Indigenous cultures for religious and spiritual ceremonies.

Within the Department of Justice (DOJ), the Drug Enforcement Administration (DEA) is the primary federal law enforcement agency responsible for investigating and enforcing potential violations of the Controlled Substances Act. DEA reported that the use of psilocybin is associated with negative physical and psychological consequences— effects are similar to other hallucinogens, such as mescaline and lysergic acid diethylamide (LSD).[5] According to DEA, the physical effects may include nausea, vomiting, muscle weakness, drowsiness, and lack of coordination. The psychological consequences of psilocybin use may include hallucinations, the inability to discern fantasy from reality. DEA officials also stated that the psychological consequences may include fear, paranoia, anxiety, and depression that may last for days, weeks, or years after use. In addition, suicide, suicide ideation, and suicidal attempts have been reported after psilocybin use, according to DEA officials.

Some medical researchers have found that applications of psilocybin may provide therapeutic options for neuropsychiatric conditions, like depression and anxiety, often in conjunction with psychotherapy. Some researchers are examining psilocybin use for post-traumatic stress disorder, substance use disorders, pain, and eating disorders, among other things. Federal authorization to conduct a study involving a Schedule I controlled substance is required for individuals or entities.

In addition, psilocybin has reportedly been used historically for certain religious and spiritual ceremonies. Federal law requires a heightened level of scrutiny for government actions that substantially burden an individual's religious exercise.[6] Pursuant to this federal law, DEA has a process to evaluate whether the enforcement of the Controlled Substances Act substantially burdens the religious exercise of an individual or entity based upon a petition for a religious exemption to the Controlled Substances Act. Concerns have been raised by numerous stakeholders regarding the timeliness of DEA

---

[5] Hallucinogens are drugs that alter awareness of perception, thoughts, and feelings. Psilocybin, mescaline, and LSD are all psychedelic hallucinogens, often just called psychedelics, which means "mind-manifesting." These substances share a similar mechanism of action, which involves activating receptors for the brain chemical serotonin. Mescaline is a psychedelic hallucinogen obtained from the small, spineless cactus Peyote, the San Pedro cactus, Peruvian torch cactus, and other mescaline-containing cacti. LSD is a synthetic hallucinogen originally derived from ergot fungus.

[6] Religious Freedom Restoration Act of 1993, Pub. L. No. 103-141, 107 Stat. 1488.

determinations for religious exemptions as well as clarity on the type of information petitioners should provide to support petitions.

The Joint Explanatory Statement accompanying the Consolidated Appropriations Act, 2023,[7] incorporates House Report 117-395, which includes a provision for GAO to report to Congress on the barriers to tribal, state, and local governments that incorporate psilocybin products, including for therapeutic use and religious, indigenous, or spiritual practices. This report addresses: (1) What federal data show about psilocybin's enforcement under the Controlled Substances Act; (2) The processes to obtain federal authorization to conduct research with psilocybin; and stakeholders' perspectives on them; and (3) The process and reported barriers that exist in the legal access and use of psilocybin for religious practices under the Religious Freedom Restoration Act of 1993.

To address our first objective, we analyzed enforcement data from DEA's CONCORDE/IMPACT Case Management System (CONCORDE System) to identify the number of closed and open investigations related to Schedule I controlled substances (including psilocybin) for each fiscal year—2018 through 2023.[8] DEA identifies an investigation as closed when all investigative and prosecutorial related activities are completed. According to DEA officials, the CONCORDE System cannot account for all closed and open investigations involving psilocybin because the system only tracks investigations by the "harshest" controlled substance involved in a seizure.[9]

We also analyzed data from DEA's National Forensic Laboratory Information System, which is comprised of data voluntarily reported by forensic laboratories on the results of its testing and analysis conducted on substances seized through federal, state, and local law enforcement operations. We also analyzed the U.S. Customs and Border Protection's (CBP) seizure data related to Schedule I controlled substances (including psilocybin) for each fiscal year—2018 through 2023. We assessed the reliability of DEA and CBP data by reviewing existing information and documentation about the data and the system that produced them and determined that they were sufficiently reliable for our purposes of presenting enforcement trends over time.

[7] Pub. L. No. 117-328, 136 Stat. 4459.

[8] According to DEA officials, the CONCORDE System is used to record and track DEA's criminal investigations.

[9] For example, DEA officials stated that if a DEA investigation involves a seizure with two controlled substances (i.e., heroin and psilocybin) the CONCORDE System may only identify heroin, because heroin may be considered to be the "harshest" controlled substance, or primary drug of concern in this instance based upon the judgment of DEA officials.

To address our second objective, we identified and analyzed DEA's policies and procedures, and other documentation that outlined the process new and existing researchers use to apply for federal authorization to conduct research with Schedule I controlled substances—including psilocybin. We interviewed DEA and Food and Drug Administration (FDA) officials to identify their perspectives on improvements needed, if any, to the federal authorization process related to conducting research with Schedule I controlled substances—including psilocybin. We also interviewed a non-generalizable sample of researchers to represent a range of perspectives on the process used to obtain federal authorization to conduct research with psilocybin and other Schedule I controlled substances, and the extent to which the process could be improved, if any.[10]

To address our third objective, we reviewed federal law and court cases involving the Religious Freedom Restoration Act; and assessed DEA's policies and procedures, and other documentation that outlined the agency's process for reviewing religious exemption petitions from the Controlled Substances Act under the Religious Freedom Restoration Act. We also analyzed DEA's information on the number of petitions filed and processing status (i.e., approved, denied, withdrawn, or pending) for applicants who submitted petitions to use psilocybin and other controlled substances for religious practices for fiscal year 2016 through January 2024. We interviewed DEA officials to identify their perspectives on the agency's process to review petitions for a religious exemption.

We also interviewed a non-generalizable sample of nine individuals from law firms and advocacy organizations selected to represent a range of perspectives on the process and reported barriers, if any, that exist in the legal access to and use of psilocybin for religious, Indigenous, or spiritual practices under the Religious Freedom Restoration Act. In addition, we attempted to meet with officials representing various Tribal Nations to obtain their perspectives on DEA's petition process for the use of psilocybin for religious or spiritual purposes. A representative from one of the eleven Tribal Nations we contacted responded to our request and stated the Tribe has no history of psilocybin use for religious, Indigenous, spiritual or any other practices.

To address all three objectives, we attended the 2023 Psychedelic Science Conference, held in Denver, Colorado and met with stakeholder

---

[10] We selected four organizations that represent a range of perspectives and expertise in the research community, including advocacy organizations, research institutions, and medical researchers.

representatives from diverse groups that represented various government, medical, spiritual, tribal, and other psychedelic related organizations. We also attended panel discussions and presentations that focused on the policy and legislation, clinical research, the Religious Freedom Restoration Act, and Indigenous and historical uses of psilocybin.

To obtain various perspectives on psilocybin use, we selected and interviewed six of the conference participants (i.e., attorneys, researchers, and faculty researchers) who were identified and considered as knowledgeable on the legal and therapeutic aspects of psilocybin use.

Based upon a review of states' laws related to psilocybin, we identified Oregon and Colorado as the two states that had legalized the adult use of psilocybin under state laws as of July 2023 and interviewed relevant and knowledgeable program officials from Oregon and Colorado to obtain their perspectives on state legalization of psilocybin—including the challenges experienced with implementing their recently passed psilocybin laws.

For background purposes to report on scientific research indicating potential uses for psilocybin, we conducted a literature review identifying sources published from January 2013 through August 2023 that related to the applications of psilocybin therapy. GAO then identified any sources that provided or cited evidence regarding psilocybin's efficacy to treat medical and mental health conditions and reviewed the methodology of the studies and the outcomes.

We conducted this performance audit from February 2023 to May 2024 in accordance with generally accepted government auditing standards.

Those standards require that we plan and perform the audit to obtain sufficient, appropriate evidence to provide a reasonable basis for our findings and conclusions based on our audit objectives. We believe that the evidence obtained provides a reasonable basis for our findings and conclusions based on our audit objectives.

Background

Federal and State Psilocybin Laws

Psilocybin is a naturally occurring hallucinogenic substance found in certain types of mushrooms. Psilocybin is a controlled substance under federal law and is classified as a Schedule I controlled substance—the most restrictive of categories of controlled substances by the federal government. The Controlled Substances Act, as amended, does not allow Schedule I controlled substances, including psilocybin, to be dispensed with a prescription,[11] and generally provides federal sanctions for the unauthorized possession, manufacture, distribution, or dispensing of such controlled substances.[12]

For a number of years, the 50 states generally had uniform drug control laws or similar provisions that mirrored the Controlled Substances Act, making their violation a state criminal offense. However, since 2017, despite the federal government's prohibition on psilocybin, a few states and localities have legalized, decriminalized, or deprioritized psilocybin use under state or local law. According to Department of the Interior's Bureau of Indian Affairs officials, based on their knowledge, no federallyrecognized Indian Tribes have legalized the use of psilocybin for religious or spiritual purposes.[13]

Legalization. As of July 2023, two states—Colorado and Oregon—passed state laws generally legalizing the adult use of psilocybin. In November 2020, Oregon passed a state ballot initiative, also known as the Oregon Psilocybin Services Act, to permit persons licensed, controlled, and regulated by the state to legally manufacture psilocybin products and provide psilocybin services to persons 21 years of age and older, subject to state law; and establish a comprehensive regulatory framework concerning psilocybin products and psilocybin services under state law, after a two-year program development period.[14] On December 31, 2022, Oregon adopted final administrative rules for the regulated framework codified in Oregon law, in Oregon Revised Statutes Chapter 475A. Beginning January 2, 2023, Oregon began reviewing applications for licensure, issuing licenses, and regulating licensees.

In 2022, Colorado passed a state ballot initiative to generally decriminalize the personal use and possession of certain hallucinogenic and entheogenic plants and fungi, including psilocybin. In addition, the initiative provided for the establishment of a natural medicine services program for the

---

[11] See 21 U.S.C. § 829.

[12] Generally, the Controlled Substances Act, as amended, allows for the limited use of Schedule I drugs in the context of a government approved research project. 21 U.S.C.§§ 823(g)(2)(A), 841, 844.

[13] As of January 2024, there were 574 federally recognized Indian Tribes in the United States. The Indian Tribes in the U.S. vary greatly in terms of culture, language, population size, land base, location, and economic status. These Tribal Nations are distinct political entities whose inherent sovereignty predates the United States and is reflected in the government-to-government relationship between Tribal Nations and the federal government. Tribal Nations are subject to federal law, but as sovereign entities, they operate under their own constitutions, enact their own laws, and provide services to their citizens.

[14] 2021 Or. Laws Ch. 1 (B.M. 109). Or. Rev. St. §§ 475A.210-722.

supervised administration of these substances, a regulatory framework for the growth, distribution, and sale of these substances, and a natural medicine advisory board to promulgate rules and implement the regulated access program. In May 2023, Colorado passed an act concerning natural medicine (referred to as the Natural Medicine Regulation and Legalization), which sets the regulatory framework for a natural medicine program in Colorado. In addition, the Act generally decriminalizes the possession, consumption, cultivation, manufacture, and sharing of natural medicine or natural medicine product for the purpose of personal use without remuneration for persons 21 years of age and older.[15]

See appendices I and II, for additional information on the legalization and regulation of psilocybin in Oregon and Colorado.

Deprioritization. The District of Columbia has not legalized or decriminalized the use of psilocybin,[16] but under the D.C. Code, generally, the Metropolitan Police Department is to make the investigation and arrest of persons 18 years of age or older for non-commercial planting, cultivating, purchasing, transporting, distributing, or possessing certain entheogenic plants and fungi, including psilocybin, as among its lowest enforcement priorities—as of March 2021.[17] In addition, pursuant to D.C. Code § 48-921.53, "[t]he people of the District of Columbia call upon the Attorney General of the District of Columbia and the United States Attorney for the District of Columbia to cease prosecution of residents of the District of Columbia for non-commercial planting, non- commercial cultivating, purchasing, transporting, distributing, engaging in practices with, and/or possessing entheogenic plants and fungi as defined in [D.C. Code] § 48-921.52."

State-level initiatives. Some states have not decriminalized, deprioritized, or legalized psilocybin but have state laws establishing state-level pilot research programs and studies. For example, Connecticut required the Department of Mental Health and Addiction Services to establish, within available appropriations, a psychedelic-assisted therapy pilot program,[18] to be

---

[15] 2023 Colo. Legis. Serv. Ch. 249.

[16] D.C. Code § 48-902.04(3)(R).

[17] D.C. Code § 48-921.52. Generally, the term "entheogenic plant and fungus" means any plant or fungus of any species in which there is naturally occurring any of the following substances in any form, which would cause such plant or fungus to be described as a Schedule I controlled substance under D.C. Code § 48-902.04(3): ibogaine, dimethyltryptamine (DMT), mescaline, psilocybin, or psilocyn.

[18] The pilot program is required to provide qualified patients with 3,4- Methylenedioxymethamphetamine (MDMA)-assisted or psilocybin-assisted therapy as part of a research program approved by FDA pursuant to 21 C.F.R. pt. 312.

administered by a medical school in the state by January 1, 2023.[19] In addition, Maryland established the Post-Traumatic Stress Disorder and Traumatic Brain Injury Alternative Therapies Fund to study the use of and provide cost-free access to alternative therapies, including the use of psilocybin, for post-traumatic stress disorder and traumatic brain injuries in veterans.[20] For an overview of some of the characteristics of selected states with legislation establishing a pilot program or study of psilocybin for therapeutic use, see appendix III.

Local-level decriminalization/deprioritization. Some localities and a municipal government have allowed for use of psilocybin even though the respective state has not decriminalized or deprioritized enforcement of psilocybin. For example, in June 2019, the City Council in Oakland, California, voted unanimously to decriminalize the adult use and possession of psilocybin and other entheogenic, or psychoactive, plants, and fungi. As a result, the city's funds are not allowed to be used to enforce laws criminalizing such substances—the Alameda County District Attorney stopped prosecuting people who have been apprehended for use or possession of such substances.

Even though some states and localities have taken steps to legalize, decriminalize, or deprioritize the personal use or possession of psilocybin, the Controlled Substances Act generally provides federal sanctions for the unauthorized possession, manufacture, distribution, or dispensing of Schedule I controlled substances, including psilocybin.[21] In addition, pursuant to federal law, it is generally unlawful to knowingly open, lease, rent, use, or maintain any place for the purpose of manufacturing, distributing, or using any controlled substance.[22]

---

[19] Conn. Gen. Stat. § 17a-484g.

[20] Md. Code Ann. Health-Gen. § 24-2102. Pursuant to Md. Code Ann. Health-Gen. § 24-2101(b), "'alternative therapies' includes hyperbaric oxygen therapy and psychedelics including 3,4—Methylenedioxymethamphetamine (MDMA), psilocybin, and ketamine." Pursuant to Md. Code Ann. Health-Gen. § 24-2101(d), "veteran" means a former member of the following entities who was discharged from active duty: the armed forces of the United States; a reserve component of the armed forces of the United States; or the National Guard of any state.

[21] 21 U.S.C. §§ 841, 844.

[22] 21 U.S.C. § 856.

Federal Roles and Responsibilities Enforcing the Controlled Substances Act

DEA is the primary federal law enforcement agency responsible for conducting criminal and regulatory investigations of potential violations of the Controlled Substances Act and works to disrupt and dismantle the leadership, command, control, and financial infrastructure of major drug- trafficking organizations. DEA uses a multifaceted approach that includes:

- investigating narcotics cases and preparing them for prosecution;
- managing a national drug intelligence program to collect, analyze, and disseminate drug intelligence;
- enforcing counternarcotics laws involving the diversion of legally produced substances for illegal purposes; and
- coordinating with and leveraging the resources of international, federal, state, and local partners.

DEA is also responsible for investigating and enforcing potential violations of the Controlled Substances Act in Indian country.[23] The Federal Bureau of Investigation (FBI) also investigates cases related to violations of the Controlled Substances Act.[24] DEA coordinates and collaborates with state and local law enforcement agencies to implement or enforce the Act by sharing information and partnering in investigations and enforcement actions. DEA also manages and reviews petitions seeking religious exemptions from the Controlled Substances Act under the Religious Freedom Restoration Act to permit the use of controlled substances, including psilocybin. Within DEA, the Diversion Control Division's Diversion Regulatory Section and the

---

[23] Pursuant to 18 U.S.C. § 1151, the term "Indian country" generally means "(a) all land within the limits of any Indian reservation under the jurisdiction of the United States Government, notwithstanding the issuance of any patent, and, including rights-of-way running through the reservation, (b) all dependent Indian communities within the borders of the United States whether within the original or subsequently acquired territory thereof, and whether within or without the limits of a state, and (c) all Indian allotments, the Indian titles to which have not been extinguished, including rights-of-way running through the same." Generally, DEA's jurisdiction for narcotics investigations in Indian country is based on the Controlled Substances Act, 21 U.S.C. §§ 801-971, which applies throughout the United States, including in Indian country.

[24] Under 28 C.F.R. § 0.85, the FBI has the authority to investigate violations of the laws, including the criminal drug laws, of the United States and collect evidence in cases in which the United States is or may be a party in interest, except in cases in which such responsibility is by statute or otherwise exclusively assigned to another investigative agency.

Import/Export Section are the two main components that carry out this process.

In addition to DEA and FBI, several other federal departments and agencies are involved in efforts to address controlled substances, including psilocybin, in the United States. Appendix IV provides some examples of the key federal agencies involved in these efforts.

The DEA is the principal agency that oversees the process for researchers to apply for authorization to study Schedule I controlled substances. However, FDA also has responsibilities in this process, which we discuss in more detail later in the report.

Federal Process to Obtain Permission to Study Psilocybin

Individuals or entities interested in working with Schedule I controlled substances, such as psilocybin, must meet DEA requirements for registration, ordering, recordkeeping, inventory, storage, and disposal of the controlled substances. Such individuals or entities include manufacturers, distributors, researchers, practitioners, and pharmacists. An individual or entity's registration lasts between 1 and 3 years.

Separate registrations are required for each place of business where a controlled substance is involved in a study, manufactured, distributed, imported, exported, or dispensed.

Registrants are to follow guidelines related to recordkeeping and reporting of the inventory and distribution of the controlled substances they have been approved to study. Additionally, they are subject to DEA inspection of the place of business, and they must implement controls to guard against theft or diversion of controlled substances. Specifically, nonpractitioners-such as researchers-must follow certain requirements when storing controlled substances and have adequate security measures to provide effective controls and procedures to guard against theft and diversion of controlled substances.

Generally, the Attorney General may deny, suspend, or revoke a registration for a practitioner to conduct research with Schedule I controlled substances upon a finding that the registrant has:

1) materially falsified any application;
2) been convicted of a felony relating to a controlled substance or certain chemicals;

3) had a state license or registration suspended, revoked, or denied by a competent state authority, or has had a suspension, revocation, or denial of a registration recommended by a competent state authority;
4) committed acts which would render the registration inconsistent with the public interest; or
5) been excluded (or directed to be excluded) from participation in certain federal health care programs.[25]

In 2021, we reported an interagency workgroup, that was facilitated by the Office of National Drug Control Policy (ONDCP) and included DEA, had developed recommendations to enact legislation to accomplish several goals, including: requiring the Attorney General and the Secretary of Health and Human Services conduct a review of the process for obtaining or modifying a research registration under the Controlled Substances Act to identify redundancies, inefficiencies, or burdens on persons seeking registrations that can be reduced while ensuring public safety; and subsequently requiring the Attorney General and the Secretary of Health and Human Services to issue joint guidance clarifying the registration process, among other recommendations.[26]

Federal Pathways Permitting Religious, Spiritual, or Medical Use of Controlled Substances

Various pathways allow for individuals or organizations to apply for exemptions which would allow for the religious or spiritual use, in limited circumstances, of psilocybin, or the use of controlled substances for medical advances, research, and treatment.

Religious Exemptions. Generally, the Religious Freedom Restoration Act provides for an individual or entity the opportunity for judicial review of government action that substantially burdens a person's religious exercise. The Act provides that the "[g]overnment shall not substantially burden a person's exercise of religion" unless the Government can demonstrate "that application of the burden to the person is in furtherance of a compelling

---

[25] 21 U.S.C. §§ 823(g)(2)(A), 824(a).

[26] The workgroup recommendations also addressed allowing registered researchers to store, administer, and otherwise work with any substances for which they hold a researcher registration at multiple practice sites on a single contiguous campus. GAO, *Synthetic Opioids: Considerations for the Class-Wide Scheduling of Fentanyl-Related Substances,* GAO-21-499 (Washington, D.C. Apr. 2021).

governmental interest and is the least restrictive means of furthering that compelling governmental interest."[27]

Generally, a person claiming that the government has placed a substantial burden on the person's practice of religion for purposes of the Religious Freedom Restoration Act must establish that the government action: (1) substantially burdens; (2) a religious belief, not just a philosophy or way of life; (3) which belief is sincerely held. Once the person has demonstrated that the government has burdened the person's exercise of religion, the government must demonstrate the government action being challenged furthers a compelling governmental interest by the least restrictive means.

In general, the Religious Freedom Restoration Act provides for a heightened standard of review for government actions, including rules of general applicability, that "substantially burden" a person's religious exercise. Typically, this burden exists when an individual must choose between refraining from following the individual's religious beliefs to avoid facing legal penalties from the government or following the individual's religious beliefs and foregoing the receipt of a government benefit. A person whose religious exercise has been burdened in violation of the Religious Freedom Restoration Act may assert that violation as a claim or defense in a judicial proceeding and obtain appropriate relief against a government.[28] This includes actions taken by the federal government pursuant to the Controlled Substances Act.[29] For example, an individual or entity may bring a suit to prohibit the federal government from enforcing the Controlled Substances Act to ban the use of a controlled substance in religious ceremonies under the Religious

---

[27] Pub. L. No. 103-141, § 3, 107 Stat. 1488, 1488-89 (codified at 42 U.S.C. § 2000bb-1). The Religious Freedom Restoration Act was enacted in response to a 1990 Supreme Court case, *Employment Division v. Smith*, 494 U.S. 872 (1990), where the Court held, in part, that generally applicable, religion-neutral criminal laws that have the effect of burdening a particular religious practice need not be justified, under the free exercise of religion clause, by a compelling governmental interest. In this case, two drug rehabilitation counselors, both of whom were members of the Native American Church, were fired from their jobs with a private corporation in Oregon because they had ingested peyote, a hallucinogenic drug, for sacramental purposes at a ceremony of the Church. The counselors applied to the Employment Division of Oregon's Department of Human Resources for unemployment compensation, but the department's Employment Appeals Board ultimately denied their applications on the ground that the counselors had been discharged for misconduct connected with work. Section 2 of the Religious Freedom Restoration Act, Pub. L. No. 103-141, § 2, 107 Stat, 1488 specifically addressed the Supreme Court's holding in *Employment Division v. Smith*, 494 U.S. 872 (1990) with the purposes of the Act to restore the compelling interest test and to guarantee its application in all cases where free exercise of religion is substantially burdened.

[28] 42 U.S.C. § 2000bb-1(c).

[29] Gonzales v. O Centro Espirita Beneficente Uniao do Vegetal, 546 U.S. 418 (2006).

Freedom Restoration Act. In addition, an individual or entity prosecuted under the Controlled Substances Act may raise as a defense to such prosecution that the federal government has placed a substantial burden on the individual or entity's practice of religion for purposes of the Religious Freedom Restoration Act.

In order to reconcile and balance the interests of the Controlled Substances Act and Religious Freedom Restoration Act, in 2009, DEA first promulgated a guidance document establishing a procedure for seeking religious exemptions from the Controlled Substances Act from DEA. In November 2020, this guidance was updated and provides a process for individuals or entities to petition for an exemption from the Controlled Substances Act to use certain controlled substances for religious circumstances.[30] We discuss DEA's establishment of a process to review religious exemptions to the Controlled Substances Act under the Religious Freedom Restoration Act later in the report.

Clinical Trials. The development and approval of a new drug is a complex and costly process that can take several years. Typically, the drug development process involves a number of stages, including basic research,[31] drug discovery,[32] preclinical research,[33] clinical trials, and review and approval.[34] Clinical trials involve the testing of the drug in human volunteers for safety and efficacy which is conducted in phases. Clinical trials are usually conducted in phases that build on one another, though the phases may overlap. Phase one trials generally test the safety of a drug with a small group of healthy volunteers (usually fewer than 100) to determine the drug's initial safety profile and find the highest dose of the new drug or treatment that can be given safely without causing severe side effects. If the drug does not show

---

[30] According to DEA officials, DEA's Diversion Regulatory Section and the Import/Export Section are the two components within DEA's Diversion Control Division that process Religious Freedom Restoration Act applications for the use of psilocybin. The Diversion Regulatory Section typically coordinates with the Office of Chief Counsel, DEA field offices, and any other Diversion Control Division sections where information can be gained to further assist with the processing of petitions under the Religious Freedom Restoration Act.

[31] Basic research may involve the scientific investigation of the molecular, cellular, or biological mechanisms of a disease that lays the foundation for the development of new drugs.

[32] Drug discovery may involve the screening of thousands of compounds in the laboratory to identify promising candidates to treat the disease.

[33] Preclinical research may involve laboratory and animal testing to further narrow the list of compounds and answer basic questions about safety and proof of concept.

[34] Review and approval involve the FDA conducting a regulatory review and approval of the drug for marketing and sales in the United States if it is found to be safe and effective for its intended use.

unacceptable toxicity in phase one clinical trials, phase two clinical trials are conducted in a larger group of volunteers (usually dozens to hundreds) to assess the drug's safety and effectiveness for a particular disease or condition and determine common short-term side effects and risks.

In phase two clinical trials, generally some volunteers receive the drug and others receive a control, such as a placebo. If there is evidence that the drug is effective in phase two clinical trials, phase three clinical trials are conducted to gather additional information on the drug's safety and effectiveness in several thousand volunteers. According to GAO's review of the National Institutes of Health's clinicaltrials.gov database, current research is investigating the effects of psilocybin on conditions such as depression, anxiety, headaches, fibromyalgia and other pain, substance use (including alcohol, tobacco, and opioids), eating disorders, obsessive- compulsive disorder, and post-traumatic stress disorder, among other things.[35]

Access to Investigational Drugs. Patients who are unable to participate in clinical trials may seek access to investigational drugs through two pathways: (1) expanded access and (2) the Right to Try Act.[36] Under either pathway, patients may only access the investigational drug if the drug sponsor agrees to provide access. Expanded access is the use of an investigational drug outside of clinical trials to treat patients with serious or immediately life-threatening diseases or conditions when there are no comparable or alternative satisfactory options.[37] Requests for expanded access must be reviewed by FDA and an Institutional Review Board. Patients diagnosed with life-threatening diseases or conditions who have exhausted approved treatment options may also be able to access investigational drugs through the Right to Try Act.[38] Unlike expanded access, the Right to Try Act does not require FDA or an institutional review board to review individual requests. The treating physician is responsible for requesting access to the investigational drug and for obtaining informed consent from the patient. FDA's role in implementing this Act is limited to receiving and posting certain information submitted to the agency.

---

[35] The National Institutes of Health's National Library of Medicine manages ClinicalTrials.gov, a website and online database of clinical research studies from around the world, including psilocybin-related clinical trials. The purpose of ClinicalTrials.gov is to provide information about clinical research studies to the public, researchers, and health care professionals. We reviewed the data including summaries and conditions studied for 139 clinical trials, as of September 18, 2023.

[36] Investigational drugs have not yet been approved by FDA.

[37] See 21 U.S.C. § 360bbb and 21 C.F.R. Part 312, Subpart I (2023).

[38] Trickett Wendler, Frank Mongiello, Jordan McLinn, and Matthew Bellina Right to Try Act of 2017, Pub. L. No. 115-176, 132 Stat. 1372 (2018) (codified at 21 U.S.C. § 360bbb-0a).

Breakthrough Therapies. Breakthrough therapy designation was established by the Food and Drug Administration Safety and Innovation Act and is a process designed to expedite the development and review of drugs intended to treat a serious or life-threatening disease or condition.[39] A sponsor of a drug may request FDA to designate the drug as a breakthrough therapy.[40] Not later than 60 calendar days after the receipt of a sponsor's request, FDA is required to determine whether the drug that is the subject of the request is intended, alone or in combination with one or more other drugs, to treat a serious or life-threatening disease or condition and preliminary clinical evidence indicates that the drug may demonstrate substantial improvement over existing therapies on one or more clinically significant endpoints, such as substantial treatment effects observed early in clinical development.[41] If FDA finds that the drug meets these criteria, FDA is required to designate the drug as a breakthrough therapy and take appropriate actions to expedite the development and review of the application for approval of such drug.[42] Two entities reported that FDA has granted breakthrough therapy designations: COMPASS Pathways for its psilocybin therapy treating treatment-resistant depression and Usona Institute for its psilocybin program treating major depressive disorder.[43]

Psilocybin Investigations, Forensic Laboratory Reports, and Seizures Are Few Relative to Other Schedule I Drugs

DEA Closed 24 Criminal Investigations in Which Psilocybin Was the Harshest Drug Involved During Fiscal Years 2018 through 2023

Over a 6-year period—fiscal years 2018 through 2023—the DEA closed a total of 24 investigations where psilocybin was the harshest drug involved, which

[39] Pub. L. No. 112-144, § 902, 126 Stat. 993, 1086-88 (2012).

[40] 21 U.S.C. § 356(a)(2).

[41] 21 U.S.C. § 356(a)(1), (a)(3)(A).

[42] 21 U.S.C. § 356(a)(3)(A).

[43] Compass Pathways is a biotechnology company dedicated to accelerating patient access to evidence-based innovation in mental health. The company studies investigational psilocybin therapy (also known as psilocybin treatment), administered with psychological support, as a treatment for certain mental health conditions. The Usona Institute is a medical research organization dedicated to supporting and conducting basic, pre-clinical and clinical research to further the scientific understanding and therapeutic application of consciousness-expanding medicines.

represents less than one percent of closed investigations involving all Schedule I controlled substances, according to DEA officials.[44] DEA officials added that because its data management system only records the drug involved in an investigation that is designated as the harshest, psilocybin may be involved in other DEA investigations but may be underreported due to the presence of harsher drugs, such as heroin or methamphetamine.[45] According to DEA officials, as of July 2023, the agency had 609 open investigations involving Schedule I controlled substances and psilocybin was the harshest drug in 16 of the investigations—representing about three percent of the total open investigations.[46] DEA officials said the agency usually focuses its investigative resources on controlled substances related cases that involve high-level drug trafficking organizations or are considered significant to the agency's enforcement efforts. Table 1 identifies the number of DEA closed investigations involving Schedule I controlled substances (including psilocybin) for each fiscal year—2018 through 2023.

Psilocybin-Related Reports Voluntarily Reported by Laboratories Increased but Were Less than One Percent of Overall Drug Reports from 2018 through 2022

According to our analysis of DEA's National Forensic Laboratory Information System drug component data,[47] the number of psilocybin-related reports (reports of psilocybin; psilocin, another Schedule I controlled substance derived from certain types of psychedelic mushrooms; and a combination of psilocybin and psilocin) increased from 1,598 in calendar year 2018 to 3,143

---

[44] DEA considers closed investigations to include cases where DEA has concluded all investigation and prosecutorial related activities.

[45] According to DEA officials, the harshest drugs include controlled substances considered to pose more serious public health and safety threats.

[46] According to DEA officials, the FBI has not initiated investigations exclusively related to psilocybin during fiscal years 2018 through 2023; however, it has encountered psilocybin in numerous investigations during the time period.

[47] The data in DEA's National Forensic Laboratory Information System is made up of data reported by forensic laboratories that voluntarily report the results of forensic testing and analysis conducted on substances seized by law enforcement operations. The term "report" is used to represent an item or exhibit that was secured in law enforcement operations and positively identified by a forensic laboratory to contain a particular substance, such as psilocybin.

in calendar year 2022.[48] This represented less than one percent of the total annual reports for each of the calendar years from 2018 through 2022. During this period, California, Illinois, Kansas, and Pennsylvania saw the largest increase in the number of psilocybin-related reports.

Table 1. Drug enforcement administration's closed investigations involving schedule i controlled substances for each fiscal year—2018 through 2023

Schedule I controlled substances[a]	Drug Enforcement Agency: Closed Investigations by Fiscal Year (FY)						
	FY 2018	FY 2019	FY 2020	FY 2021	FY 2022	FY 2023	Total closed investi-gations
Psilocybin	3	2	1	4	8	6	24
All other Schedule I controlled substances	1,602	2,587	2,526	2,721	2,582	1,847	13,865
Total closed investigations	1,605	2,589	2,527	2,725	2,590	1,853	13.889

Source: GAO analysis of DEA's enforcement data. | GAO-24-106630.

Note: According to DEA officials, DEA tracks its investigations by one drug type—typically the drug involved in the investigation that is considered the harshest by the agency.

[a] The Controlled Substances Act, Pub. L. No. 91-513, 84 Stat. 1242, places all federally controlled substances in one of five "schedules" depending, among other things, on the drug's likelihood for abuse or dependence, and whether the drug has an accepted medical use. These schedules range from I through V – with Schedule I having the greatest restrictions. Schedule I controlled substances are those that have been found to have a high potential for abuse, no currently accepted medical use in treatment in the United States, and a lack of accepted safety for use under medical supervision.

DEA's National Forensic Laboratory Information System systematically collects drug identification results and associated information from drug reports submitted to and analyzed by federal, state, and local forensic laboratories. The laboratory system includes voluntary participation from 50

[48] According to DEA officials, the data presented are sums of reports of psilocybin, psilocin, and psilocin and/or psilocybin. Psilocin (or "psilocyn") is a schedule I controlled substance found in psychedelic mushrooms. 21 U.S.C. § 812(c), Schedule I (c)(16).

state systems and 111 local or municipal laboratories, representing a total of 286 individual laboratories. DEA data include results for drug reports submitted by DEA agents, other federal law enforcement agencies, and select local police agencies. In addition to drug reports from DEA, reports from seven CBP laboratories are also included.

According to DEA officials, the forensic laboratories exist to support investigations and court cases. Figure 1 identifies the number of psilocybin-related drugs voluntarily reported by forensic laboratories in the various states for calendar years 2018 through 2022.

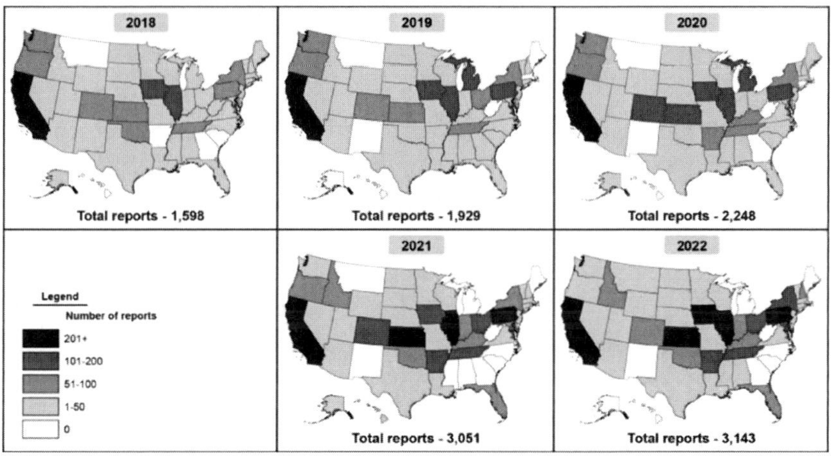

Source: GAO analysis of Drug enforcement Administration's National Forensic Laboratory Information System Data. | GAO-24-106630.

Note: The term "report" is used to represent an item or exhibit that was secured in law enforcement operations and positively identified by a forensic laboratory to contain a particular substance, such as psilocybin, psilocin, and psilocybin and/or psilocin. Psilocin (or "psilocyn") is a Schedule I controlled substance found in psychedelic mushrooms. 21 U.S.C. § 812(c), Schedule I (c)(16).

Figure 1. Number of Psilocybin-Related Reports Voluntarily-Reported by Forensic Laboratories by State, Calendar Years 2018 through 2022.

Federal Prosecution Data Do Not Track Psilocybin

For fiscal years 2018 through 2023, Executive Office for United States Attorneys (EOUSA) officials stated that it is unable to identify the number of cases prosecuted by U.S. Attorneys' offices related to psilocybin under the

Controlled Substances Act, including cases for simple possession, manufacturing, distributing, or dispensing of psilocybin, because this drug type is not specifically identified in CaseView or other database systems the U.S. Attorneys' offices use to manage cases.[49] However, according to EOUSA officials, the inability to identify these types of cases does not mean that DOJ has not and does not prosecute Controlled Substances Act violations related to psilocybin.

CBP Seizures Involving Psilocybin Accounted for About 2 Percent of the Agency's Total Drug Seizures During Fiscal Years 2018 through 2023

DHS's CBP reported the seizure of 49 different drug types—representing a total of 371,088 drug seizures—over the last 6-years (fiscal years 2018 through September 18, 2023). During this period, psilocybin accounted for 8,349 drug seizures—representing about 2 percent of the total seizures reported by CBP. Another Schedule I controlled substance that is classified as a hallucinogen, LSD,[50] accounted for 13,489 drug seizures—representing 4 percent of the total seizures reported by CBP during the same period. CBP's drug seizures most often involved marijuana[51] (80,583 seizures—representing about 22 percent of CBP's total seizures) during the 6-year time frame.

During fiscal years 2018 through September 18, 2023, CBP's seizure data show that the number and weight of its drug seizures involving psilocybin generally increased—accounting for about a 400 percent increase in the number of psilocybin seizures and over a 1,000 percent increase in the weight (in pounds) of the seizures. Over this six-year period, CBP's Chicago Field Office location accounted for about 37 percent (3,081), which is the CBP field office with the largest number of the seizures related to psilocybin. Figure 2 identifies the number and weight of CBP's drug seizures involving psilocybin for each fiscal year— 2018 through September 18, 2023.

---

[49] CaseView is the case management system for the U.S. Attorneys' offices.
[50] 21 U.S.C. § 812(c), Schedule I (c)(9).
[51] 21 U.S.C. § 812(c), Schedule I (c)(10) (referred to as "marihuana").

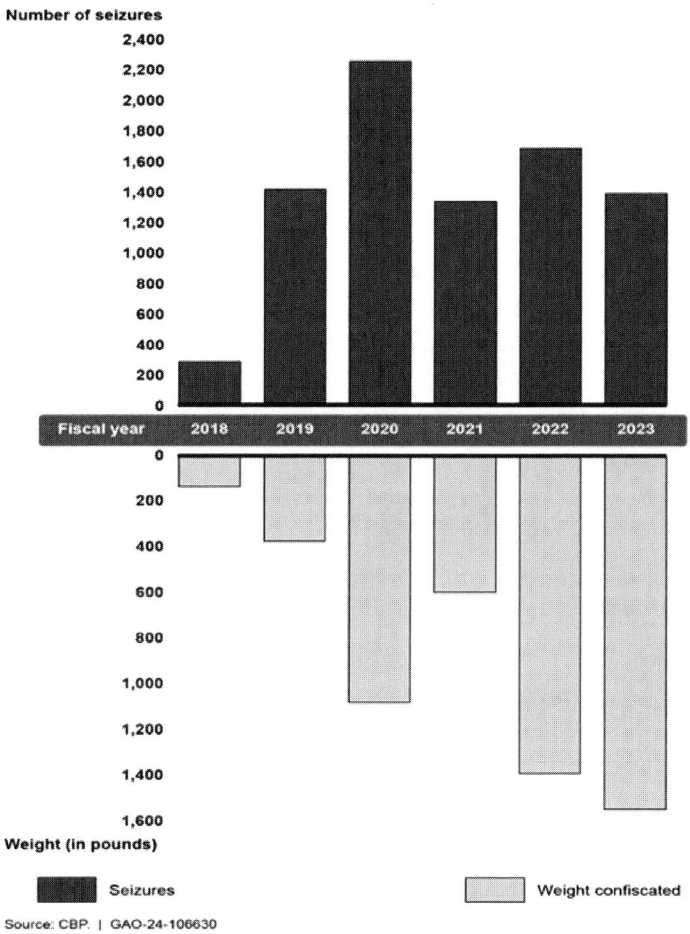

Source: GBP. | GAO-24-106630.

Figure 2. Number and Weight of U.S. Customs and Border Protection's Drug Seizures Involving Psilocybin for Each Fiscal Year, 2018 through September 18, 2023.

Application Process to Conduct Psilocybin Research and Stakeholders' Perspectives

To conduct research involving psilocybin, researchers must (1) obtain approvals from their respective states and institutions, (2) be registered with DEA to conduct research with schedule I controlled substances and be authorized to carry out a specific research protocol involving psilocybin,[52] and (3) if the research involves human subjects (clinical trials), submit to FDA an investigational new drug (IND) application, which must be in effect at the time the research is being conducted.[53] In 2022, DEA updated its Researcher's Manual, which provides guidance for new and current research registrants who intend to conduct research with Schedule I controlled substances, such as psilocybin.[54] The guidance outlines DEA's requirements for researchers related to registration, ordering, recordkeeping, inventory, storage, and disposal of controlled substances. Based on the guidance, a researcher's registration must be renewed annually. Figure 3 provides an overview of the process to obtain authorization to conduct research on Schedule I controlled substances.

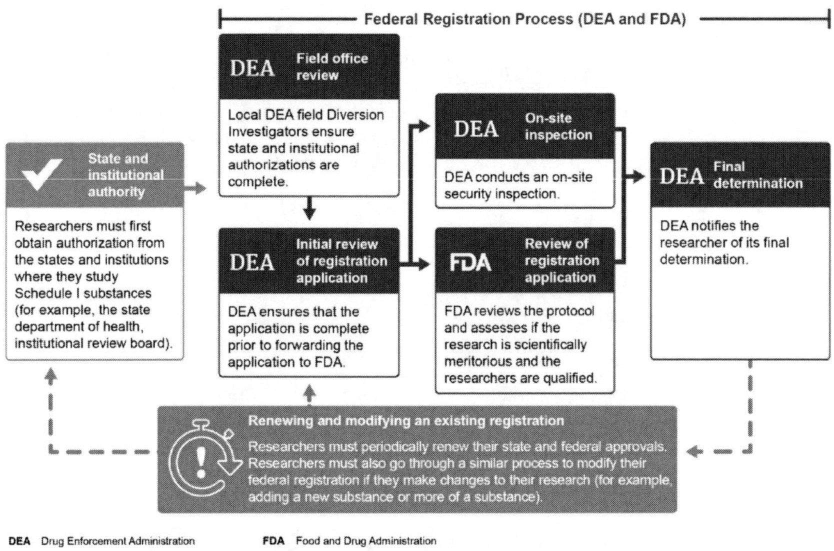

Source: GAO analysis of DEA and FDA information; agency logos courtecy of respective agencies; GAO adaptation of AtScene/stock.adobe.com illustration (clock); GAO (icon). | GAO-24-106630.

Figure 3. The Process to Obtain Authorization to Conduct Research on Schedule I Controlled Substances.

---

[52] 21 U.S.C. § 823(g)(2); 21 C.F.R. §§ 1301.18, 1308.32.

[53] 21 U.S.C. § 355(i); 21 C.F.R. Part 312 (2023).

[54] DOJ, Drug Enforcement Administration, Diversion Control Division, *Researcher's Manual: An Informational Outline of the Controlled Substances Act* (Revised 2022) DEA- DC-057, EO-DEA217 (Springfield, VA.: June 15, 2022).

State and institutional authorization. Before applying for DEA registration, researchers must obtain authorization from their sponsoring institution and the state in which the institution is registered with the DEA. Specific requirements vary by state and institution, and applicants may contact their local diversion field office on clarification on state laws and regulations before completing their application, according to DEA's research manual.

Initial DEA review of registration application. After obtaining the necessary state and institutional authorization, a researcher must apply to receive a registration from DEA. DEA's Registration and Program Support Section receives registration applications and DEA's Drug and Chemical Evaluation Section reviews the applications for completeness.

Applications are to include information such as the researcher's professional curriculum vitae, substances being studied and their amounts, and the location(s) where the research will take place.

FDA review of investigational new drug application. Before obtaining a DEA registration, researchers who intend to conduct investigations involving human subjects (clinical trials) are required to submit an IND application to FDA.[55] During this time, FDA has an opportunity to review. Generally, an IND application goes into effect 30 days after it has been submitted, unless FDA issues a clinical hold to delay the proposed trial. During this time, FDA has an opportunity to review the application to ensure the safety and rights of trial participants.

FDA review of registration application and DEA onsite inspection. Once DEA completes its initial review to ensure the application is complete, it sends the application to FDA for review and determination on whether applicants are qualified and the research protocol has scientific merit.[56] Simultaneously, DEA's field offices conduct an on-site inspection of research facilities for security of the controlled substances and a background inspection of the researcher and individuals handling the controlled substances.

DEA final review and determination. Following FDA advisement to DEA on the research protocol merits and investigator qualifications, the diversion investigator assigned to the registration application can make the final determination to approve or deny the application. Once the on- site inspection and all related matters are complete, DEA notifies the researcher of its final determination.

---

[55] 21 U.S.C. § 355(i); 21 C.F.R. Part 312 (2023).

[56] 21 U.S.C. § 823(g)(2); 21 C.F.R. § 1308.32.

DEA uses the Registrant Information Consolidated System to review applications requesting authority to conduct Schedule I-based research and manages DEA's research registrant data for those approved to work with controlled substances.[57] Based on DEA's data, in fiscal year 2018, the new registrations approved for psilocybin studies represented about 3 percent (4 out of 153 approvals) of the new research registrations for all Schedule I controlled substances. In fiscal year 2022, the new registrations approved for psilocybin studies increased to about 29 percent (39 out of 134 approvals) of the new research registrations for all Schedule I controlled substances. See table 2 for additional information on DEA's new research registration approvals for each fiscal year—2018 through 2023.

Table 2. Drug Enforcement Administration's (DEA) new research registrations for each fiscal year—2018 through 2023

New research registrations	Number of DEA's New Research Registrations by Fiscal Year (FY)					
	FY 2018	FY 2019	FY 2020	FY 2021	FY 2022	FY 2023 (partial)[a]
	4	11	16	26	39	28
Psilocybin approvals						
	153	*189*	*113*	*120*	134	71
Total Schedule I drug approvals						

Source: Data from DEA's Registrant Information Consolidated System. | GAO-24-106630.

Note: The new research registrations approvals for the psilocybin category are a subset of the category for the total new research registrations for Schedule I drug approvals.

[a] The fiscal year 2023 data represent the period covering October 1 through March 31. The data for the remaining fiscal years represent the period covering October 1 through September 30.

Based on DEA's data, in fiscal year 2018, the active registrations for psilocybin studies represented about 5 percent (32 out of 693 approvals) of the active research registrations for all Schedule I drugs. In fiscal year 2022, the active registrations approved for psilocybin studies increased to about 18 percent (148 out of 819 approvals) of the active research registrations for all

[57] The Registrant Information Consolidated System is a database that consolidates several of DEA's internal systems, each with its own uniquely different functions, that DEA uses to manage all registrant actions and information records. In addition, the system allows DEA field divisions to know when registrants are being investigated at the national level to avoid duplicate efforts.

Schedule I controlled substances. See table 3 for additional information on DEA's active approved research registrations for each fiscal year—2018 through 2023.

Table 3. Drug Enforcement Administration's (DEA) active approved research registrations for each fiscal year—2018 through 2023

Active approved research registrations	Number of DEA's Active Research Registrations by Fiscal Year (FY)					
	FY 2018	FY 2019	FY 2020	FY 2021	FY 2022	FY 2023 (partial)[a]
	32	47	65	100	148	181
Psilocybin registrations						
	693	820	832	804	819	842
All Schedule I drug registrations						

Source: Data from DEA's Registrant Information Consolidated System. | GAO-24-106630.

Note: The active research registrations approvals for the psilocybin category are a subset of the category for the total active research registrations for Schedule I drug approvals.

[a] The fiscal year 2023 data represent the period covering October 1 through March 31. The data for the remaining fiscal years represent the period covering October 1 through September 30.

Selected stakeholders we interviewed provided feedback on DEA's process for authorizing research to study a Schedule I controlled substance.[58] We also obtained comments from DEA officials regarding some of the concerns shared by these stakeholders.

License requirements. According to a selected stakeholder from a large university, they must obtain a DEA license for each building included in a psilocybin-related study. The stakeholder said that these steps are redundant and time consuming for a registrant with one study across multiple buildings. By regulation, a separate registration is required for each principal place of business or professional practice at one general physical location where

---

[58] We interviewed four stakeholder organizations representing two universities and two research institutes that sponsor psilocybin-based research. We selected these stakeholders based on the literature reviews we conducted, and comments received from individuals regarded as knowledgeable and considered to have a high-level of experience in psilocybin-based clinical research.

controlled substances are manufactured, distributed, imported, exported, or dispensed by a person.[59] DEA officials explained that this requirement is intended to prevent diversion as the transport of a controlled substance from one location to another can be a security risk.[60]

Time requirements. According to a selected stakeholder who represented an organization involved in psilocybin-related research, the DEA registration process has detailed requirements that take up staff time and lead to delays without adding significantly to preventing the misuse of a controlled substance. DEA officials stated the longest delay in processing an application is typically when waiting for an applicant to provide all the necessary information to complete their application package. The officials added that the research protocols (i.e., Institutional Review Board, Institutional Animal Care and Use Committee approval documentation, investigational new drug application, drug amount/quantity/source, security, and storage specifications) are all documents and information that the researchers should have in place before applying for a DEA registration. The DEA officials said the application package does not require new or novel information; rather, it simply requires the transmission of information the researchers should already have or know. DEA cannot transmit the application package to FDA for review until all the necessary information is obtained. According to DEA officials, DEA staff work with researchers to gather all the necessary documentation to assure compliance with the Controlled Substances Act.

DEA headquarters communication. According to a selected researcher who represented an organization involved in psilocybin-related research, researchers' communication with DEA headquarters is challenging unless working with a specific point of contact. For example, some emails sent to DEA headquarters' general email inboxes either bounce back or go unanswered. DEA officials noted that it could not speak to all the agency's general email inboxes but described the inbox for Schedule I research inquiries as being regularly monitored, and that its messages are swiftly responded to by staff.

---

[59] 21 C.F.R. § 1301.12(a).

[60] According to DEA, many problems associated with drug abuse are the result of legitimately made controlled substances being diverted from their lawful purpose into illicit drug traffic. DEA's Diversion Control Division is tasked to prevent, detect, and investigate the diversion of controlled pharmaceuticals and listed chemicals from legitimate sources while ensuring an adequate and uninterrupted supply for legitimate medical, commercial, and scientific needs.

DEA not communicating with sponsors. One selected stakeholder operating as a sponsor of psilocybin-based research explained that DEA's refusal to communicate directly with sponsors prolonged the challenges one of their researchers had been experiencing. In this instance, the researcher had questions regarding DEA Form 222 but had not received support from DEA, leaving the researcher to approach their sponsor for guidance which forced the two parties to spend time screen- sharing to trouble-shoot the issue.[61]

DEA officials explained that all agency communications be made directly with research registrants due to privacy concerns. The DEA referenced that research registrants may provide explicit permission for DEA to communicate with an approved party, like a sponsor. According to DEA officials, sponsors and contractors who represent sponsors are not registrants. DEA staff do work with sponsors in general terms to help them prepare for large, multi-site studies to assure the approval process goes as smoothly as possible. The DEA officials stated that when dealing with specific registrations and applications, communications are directed to the researcher. In addition, researchers can seek clarification and help through their assigned diversion investigator and the DPEScheduleIResearch@dea.gov mailbox.

The same selected stakeholders we spoke with also provided general perspectives on the process to obtain federal authorization to conduct research with a Schedule I controlled substance.

Working with FDA. One selected stakeholder described FDA as being very involved and communicative throughout the process, while characterizing FDA's involvement as friendly and helpful. Additionally, this selected stakeholder noted that the requirements set by FDA were relevant to the safety of research participants and appeared to be appropriate for such research to take place. According to DEA officials, this comment may be relevant to the IND application review process, which is different from the Schedule I research review process. FDA's controlled substances personnel do not communicate directly with researchers, instead communicating back to DEA to address any concerns.

Local DEA offices. Another selected researcher highlighted their local DEA office as being very responsive and accessible, which has enabled them to receive timely responses to questions throughout the process.

---

[61] DEA's Office of Diversion Control will accept requests from distributors that require a large volume of Order Forms (DEA Form 222)—the forms are used for the distribution of a Schedule I or II controlled substance.

Inventory record-keeping requirements. One selected stakeholder stated that the federal requirements set for the record-keeping of its inventory were not too burdensome as they are considered standard requirements for research laboratories to uphold. With respect to researchers, generally, each person registered or authorized to dispense or conduct research with controlled substances is required by regulation to include in the inventory a complete and accurate record of all controlled substances on hand on the date the inventory is taken. For example, this inventory is required to include for each controlled substance in finished form, the name of the substance; each finished form of the substance; the number of units or volume of each finished form in each commercial container; and the number of commercial containers of each such finished form.[62]

Aspects of DEA's Religious Freedom Restoration Act Exemption Review Process Are Unclear to Petitioners

DEA Established a Petition for Religious Exemption to Meet Legal Requirements

DEA established a process for individuals and entities to apply for religious exemption to the Controlled Substances Act under the Religious Freedom Restoration Act in response to a Supreme Court case. The Supreme Court held that government action taken pursuant to the Controlled Substances Act is subject to the Religious Freedom Restoration Act. Under the Religious Freedom Restoration Act, the federal government may not substantially burden a person's exercise of religion, even if the burden results from a rule of general applicability.[63]

DEA Established a Process for Applying for Religious Exemption to the Controlled Substances Act Under the Religious Freedom Restoration Act in Response to a Supreme Court Case

Gonzales v. O Centro – Compelling Interest Test

[62] 21 C.F.R. § 1304.11.
[63] 42 U.S.C. § 2000bb-1(a).

In O Centro, a religious sect brought suit, seeking to preliminarily enjoin the federal government from enforcing the Controlled Substances Act to ban the sect's use of hoasca (or ayahuasca), a tea containing a Schedule I controlled substance, dimethyltryptamine (DMT), in religious ceremonies. After U.S. Customs inspectors seized a hoasca shipment to the religious sect and threatened prosecution, the sect filed a suit for declaratory and injunctive relief, alleging that applying the Controlled Substances Act to the sect's sacramental hoasca use violated the Religious Freedom Restoration Act. The federal government conceded that the challenged application would substantially burden a sincere exercise of religion but argued that this burden did not violate the Religious Freedom Restoration Act because applying the Controlled Substances Act was the least restrictive means of advancing three compelling governmental interests and does not allow exceptions.

Source: Gonzales v. O Centro Espirita Beneficente Uniao do Vegetal, 546 U.S. 418 (2006). | GAO-24-106630.

The only exception recognized by the statute requires the government to satisfy the compelling interest test. This means the government must show that the application of the burden to the person is in furtherance of a compelling governmental interest and is the least restrictive means of furthering that compelling governmental interest.[64] A person whose religious exercise has been burdened in violation of the statute may assert that violation as a claim or defense in a judicial proceeding and obtain appropriate relief against a government.[65]

The Controlled Substances Act generally prohibits the unauthorized handling of controlled substances. Thus, for individuals and entities who want to engage in the use, manufacture, importation, or dispensing of controlled substances for religious purposes or ceremonies, the Controlled Substances Act may conflict with the Religious Freedom Restoration Act. This is because, as held by the Supreme Court, the Religious Freedom Restoration Act prohibits DEA from burdening an individual's free exercise of sincerely held religious beliefs through action taken pursuant to the Controlled Substances Act unless DEA can demonstrate that the burden advances a compelling governmental interest and is carried out with the least restrictive means.[66]

---

[64] 42 U.S.C. § 2000bb-1(a)-(b).

[65] 42 U.S.C. § 2000bb-1(c).

[66] Gonzales v. O Centro Espirita Beneficente Uniao do Vegetal, 546 U.S. 418 (2006).

DEA Established a Process for Applying for Religious Exemption to the Controlled Substances Act Under the Religious Freedom Restoration Act in Response to a Supreme Court Case

The Supreme Court indicated that under the more focused inquiry required by the Religious Freedom Restoration Act and the compelling interest test, the government's mere invocation of the general characteristics of Schedule I substances, as set forth in the Controlled Substances Act, was not sufficient. Rather, the Supreme Court indicated that the Religious Freedom Restoration Act and its strict scrutiny test required the federal "[g]overnment to demonstrate that the compelling interest test is satisfied through application of the challenged law 'to the person'—the particular claimant whose sincere exercise of religion is being substantially burdened."

Source: Gonzales v. O Centro Espirita Beneficente Uniao do Vegetal, 546 U.S. 418 (2006). | GAO-24-106630.

According to DEA, it recognized that the Supreme Court decision required DEA to engage in a case-by-case analysis of religious exemptions to the Controlled Substances Act in order to strike sensible balances of interests based on desired religious uses of controlled substances.[67] As such, DEA first promulgated a guidance document in 2009 to establish a procedure for seeking religious exemptions from the Controlled Substances Act pursuant to the Religious Freedom Restoration Act. This guidance, entitled *Guidance Regarding Petitions for Religious Exemption from the Controlled Substances Act Pursuant to the Religious Freedom Restoration Act (Revised)*, was most recently updated in November 2020.[68]

---

[67] In Soul Quest Church of Mother Earth, Inc. v. Attorney General, No. 22-110722, 2023 WL 8714320 (11th Cir. 2023), the Eleventh Circuit Court of Appeals found that "[t]he DEA's religious exemption process and the accompanying Religious Freedom Restoration Act Guidelines were a direct response to the Supreme Court's warning in O Centro that [the Religious Freedom Restoration Act] may warrant accommodations to the Controlled Substances Act," and "[t]herefore, it was entirely appropriate that the DEA seek to reconcile the two statutes and that the agency consider [individuals'] rights under [the Religious Freedom Restoration Act] when implementing the Controlled Substances Act."

[68] DEA, Guidance Regarding Petitions for Religious Exemption from the Controlled Substances Act Pursuant to the Religious Freedom Restoration Act (Revised). Accessed November 16, 2023.

DEA's guidance generally sets forth a process for obtaining a religious exemption for the use of controlled substances. Parties requesting religious exemptions from the Controlled Substances Act must submit a petition in writing or email to DEA's Diversion Control Division. The guidance indicates that a petition may include both a written statement and supporting documents and a petitioner should provide as much information as the petitioner deems necessary to demonstrate that application of the Controlled Substances Act to the party's activity would (1) be a substantial burden on (2) the petitioner's sincere (3) religious exercise. The guidance also indicates the record should include detailed information about, among other things, (1) the nature of the religion; (2) each specific religious practice that involves the manufacture, distribution, dispensing, importation, exportation, use or possession of a controlled substance; (3) the specific controlled substance that the party wishes to use; and (4) the amounts, conditions, and locations of its anticipated manufacture, distribution, dispensing, importation, exportation, use or possession. In addition, the guidance provides that the petitioner may submit any and all information they believe to be relevant to DEA's determination under the Religious Freedom Restoration Act and the Controlled Substances Act.

In a recent decision, the Court of Appeals for the Eleventh Circuit held that this "petition [is] the first step, a prerequisite to obtaining permission to handle a controlled substance."[69] In accordance with that holding, should the petition be granted, the second step under the guidance is for the petitioner to apply for and receive a DEA Certificate of Registration.[70] The guidance directs that no petitioner may engage in any activity prohibited under the Controlled Substances Act or its regulations unless the petition has been granted and the petitioner has applied for and received a DEA Certificate of Registration.

This means that even a petitioner whose petition for a religious exemption from the Controlled Substances Act is granted remains bound by all applicable laws and Controlled Substances Act regulations governing registration,

---

[69] Soul Quest Church of Mother Earth, Inc. v Attorney General, No. 22-110722, 2023 WL 8714320 (11th Cir. 2023).

[70] Generally, pursuant to 21 U.S.C. § 823(a), DEA considers whether the requested registration is consistent with the public interest. In evaluating the public interest, DEA generally considers various factors, including: (1) the need to maintain effective control against diversion of the controlled substances into non-legitimate channels; (2) the applicant's compliance with applicable state and local law regarding use of the controlled substance; (3) whether the applicant has any prior convictions relating to controlled- substance manufacture, distribution, or dispensing; (4) the applicant's past experience in manufacturing controlled substances; and (5) other factors that may be relevant to and consistent with the public health and safety.

labeling and packaging, quotas, recordkeeping and reporting, security and storage, and periodic inspections, among other things.[71] The guidance states that a petitioner seeking exemption from these Controlled Substances Act regulations may petition under 21 C.F.R. § 1307.03, and the "petition must separately address each regulation from which the petitioner seeks exemption and provide a statement of the reasons for each exemption sought."[72] The regulation provides for those petitions to be submitted to DEA's Office of Diversion Control.

Court of Appeals for the Eleventh Circuit Recognition of DEA's Process for Religious Exemptions to the Controlled Substances Act under the Religious Freedom Restoration Act

Soul Quest Church of Mother Earth, Inc. – Appeal

In December 2023, the Eleventh Circuit Court of Appeals, in response to an appeal filed by Soul Quest Church of Mother Earth, Inc. ("Soul Quest") seeking to legally use and handle a sacramental tea known as ayahuasca, described the two-step process for obtaining a religious exemption for the use of controlled substances from DEA's guidance. The court said that the petition was the first step, a prerequisite to obtaining a permission to handle a controlled substance. The court further stated that even if the DEA granted a petition, a petitioner must continue to refrain from engaging in any activity prohibited under the Controlled Substances Act or its regulations until the petitioner has applied for and received a Certificate of Registration. The court also noted that the Controlled Substances Act and its attendant regulations permit a waiver of Controlled Substances Act provisions, including registration, as a potential alternative route to lawful use of controlled substances.

Source: Soul Quest Church of Mother Earth, Inc. v. Attorney General, No. 22-110722, 2023 WL 8714320 (11th Cir.2023). | GAO-24-106630.

According to DEA officials, in 2019, DEA initiated the drafting of a notice of proposed rulemaking related to DEA's process for petitioning for

[71] See 21 C.F.R. pts. 1300-1316.

[72] 21 C.F.R. § 1307.03. See also 21 U.S.C. § 822(d) (permitting the Attorney General, by regulation, to waive the requirement for registration of certain manufacturers, distributors, or dispensers if he finds it consistent with the public health and safety).

religious exemptions to the Controlled Substances Act under the Religious Freedom Restoration Act. According to DEA, the draft notice was developed and drafted by DEA's Diversion Control Division and the Office of Chief Counsel. In addition, the notice of proposed rulemaking is listed on the Fall 2023 Unified Agenda of Regulatory and Deregulatory Actions as a DEA priority. According to the Unified Agenda, DEA proposes to amend its regulations to accommodate religious entities who seek to apply for a DEA registration based on the terms of the Religious Freedom Restoration Act. Additionally, DEA also proposes regulatory amendments to incorporate and accommodate religious entities under the regulatory framework and proposes certain related, but generally applicable changes to regulatory definitions, application procedures, and hearing procedures. However, DEA has no estimated timeline for issuing the notice of proposed rulemaking, according to DEA officials.

Court of Appeals for the Eleventh Circuit Recognition of DEA's Process for Religious Exemptions to the Controlled Substances Act under the Religious Freedom Restoration Act

In the case of Soul Quest, the court found that Soul Quest did not seek a waiver of any provision, and that DEA classified Soul Quest as an applicant for registration, deeming its petition for exemption to be commensurate with an application for registration. DEA denied Soul Quest's petition. DEA found that Soul Quest's promotion of ayahuasca to the public for self-help and therapeutic reasons was not a sincere exercise of religion under the Religious Freedom Restoration Act. In addition, DEA determined that even assuming Soul Quest had proven the sincerity of its religious belief and that Controlled Substances Act enforcement would be a substantial burden on its religious exercise, Soul Quest's religious practices could not be accommodated in a manner that would allow DEA to preserve its compelling interests in public health and safety and in preventing the illegal diversion of ayahuasca. The court found that DEA's denial of Soul Quest's petition for religious exemption to the Controlled Substances Act was a denial at the first step of the two-step process; however, the court also said that because this denial precluded Soul Quest from applying for registration, it was also a decision made under the Controlled Substances Act. In addition, the court found that DEA discussed whether Soul Quest's handling of ayahuasca was consistent with public health and safety and whether the church maintained effective controls against diversion, which are relevant to the Controlled Substances Act's registration process. As such, the court held that "DEA's final decision adjudicated both [the church's Religious Freedom Restoration Act] right and its ultimate right to a Certificate of Registration under the [Controlled Substances Act]."

Source: Soul Quest Church of Mother Earth, Inc. v. Attorney General, No. 22-110722, 2023 WL 8714320 (11th Cir. 2023). | GAO-24-106630.

DEA Has a Process to Review Petitions and Conduct Investigations

DEA's assessment process for petitions submitted under the Religious Freedom Restoration Act is applied across all petitions to include the use of an internal tracking system to identify where each petition is in the review process, according to DEA. Further, DEA indicated that it ensures that all petitions are handled using consistent procedures, which are outlined in the guidance posted on the Diversion Control Division website.

According to DEA officials, DEA also is responsible for conducting on-site visits and interviews which, according to DEA officials, also serve an educational purpose to inform the petitioner about DEA's regulatory requirements. In addition, DEA investigates a petitioner's past conduct, as it may indicate the ability to properly handle controlled substances.

According to DEA, following the on-site visits and interviews with the petitioner, a field report is submitted. DEA's Diversion Control Division reviews the petition in its entirety and all information provided by the field office. According to DEA officials, these reviews are to be done on a case-by-case basis, and the facts and information pertaining to the Religious Freedom Restoration Act petition will be assessed in light of public health and welfare interest factors, as well as religious sincerity considerations. If necessary, the Diversion Control Division may direct the field to request further information from the petitioner, or to conduct additional interviews or investigations with the petitioner or related third- parties. As a result of this review, the Diversion Control Division is to make a decision to grant or deny the petition.

According to DEA officials, the agency's processing times for religious exemption petitions may vary greatly based on various factors. For example, DEA officials stated that common issues with these petitions may include unsuccessful attempts to locate a petitioner, insufficient information to determine whether a religious belief is sincerely held, unsafe practices that may threaten the public health and safety, prior criminal convictions, and inability of a petitioner to meet reasonable/minimum security requirements to prevent the diversion of controlled substances. Figure 4 provides an overview of the process to obtain a Religious Freedom Restoration Act exemption to the Controlled Substances Act to permit the use of controlled substances.

Petition is submitted. A petitioner submits a petition for a religious exemption from the Controlled Substances Act under the Religious Freedom Restoration Act that would permit the use of controlled substances. The guidance indicates that a petition may include both a written statement and supporting documents and a petitioner should provide as much information as the petitioner deems necessary to demonstrate that application of the Controlled Substances Act to the party's activity would (1) be a substantial burden on (2) the petitioner's sincere (3) religious exercise. According to the guidance, the petition is to be submitted in writing or email to the Assistant Administrator, Diversion Control Division, DEA. In addition, the petition must be signed by the petitioner, who must declare under penalty of perjury that the information provided therein is true and correct.

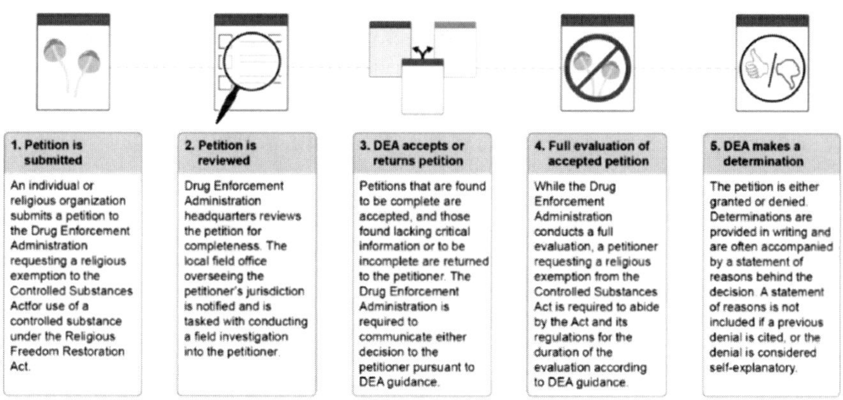

Source: GAO analysis of DEA documentation; GAO (icons), Myurent/adobestock.com. | GAO-24-106630.

Figure 4. Drug Enforcement Administration's Religious Freedom Restoration Act Review Process.

Petition is reviewed. According to DEA, DEA's Diversion Regulatory Section reviews the petition, checking for the following information:

- the nature of the religion (e.g., its history, belief system, structure, practice, membership policies, rituals, holidays, organization, leadership, etc.);
- each specific religious practice that involves the manufacture, distribution, dispensing, importation, exportation, use or possession of a controlled substance;
- the specific controlled substance that the party wishes to use; and
- the amounts, conditions, and locations of its anticipated manufacture, distribution, dispensing, importation, exportation, use or possession.

DEA accepts or returns petition. According to DEA guidance, if a petition is found to be incomplete or have insufficient information, it will be returned with a statement of the reason explaining why it was not accepted. The petitioner may correct and resubmit a deficient petition. It is the petitioner's responsibility to provide DEA with accurate contact information. If a petitioner does not respond to a request for additional information within 60 days from the date of DEA's request, the petition will be considered to be withdrawn, according to the guidance.

Full evaluation of accepted petition. The DEA guidance indicates that the petitioner must not engage in any activity prohibited under the Controlled Substances Act or its regulations during the review period.

Two attorneys we spoke with said that included petitioners refraining from any religious sacraments that involve the controlled substance referenced in the petition.

DEA makes a determination. Once the full evaluation has been completed, including all submissions in response to any requests for additional information, the Assistant Administrator of the Diversion Control Division will provide the petitioner with a written response on the outcome, according to DEA. According to DEA guidance, the written response is a final determination under 21 U.S.C. § 877 and as such can then be reviewed in the United States Court of Appeals for the District of Columbia or for the circuit in which the principal place of business is located. Under that statutory provision, the petitioner has thirty days after notice of the decision to file their petition for review.

Aspects of Process and Timeframes for Review of Petitions Were Unclear to Selected Stakeholders

A select group of nine individuals from law firms and advocacy organizations told us the DEA's religious freedom exemption review process is difficult to navigate and lacks clear guidance in some instances.[73] Specifically, they found challenges with burdensome requirements, lack of clarity and communication related to processing time, and general lack of faith in the DEA's review process. See appendix V for additional perspectives we obtained related to the challenges and barriers that exist in the legal access and use of psilocybin for religious practices under the Religious Freedom Restoration Act.

Burden of DEA requirements for Religious Freedom Restoration Act exemptions. According to three of nine selected stakeholders, the amount of information required throughout the Religious Freedom Restoration Act petition process can be overly burdensome. For example, a stakeholder told us that they do not know how much and what type of information DEA would consider to be proof of religious sincerity. Such a requirement can be especially true for those petitioners who come from cultures where psilocybin has been used for generations and do not maintain documentation to prove their use of psilocybin is sincere, according to stakeholders.

In adjudicating a petition that was made public pursuant to litigation, DEA applied the "compelling interest test" from the Religious Freedom Restoration Act and the Supreme Court case *O Centro.* DEA further applied the case law interpreting it, in addition to relying upon its investigation of the petitioner. This is consistent with internal DEA guidance we reviewed that draws upon relevant factors from case law related to the Religious Freedom Restoration Act to be considered in making a threshold determination under the Act, as well as the various kinds of information that investigators should seek to collect. However, DEA's guidance does not provide the standard the agency will use to assess "religious sincerity" or other aspects of the application. DEA officials told us the agency continuously reevaluates certain areas to prevent any unnecessary burden on the petitioner and its internal processes.

Lack of clarity and communication. According to five of nine selected stakeholders we spoke with, DEA's Religious Freedom Restoration Act guidance and lack of communication make the process to obtain a religious

---

[73] We selected nine individuals from law firms and advocacy organizations that represent a range of perspectives on the barriers, if any, that exist in the legal access to and use of psilocybin for religious, indigenous, or spiritual practices under the Religious Freedom Restoration Act.

exemption to the Controlled Substances Act under the Religious Freedom Restoration Act confusing. For example, the DEA guidance requires petitioners to provide documentation on a belief system, structure, and practice, but the guidance does not explicitly state what type of documentation would sufficiently address this requirement. And while the guidance provides a petition process for a "religious exemption" from the Controlled Substance Act, it states that successful petitioners remain bound by all applicable laws and Controlled Substances Act regulations without indicating that petitioners may have additional claims under the Religious Freedom Restoration Act for exemptions from those regulations.[74]

Additionally, stakeholders shared that DEA does not answer petitioners' questions after a petition has been submitted, leaving petitioners unaware of their petition's status, potentially for years. The lack of petition review updates and expected dates for processing outcomes in the DEA's guidance were specifically cited as challenges in the DEA's processing of petitions. Such status updates may involve DEA determining a petition as having insufficient information. DEA officials stated that generally local field offices are the primary point of contact for petitioners, unless specific circumstances are in place requiring input from DEA's Office of Chief Counsel. Officials added that a petitioner may communicate with their local DEA field office to receive an update on the processing status of their petition at any time. However, DEA's guidance does not identify local DEA offices as a point of contact for petitioners. Additionally, DEA officials noted that they are aware of public comments on the need to better understand DEA's policies and processes that impact their petitions. In response, DEA stated it has conducted an assessment resulting in possible resolutions to address these needs.[75]

Processing timelines for petitions. Five of nine selected stakeholders highlighted that the absence of a clear benchmark for processing has enabled the petitioning process to become a lengthy procedure. Another selected stakeholder further illustrated this by describing the processing period as an activity lasting for an undetermined time. Over an 8-year period—fiscal year 2016 through January 2024—DEA reported that 24 petitioners requested a religious exemption from the Controlled Substances Act under the Religious Freedom Restoration Act. As of January 2024, DEA's information indicated

---

[74] As noted above, DEA's guidance states that a petitioner seeking exemption from Controlled Substances Act regulations may petition under 21 C.F.R. § 1307.03.

[75] DEA's possible resolutions include but are not limited to, streamlining internal processes, regulatory drafting, and revision of online guidance and additional investigative guides to field investigators.

that none of these petitioners were granted a religious exemption. Specifically, based on DEA's information, two of the 24 petitioners were denied a religious exemption.[76]

There are also 14 petitioners that are pending a determination related to a religious exemption and 8 petitioners that withdrew from consideration, according to DEA's information. Of the 24 petitioners requesting a religious exemption, DEA reported that 6 petitioners requested a religious exemption related to psilocybin—three withdrawing and three pending a determination from DEA. Based on DEA's information, the "date of receipt" to "date of action(s)" for petitioners that withdrew their requests related to psilocybin ranged from about 7 months to over 4 years.

Additionally, petitioners' exemption requests related to psilocybin that are pending a DEA determination ranged from about 8 months to over 3 years from the date of receipt. Over the 8-year period, based on DEA's information, we identified instances where DEA's finalized actions regarding petitions related to other controlled substances have been pending a DEA determination for an extensive period—one almost 5 years and one almost 8 years.[77] Figure 5 identifies DEA's processing time(s)—"date of receipt" to "date of action"—for each of the 24 petitioners that requested a religious exemption from the Controlled Substances Act under the Religious Freedom Restoration Act, fiscal year 2016 through January 2024.

In 2017, petitioners from the Soul Quest Church requested a religious exemption from the Controlled Substances Act. After three years without a response from DEA, the petitioner, Soul Quest, filed a complaint against the DEA in federal district court and an accompanying motion seeking declaratory and injunctive relief. Soul Quest claimed that through the DEA's failure to respond to its petition, the agency violated Soul Quest's right to the free exercise of religion and its rights under the Religious Freedom Restoration Act. According to the Eleventh Circuit decision, shortly afterward, DEA responded to Soul Quest with an undated letter confirming receipt of the petition.

---

[76] Based on DEA's information, one petitioner was denied a religious exemption after nearly 9 months, while the other petitioner was denied a religious exemption after more than 3 years.

[77] Based on DEA's guidance, the agency's final determination or action regarding a petition for a religious exemption is categorized as either granted (approved), or denied.

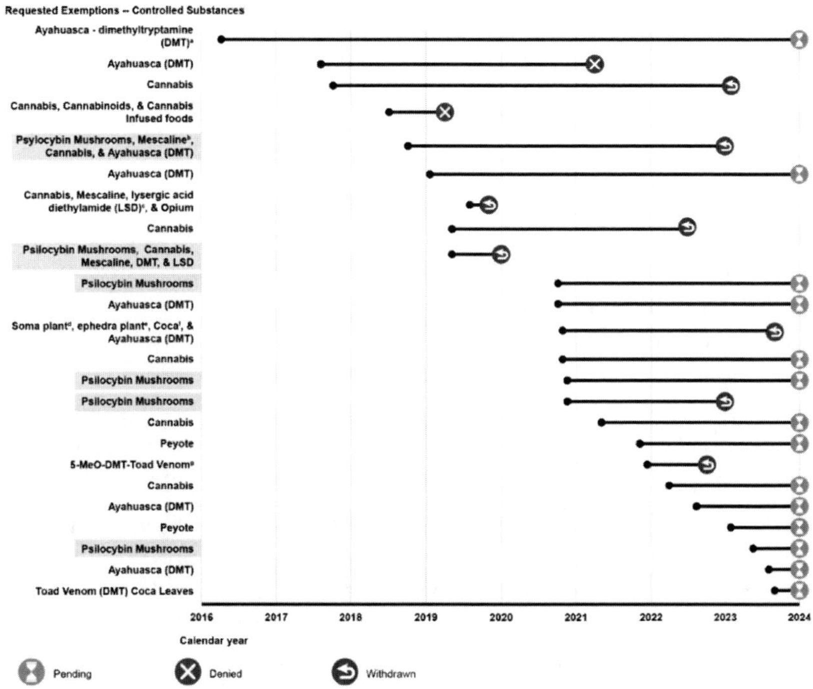

Source: GAO analysis of DEA information. | GAO-24-106630.

Note: The DEA processing times information presented reflects the fiscal year 2016 through January 2024 time frame.

[a] Ayahuasca is a tea containing a Schedule I controlled substance, dimethyltryptamine (DMT). DMT is a hallucinogen that is found in a number of plant materials and can be extracted or synthetically produced.

[b] Mescaline is the active hallucinogen ingredient in peyote—a small, spineless cactus. Mescaline is a Schedule I controlled substance.

[c] Lysergic acid diethylamide (LSD) is a potent hallucinogen that has a high potential for abuse and currently has no accepted medical use in treatment in the United States. LSD is a Schedule I controlled substance.

[d] Soma plant contains a psychoactive stimulant similar to ephedra used to produce a hallucinogenic stimulant drink made from the juice of the plant.

[e] Ephedra plant species grow as low, shrubby plants and considered a stimulant. Certain ephedra plant species contain ephedrine or pseudoephedrine which are precursor chemicals that may be used to produce methamphetamine and amphetamine. Ephedrine and pseudoephedrine are scheduled listed chemical products pursuant to 21 U.S.C. § 802(45). Methamphetamine is a Schedule II controlled substance and amphetamine is a Schedule III controlled substance.

[f] Coca is a common name for cocaine and is derived from coca leaves. Cocaine is a stimulant drug and a Schedule II controlled substance.

[g] 5-MeO-DMT-Toad Venom is a hallucinogenic substance found in the secretion from the parotoid glands of the Bufo alvarius toad. 5-MeO-DMT is a Schedule I controlled substance pursuant to 21 C.F.R. § 1308.11(d)(15).

Figure 5. DEA's Processing Times for Religious Exemptions from the Controlled Substances Act, Fiscal Year 2016 through January 2024.

DOJ and Soul Quest seemingly reached an agreement on the procedures for handling Soul Quest's exemption request. In June 2020, the DOJ sent a follow-up letter memorializing their discussions. Soul Quest agreed to stay its litigation against the DEA and to withdraw its motion for a preliminary injunction. In return, the DEA committed to responding to Soul Quest within 14 days of receiving the information it had requested in its previous communication (an undated letter confirming receipt of Soul Quest's petition). In addition, the agency committed to providing Soul Quest with a final decision on its petition within 75 days after the completion of the factfinding process.

DEA officials acknowledged its long processing times for Religious Freedom Restoration Act petitions and explained that it had put in place processes aimed at reducing processing times, while still assessing other areas in which processing can be streamlined.[78] Further, the agency stated that it had established timelines for specific stages throughout the process,[79] and continually considers the implementation of additional timelines. Lastly, officials pointed out that DEA's necessity to request additional information from petitioners can create delays in the petition's processing timeline.

Belief that DEA will not grant religious exemptions. According to five of nine selected stakeholders, DEA is unlikely to grant a petition for religious exemption for psilocybin use. Selected stakeholders cited reasons such as DEA's record of granting zero exemptions for protected psychedelic use through the petitioning process, and DEA having to assess the sincerity of non-western religious beliefs. Selected stakeholders we spoke to also stated that the absence of processing timelines and processing updates on the part of DEA have enabled the agency to withhold determinations from applicants following their submission. As a result, clients of these stakeholders have opted to withdraw their submitted petitions, sue DEA to receive a determination, or continue their psilocybin-based practices without going through the petitioning process.

DEA officials explained that its processing of Religious Freedom Restoration Act petitions does not vary based on the controlled substance(s)

---

[78] These processes included (1) ensuring consistent procedures in the handling of petition, (2) synchronizing related processes with key offices (i.e., DEA local field office, Office of Chief Counsel, and Diversion Control Division), and (3) providing specialized training and streamlined guidance to all local field offices handling such Religious Freedom Restoration Act-related petitions.

[79] DEA did not name the stages in which timelines are in place for, nor were any benchmarks shared for these timelines.

being requested. According to DEA officials, the agency did not approve or deny any petitions related to psilocybin. As stated above, information provided by DEA shows that from fiscal year 2016 through January 2024, no exemptions for any controlled substances were granted, only two exemptions were denied, and eight exemptions were withdrawn. DEA added that the agency has no records suggesting these exemptions were withdrawn by petitioners based on DEA denying the use of psilocybin or other controlled substances for religious purposes.

DEA has posted on its Diversion Control Division website the agency's guidance which generally outlines how petitions will be processed by the agency; however, this guidance does not include key information that clearly defines the types of information DEA requires of petitioners to evaluate religious sincerity, nor the standards or relevant factors that DEA will consider in making a threshold determination on evaluating a petition for an exemption from the Controlled Substances Act under the Religious Freedom Restoration Act. DEA officials stated the guidance is meant to clearly outline the Religious Freedom Restoration Act process and requirements for petitioners, and to ensure messaging is consistent.

In addition, DEA's guidance lacks established reporting time frames for DEA to respond to petitioners regarding decisions, as well as information on a communication process for providing updates to petitioners on the status of the exemption petition review. As a result, stakeholders and petitioners have limited transparency and may continue experiencing long petition review times without any mechanisms in place to obtain status updates from DEA. In addition, it is unclear when or if the notice of proposed rulemaking will be finalized.

Standards for Internal Control in the Federal Government requires management to implement control activities through policies and effectively communicate externally to support the internal control system.[80] It is important that an organization's management document the internal control responsibilities of the organization and the operational processes, objectives, control activity and operating effectiveness of each organizational unit in its policies. These policies may further define day-to-day procedures and include the timing of when a control activity occurs and any follow-up or corrective

---

[80] Internal control is a process effected by an entity's oversight body, management, and other personnel that provides reasonable assurance that the objectives of an entity will be achieved. See GAO, *Standards for Internal Control in the Federal Government*, GAO-14-704G (Washington, D.C.: Sept. 2014).

actions to be performed.[81] Also, management should externally communicate the necessary quality information to achieve the entity's objectives. This includes communicating with and obtaining quality information from external parties using established reporting lines. Open two-way external reporting lines allow for this form of communication. Established reporting lines to communicate quality information externally may help entities achieve their objectives and address related risks.[82]

According to DEA officials, the agency's notice of proposed rulemaking related to DEA's process to petition for religious exemptions to the Controlled Substances Act under the Religious Freedom Restoration Act was being reviewed by the Office of the Administrator. It is unclear when the notice of proposed rulemaking will be published, whether any regulations will ultimately be finalized, and the extent to which, if any, these regulations will address the concerns identified in our report.

According to DEA, the agency had no estimated timeline for issuing the notice of proposed rulemaking due to the multi-step interagency review process. Better clarifying its process to petitioners and establishing a process to provide regular updates to petitioners on the status of its reviews will help ensure that petitions include the information DEA needs to appropriately adjudicate Religious Freedom Restoration Act rights.

Additionally, it will ensure that petitioners who are required by DEA guidance to refrain from any use of a controlled substance have more information on the amount of time they can expect to receive a decision on their petition from DEA.

Conclusion

DEA established a process for parties that wish to petition for an exemption from the Controlled Substances Act under the Religious Freedom Restoration Act to use certain controlled substances for religious or spiritual purposes. DEA also provides guidance on its website that outlines how petitions will be processed by the agency. However, this publicly available guidance does not include information that clearly defines the types of information DEA requires of petitioners to evaluate their religious sincerity, nor the standards or relevant

---

[81] GAO-14-704G, pg. 44, Control Activities, Principle 12, Implement Control Activities, pg. 56.

[82] GAO-14-704G, pg. 58, Information and Communication, Principle 15—Communicate Externally, pg. 62.

factors that DEA will consider in making a threshold determination on evaluating a petition.

This guidance also does not inform petitioners of review processing timeframes for a petition for an exemption from the Controlled Substances Act. In addition, the guidance lacks information for petitioners to be able to inquire about the status of any petitions that have been submitted. As a result, stakeholders and petitioners have limited transparency and may continue experiencing long petition review times without any mechanisms in place to obtain status updates from DEA. DEA officials stated that its website guidance is meant to clearly outline the Religious Freedom Restoration Act process and requirements for petitioners, and to ensure messaging is consistent.

DEA initiated a draft notice of proposed rulemaking related to DEA's process for petitioning for religious exemptions from the Controlled Substances Act under the Religious Freedom Restoration Act in 2019. The draft notice was submitted to DEA's Office of the Administrator and is being reviewed by the office, according to DEA officials. However, DEA officials stated that the agency has no estimated timeline for issuing the notice of proposed rulemaking. Therefore, it is unclear whether any regulations will be finalized and when that may occur. In addition, it is unclear the extent to which the notice of proposed rulemaking and any corresponding regulations will address the concerns identified in our report. Providing clearer guidance on the information that petitioners should provide to address the relevant factors in DEA's determination of religious sincerity and the standard DEA will use to assess religious sincerity, better clarifying its exemption petition process timeframes to petitioners, and establishing a process to provide regular updates to petitioners on the status of its reviews will help ensure that petitions include the information DEA needs to appropriately adjudicate Religious Freedom Restoration Act rights. Clearer guidance could also strengthen the quality of reviews, increase the trust among stakeholders and petitioners, provide transparency in the process, and clarify and identify DEA's standard petition review processing times for exemptions from the Controlled Substances Act.

Recommendations for Executive Action

We are making the following four recommendations to DEA:

- The DEA Administrator should more clearly communicate the types of information that Religious Freedom Restoration Act petitioners should provide to allow DEA to evaluate petitions for religious sincerity. (Recommendation 1)
- The DEA Administrator should more clearly communicate the standards and relevant factors to Religious Freedom Restoration Act petitioners in making a determination related to religious sincerity. (Recommendation 2)
- The DEA Administrator should establish timeframes for DEA to make determinations on completed religious exemption petitions to provide Religious Freedom Restoration Act petitioners with DEA's final determinations. (Recommendation 3)
- The DEA Administrator should provide Religious Freedom Restoration Act petitioners with information for petitioners to be able to receive updates on the agency's progress related to exemption reviews. (Recommendation 4)

Agency Comments and Our Evaluation

We provided a draft of this report to DHS, DOJ, DOI, and HHS for review and comment. DOJ agreed with our 4 recommendations to the DEA Administrator. DOJ did not provide written comments. DOJ and HHS provided technical comments, which we incorporated as appropriate. DHS and DOI had no comments.

If you or your staff have any questions about this report, please contact me at (202) 512-8777 or mcneilt@gao.gov. Contact points for our Offices of Congressional Relations and Public Affairs may be found on the last page of this report. GAO staff who made key contributions to this report are listed in appendix VI.

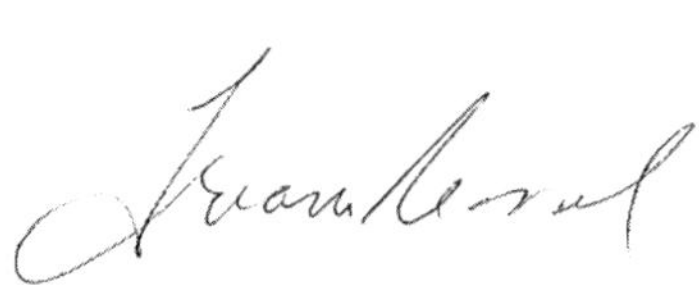

Triana McNeil
Director, Homeland Security and Justice

List of Committees

The Honorable Jeanne Shaheen
Chair

The Honorable Jerry Moran,
Ranking Member
Subcommittee on Commerce, Justice, Science, and Related Agencies
Committee on Appropriations
United States Senate

The Honorable Hal Rogers
Chairman

The Honorable Matt Cartwright
Ranking Member
Subcommittee on Commerce, Justice, Science, and Related Agencies
Committee on Appropriations
House of Representatives

Appendix I: State of Oregon's Legalization of Psilocybin

In 2017, Oregon generally reduced the penalties for knowingly or intentionally possessing a Schedule I controlled substance, including psilocybin, from a Class B felony (which generally has a maximum term of imprisonment of 10 years and a fine not to exceed $250,000)[83] to a Class A misdemeanor (which generally has a maximum term of imprisonment of 364 days and a fine not to exceed $6,250).[84] Subsequently, in 2020, Oregon passed a state ballot

[83] 2017 Or. Laws Ch. 706. Or. Rev. Stat. §§ 161.605(2), 161.625(1)(c) (2016).

[84] Or. Rev. Stat. § 475.752(3)(a) (2017). With respect to psilocybin, pursuant to Or. Rev. Stat. § 475.752(7) (2017), unlawful possession of a controlled substance in Schedule I is a Class B felony if: (a) The person possesses a usable quantity of the controlled substance and: (A) At the time of the possession, the person has a prior felony conviction; (B) At the time of the possession, the person has two or more prior convictions for unlawful possession of a

initiative which generally reduced the penalties for knowingly or intentionally possessing a Schedule I controlled substance, including psilocybin, from a Class A misdemeanor to a Class E violation, which became effective in 2021.[85] A person subject to the penalty for a Class E violation may, in lieu of the fine,[86] complete a Behavioral Health Resource Network screening by a certified addiction peer support or wellness specialists or other qualified persons, or any other equivalent or more intensive treatment contact, within 45 days of when the person receives the citation for the Class E violation. Upon verification of the screening, the court shall dismiss the citation.[87]

In April 2024, Oregon passed legislation that generally repeals the Class E violation that previously applied to possession of small amounts of a controlled substance, and replaces it with a new misdemeanor crime ofunlawful possession of a controlled substance, effective September 1, 2024.[88]

In addition, in November 2020, Oregon passed a separate state ballot initiative, also known as the Oregon Psilocybin Services Act, to permit persons licensed, controlled, and regulated by the state to legally manufacture psilocybin products and provide psilocybin services to persons 21 years of age and older, subject to state law; and establish a comprehensive regulatory framework concerning psilocybin products and psilocybin services under state law, after a two-year program development period.[89] According to the legislative findings of the Oregon Psilocybin Services Act, the State of Oregon has one of the highest prevalence rates of mental illness among adults in the nation.[90] An estimated one in every five adults in Oregon is coping with a

---

usable quantity of a controlled substance; or (C) The possession is a commercial drug offense under ORS 475.900 (1)(b); or (b) The person possesses twelve grams or more of a mixture or substance containing a detectable amount of psilocybin. Or. Rev. Stat. § 161.615(1) (maximum term of imprisonment for Class A misdemeanor). Or. Rev. Stat. § 161.615(1)(a) (maximum fine for Class A misdemeanor).

85 2021 Or. Laws Ch. 2 (B.M. 110). Or. Rev. Stat. § 475.752. Pursuant to Or. Rev. Stat. § 475.752(7), unlawful possession of a controlled substance in Schedule I is a Class A misdemeanor if the person possesses twelve grams or more of a mixture or substance containing a detectable amount of psilocybin or a Class B felony if the possession is a commercial drug offense under Or. Rev. Stat. § 475.900(1)(b); or the person possesses a substantial quantity (sixty grams or more of a mixture or substance containing a detectable amount of psilocybin) under Or. Rev. Stat. § 475.900(2)(b).

86 Pursuant to Or. Rev. Stat. § 153.018(2)(e), the maximum fine for a violation committed by an individual is $100 for a Class E violation.

87 Or. Rev. Stat. § 153.062.

88 2024 Or. HB 4002.

89 2021 Or. Laws Ch. 1 (B.M. 109). Or. Rev. St. §§ 475A.210-.722.

90 Or. Rev. Stat. § 475A.200(1).

mental health condition.[91] In addition, the 2019-2021 governor's budget proposed spending over $2.8 billion on mental health and behavioral health programs.[92] The legislative findings also reported that "studies conducted by nationally and internationally recognized medical institutions indicated that psilocybin has shown efficacy, tolerability, and safety in the treatment of a variety of mental health conditions, including but not limited to addiction, depression, anxiety disorders, and end-of-life psychological distress."[93]

Some of the purposes of the Act are to educate the people of Oregon about the safety and efficacy of psilocybin in treating mental health conditions; reduce the prevalence of mental illness among adults in the state, and to improve the physical, mental, and social well-being of all people in the state; and to develop a long-term strategic plan for ensuring that psilocybin services will become and remain a safe, accessible and affordable therapeutic option for all persons 21 years of age and older in Oregon for whom psilocybin may be appropriate.[94]

The Oregon Health Authority licenses and regulates the manufacturing, transportation, delivery, sale, and purchase of psilocybin products and the provision of psilocybin services. Although Oregon has generally legalized or decriminalized the manufacture, sale, and use of psilocybin under certain circumstances, the federal Controlled Substances Act provides federal sanctions for the possession, manufacture, distribution, and dispensing of Schedule I controlled substances, including psilocybin, except in limited circumstances.[95] Figure 6 provides an overview of the legislative and administrative components involved in the state's legalization of psilocybin.

In December 2022, the Oregon Health Authority adopted rules to regulate the production of psilocybin products and the provision of psilocybin services in Oregon. The following describes some of the features of Oregon's regulatory system.

Licensing. The Oregon Health Authority has established four types of psilocybin licenses that allow licensees to conduct specific tasks, including a

---

[91] Or. Rev. Stat. § 475A.200(2).

[92] Or. Rev. Stat. § 475A.200(4).

[93] Or. Rev. Stat. § 475A.200(5).

[94] Or. Rev. Stat. § 475A.205(1)(a)-(c).

[95] 21 U.S.C. §§ 841, 844.

manufacturer license,[96] a facilitator license,[97] a psilocybin service center operator license,[98] and a laboratory license.[99] Generally, an applicant for a license must apply to the Oregon Health Authority in the form required by the authority by rule, showing the name and address of the applicant, location of the premises that is to be operated under the license and other pertinent information required by the authority.[100] An applicant for a facility license need not show the location of any premises.[101] In addition, generally, a licensee must be 21 years of age or older and pass a criminal background check.

By law, generally, an individual who performs work for or on behalf of a licensee must have a valid permit issued by the Oregon Health Authority if the individual participates in certain psilocybin-related activities, such as the provision of psilocybin services at the premises for which a license has been issued; the possession, manufacturing, securing or selling of psilocybin products at the premises for which the license has been issued; the recording of the possession, manufacturing, securing or selling of psilocybin products at the premises for which the license has been issued; or the verification of any document for the sale or provision of a psilocybin product to another person.[102] In addition, a licensee must verify that an individual has a valid permit from the Oregon Health Authority before allowing the individual to perform any of the previous work described.[103] Figure 7 identifies the number and status of licenses and work permits submitted to the Oregon Health Authority, as of December 4, 2023.

---

96 Or. Rev. Stat. § 475A.290. Pursuant to Or. Rev. Stat. § 475A.220(7), "'[m]anufacture' means the manufacture, planting, cultivation, growing, harvesting, production, preparation, propagation, compounding, conversion or processing of a psilocybin product, either directly or indirectly by extraction from substances of natural origin, or independently by means of chemical synthesis, or by a combination of extraction and chemical synthesis, and includes any packaging or repackaging of the psilocybin product or labeling or relabeling of its container."

97 Or. Rev. Stat. § 475A.325. Generally, a facilitator provides services to a client during a preparation, administration, or integration session.

98 Or. Rev. Stat. § 475A.305. Pursuant to Or. Rev. Stat. § 475A.498, a client may purchase, possess, and consume a psilocybin product only at a psilocybin service center and only under the supervision of a psilocybin service facilitator.

99 Or. Rev. Stat. § 475A.594. A laboratory that conducts testing of psilocybin products must be accredited by the Oregon Environmental Laboratory Accreditation Program.

100 Or. Rev. Stat. § 475A.245(1).

101 Or. Rev. Stat. § 475A.245(4).

102 Or. Rev. Stat. § 475A.480(1).

103 Or. Rev. Stat. § 475A.480(2).

State of Oregon:
Oregon Psilocybin Services Act

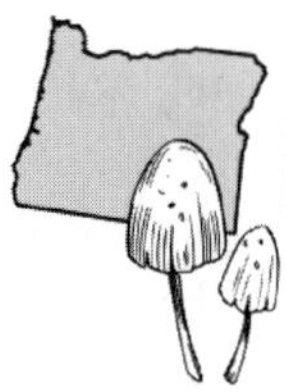

The Oregon Psilocybin Services Act was primarily codified in Oregon Revised Statutes, Title 37, Chapter 475A and generally directs the Oregon Health Authority (OHA) to license and regulate psilocybin products and the provision of psilocybin services.

By law, "psilocybin services[a]" means services provided to a client before, during, and after the client's consumption of a psilocybin product, including: a preparation session[b]; an administration session[c]; and an integration session[d]. The sale of psilocybin products and the provision of psilocybin services are available for individuals aged 21 and over and do not require a prescription or medical referral.

The Oregon Psilocybin Services (OPS) Section, within the Oregon Health Authority Public Health Division's Center for Health Protection, implements the Oregon Psilocybin Services Act. The Oregon Health Authority is responsible for licensing and regulating the manufacturing, transportation, delivery, sale, and purchase of psilocybin products and the provision of psilocybin services.

The Act established the Oregon Psilocybin Advisory Board to provide advice to the Oregon Health Authority with respect to the administration of Oregon's psilocybin program, including, but not limited to, making recommendations to the authority on available medical, psychological, and scientific studies, research, and other information relating to the safety and efficacy of psilocybin in treating mental health conditions, including but not limited to addiction, depression, anxiety disorders, and end-of-life psychological distress; making recommendations to the authority on the requirements, specifications and guidelines for providing psilocybin services to a client; and making recommendations to the authority on the education and training that psilocybin service facilitators must complete and on the examinations that psilocybin service facilitators must pass.[e]

The OPS Section began accepting applications for licensure on January 2, 2023. According to Oregon officials, psilocybin service centers began to open their doors to clients in the summer of 2023.

Source: GAO analysis of the State of Oregon Psylocibin Services Act. | GAO-24-106630.

[a] Or. Rev. Stat. § 475A.220(16).

[b] Pursuant to Or. Rev. Stat. § 475A.220(9), a preparation session "means a meeting between a client and a psilocybin service facilitator that must occur before the client participates in an administration session."

[c] Pursuant to Or. Rev. Stat. § 475A.220(1), an administration session "means a session held at a psilocybin service center at which a client purchases, consumes, and experiences the effects of a psilocybin product under the supervision of a psilocybin service facilitator."

[d] Pursuant to Or. Rev. Stat. § 475A.220(3), an integration session "means a meeting between a client and a psilocybin service facilitator that may occur after the client completes an administration session."

[e] Or. Rev. Stat. § 475A.230.

Figure 6. Overview of State of Oregon's Legislative and Administrative Components Involved Legalizing Psilocybin.

Application type	Submitted[a]	Approved[b]
Manufacturer	21	7
Facilitator	249	183
Service center operator	35	19
Testing labratory	3	2
Worker permit	594	382

Source: GAO's analysis of the state of Oregon's Psylocynin services data. | GAO-24-106630.

[a] Submitted is considered as an application that is submitted through the Training program, Licensing, and Compliance (TLC) system or by mail.

[b] Approved is considered as an application that is approved, and fees are paid and cleared.

Figure 7. Oregon Psilocybin Services Applications for Licenses and Worker Permits, as of December 4, 2023.

Facility security measures. Oregon regulations require certain security measures for facilities. A service center, manufacturer or laboratory licensee is responsible for the security of all psilocybin products on the licensed premises or in transit from the licensed premises, including providing adequate safeguards against theft or diversion of psilocybin products. Licensees must ensure that all limited access areas of a licensed premises are accessible only to licensee representatives and other personnel authorized to be present. During hours when the licensee is not operating, the licensee must ensure that all points of ingress and egress to and from indoor areas of the licensed premises are securely locked.[104] A service center, manufacturer or laboratory must have a fully operational security alarm system on the licensed premises, activated at all times when the licensed premises is closed for business. In addition, licensees must make all information related to security alarm systems, monitoring and alarm activity available to the Oregon Health Authority, upon request.[105] A licensed premises must have a fully operational video surveillance recording system.[106] The regulations specify that the video surveillance equipment, must at a minimum, consist of digital or network

[104] Or. Admin. R. 333-333-4550.

[105] Or. Admin. R. 333-333-4600.

[106] Or. Admin. R. 333-333-4620.

video recorders, cameras capable of meeting certain coverage requirements of the licensed premises, video monitors, digital archiving devices, a minimum of one monitor on the premises capable of viewing video, and interface devices such as a mouse or keyboard, if required to operate the system. In addition, the equipment must have the capability of producing and printing a still photograph from any camera image and have sufficient battery backup to support a minimum of one hour of recording time in the event of a power outage. A service center, manufacturer or laboratory licensee must have cameras that continuously record, 24 hours a day, using cameras that record at a minimum resolution of 1280 x 720 pixels and record at 10 frames per second (fps) in all areas where psilocybin products are produced or stored on the licensed premises and psilocybin waste may be present on the licensed premises, and all points of entry or exit to these areas and the indoor areas of the licensed premises.[107]

Verification of age. Pursuant to regulation, prior to completing the sale of a psilocybin product or providing psilocybin services to a client, a service center licensee representative and a facilitator must verify that the client has a valid, unexpired government-issued photo identification and must verify that the client is 21 years of age or older by viewing a particular type of government-issued client's identification, such as a passport, driver's license, or identification card issued by a federally recognized Indian tribe with photo, name and date of birth.[108]

Product tracking. A service center, manufacturer or laboratory licensee must use the psilocybin tracking system as an inventory and record keeping system, have a psilocybin tracking system account activated and functional within five business days of being licensed, and maintain an active psilocybin tracking system account while licensed.[109] Each service center, manufacturer and laboratory licensee must have at least one licensee who is a psilocybin tracking system administrator. A licensee may authorize additional licensees or licensee representatives to obtain psilocybin tracking system administrator accounts. Generally, to obtain a psilocybin tracking system administrator account, a license holder must attend and successfully complete all required psilocybin tracking system training. The Oregon Health Authority may also require additional ongoing, continuing education for individual administrators to retain his or her psilocybin tracking system administrator account.

---

[107] Or. Admin. R. 333-333-4650.
[108] Or. Admin. R. 333-333-4490.
[109] Or. Admin. R. 333-333-8200.

Preparation, Administration, and Integration Sessions with Clients. Prior to a client being able to purchase and consume a psilocybin product, a facilitator must complete a preparation session with each client who will participate in an administration session at least twenty-four hours but no more than 90 days prior to the commencement of the client's first administration session with the facilitator. For every client who will participate in an administration session, a facilitator must receive a completed client information form, complete a transportation plan in coordination with the client,[110] and coordinate with the client to complete a safety and support plan. Additionally, a facilitator must review certain documents with a client during the preparation session, such as the required informed consent document, the client bill of rights, and the product information document for any products that may be consumed during an administration session.[111] Administration sessions must be conducted by a facilitator and may only take place within a service center's designated administration area. Generally, a facilitator must always be present during administration sessions and is required to continuously monitor any client participating in the administration session. Continuous monitoring means that a facilitator must maintain visual and audio contact with clients and monitor clients for signs of physical or emotional distress. Video monitoring or other equipment may not be used to satisfy the requirement to continuously monitor clients. In addition to a facilitator conducting the administration session, at least one licensee representative of a service center license must be present on the licensed premises at all times when an administration session is taking place at a service center. If the additional licensee representative required to be present also holds a facilitator licensee, they are prohibited from transferring, selling or otherwise handling any psilocybin product while they are facilitating a preparation, administration or integration session.

Facilitators must also ensure that a back-up facilitator is available to assist in case of unforeseen circumstances that prevent the primary facilitator from completing the session. Back up facilitators must be able to reach the licensed premises within a reasonable period of time. In addition, a service center is limited in the number of clients it may have for administrative sessions at one time. A service center may not host administrative sessions for more than 100 clients at any given time regardless of whether the clients are participating in

---

[110] By regulation, the transportation plan may not approve a client to operate a motor vehicle, bicycle, or other form of self-operated transportation following the administration session.

[111] Or. Rev. Stat. § 333-333-5000.

separate individual or group administration sessions.[112] Client-facilitator ratios are required for group administration sessions depending on the dosage of psilocybin consumed. In addition, group administration sessions may not exceed a total of 25 clients, or the service center's maximum occupancy, regardless of the number of facilitators present.

Appendix II: State of Colorado's Legalization of Psilocybin

In November 2022, the voters of Colorado approved a citizen-initiated measure, the Natural Medicine Health Act of 2022, related to the use of certain plants and fungi, including psilocybin, for people 21 years of age and older. Within the legislative declaration of the Act, the voters of Colorado stated that the state's "current approach to mental health has failed to fulfill its promise. Coloradans deserve more tools to address mental health issues, including approaches such as natural medicines that are grounded in treatment, recovery health, and wellness rather than criminalization, stigma, suffering, and punishment."[113] In addition, according to the Act, "Coloradans are experiencing problematic mental health issues, including but not limited to suicidality, addiction, depression, and anxiety."[114] The legislative declaration of the Act also stated "an extensive and growing body of research is advancing to support the efficacy of natural medicines combined with psychotherapy as treatment for depression, anxiety, substance use disorders, end-of-life distress and other conditions."[115]

The purpose of the Natural Medicine Health Act of 2022 is to establish a new, compassionate, and effective approach to natural medicines by adopting a public health and harm reduction approach to natural medicines by removing criminal penalties for personal use for adults 21 years of age and older; developing and promoting public education related to the use of natural medicines and appropriate training for first responders; and establishing regulated access by adults twenty-one years of age and older to natural medicines that show promise in improving well-being, life satisfaction, and overall health.[116] In May 2023, Colorado passed an act concerning natural medicine referred to as the Natural Medicine Regulation and Legalization,

---

[112] Or. Rev. Stat. § 333-333-5200.
[113] Colo. Rev. Stat. § 12-170-102(1)(a).
[114] Colo. Rev. Stat. § 12-170-102(1)(b).
[115] Colo. Rev. Stat. § 12-170-102(1)(c)-(d).
[116] Colo. Rev. Stat. § 12-170-102(j).

which repealed and reenacted, with amendments, portions of the citizen-initiated measure. This act sets the regulatory framework for a regulated natural medicine program in Colorado.[117]

Under the law, the Director of the Colorado Division of Professions and Occupations (Director) within the Colorado Department of Regulatory Agencies has the power and duties to promulgate rules related to the requirements for the safe provision of regulated natural medicine, regulated natural medicine product, and natural medicine services to a participant.[118] For example, this includes promulgating rules related to the parameters for a preparation session,[119] administration session,[120] and integration session, for a participant to consume and experience the effects of a regulated natural medicine or product, such as psilocybin, at a licensed facility.[121] In addition, generally this includes promulgating rules on the requirements for the licensing of facilitators, practice of facilitation, and professional conduct of facilitators, including the form and procedures for applying for a new license, renewing or reinstating a license; and the educational and experiential requirements and qualifications for an individual to become a facilitator, including education and training on participant safety, drug interactions, contraindications, mental health and state, physical health and state, social and cultural considerations, preparation, administration, integration, and ethics.[122] Colorado also established a state licensing authority for the purpose of regulating and licensing the cultivation, manufacturing, testing, storage, distribution, transport, transfer, and dispensation of natural medicine or natural medicine product by and between natural medicine licensees.[123]

The Director is required to establish the federally recognized American tribes and Indigenous community working group for the purpose of engaging and creating a dialogue to identify issues related to the commercialization of

---

[117] 2023 Colo. Legis. Serv. Ch. 249.

[118] Colo. Rev. Stat. § 12-170-105.

[119] Colo. Rev. Stat. § 12-170-104(16). A preparation session means a meeting between a participant and facilitator that occurs before an administration session, but does not mean an initial consultation, an inquiry, or a response about natural medicine services.

[120] Colo. Rev. Stat. § 12-170-104(1). An "administration session' means a session conducted at a healing center, or another allowed location…during which a participant consumes and experiences the effects of regulated natural medicine or regulated natural medicine product under the supervision of a facilitator."

[121] Colo. Rev. Stat. § 12-170-104(10). An "integration session' means a meeting between a participant and facilitator that occurs after the completion of an administration session."

[122] Colo. Rev. Stat. § 12-170-105(1)(a)(II).

[123] Colo. Rev. Stat. § 44-50-201.

natural medicine, natural medicine product, and natural medicine services for tribal and Indigenous people, communities, cultures, and religions.[124]

Colorado also created the Natural Medicine Advisory Board (Board).[125] This Board's duties include, but are not limited to, examining issues related to natural medicine and natural medicine product, and making recommendations to the Director and the executive director of the state licensing authority. In addition, the Board is responsible for making recommendations to the Director and state licensing authority related to the addition of other types of natural medicine, including ibogaine, dimethyltryptamine and mescaline. These recommendations are to be based on available medical, psychological, and scientific studies, research, and other information related to the safety and efficacy of each natural medicine, with prioritization on the consideration of the addition of ibogaine.[126]

Generally, Colorado has legalized and decriminalized the personal use of natural medicines and natural medicine products, including psilocybin, under certain circumstances. Under Colorado law, unless expressly limited by the law, a person who, for the purpose of personal use and without remuneration, possesses, consumes, shares, cultivates, or manufactures natural medicine or natural medicine product, does not violate state law, or county, municipality, or city and county ordinance, rule, or resolution.[127] However, there are activities that are prohibited under Colorado law. For example, a person who is under 21 years of age who knowingly possesses or consumes natural medicine or natural medicine product commits a drug petty offense. Upon conviction, the person is subject to a fine of not more than $100 or not more than 4 hours of substance use education or counseling. A second or subsequent conviction for this violation is subject to a fine of not more than $100, not more than 4 hours of substance use education or counseling, and not more than

---

[124] Colo. Rev. Stat. § 12-170-107. In general, this community working group is required to study a number of issues, including, but not limited to avoiding the misappropriation and exploitation of the federally recognized American tribes and Indigenous people, communities, cultures, and religions; avoiding the excessive commercialization of natural medicine, natural medicine product, and natural medicine services; conservation issues associated with the legalization and regulation of natural medicines; and best practices and open communication to build trust and understanding between the certain entities for the purpose of avoiding unnecessary burdens and criminalization of traditional tribal and Indigenous uses of natural medicine.

[125] Colo. Rev. Stat. § 12-170-106.

[126] Colo. Rev. Stat. § 12-170-106(5)(f).

[127] Colo. Rev. Stat. § 18-18-434(5)(a). Pursuant to Colo. Rev. Stat. §§ 18-18-102(31) and 12-170-104(19), "'remuneration' means anything of value, including money, real property, tangible and intangible personal property, contract rights, choses in action, services, and any rights of use or employment or promises or agreements connected therewith."

24 hours of useful public service.[128] It is also unlawful for a person to openly and publicly display or consume natural medicine or natural medicine product. Under the law, this is a drug petty offense and, upon conviction, the person is subject to a fine of not more than $100 and not more than 24 hours of useful public service.[129] A person who knowingly cultivates natural medicine that cumulatively exceeds an area of more than 12 feet wide by 12 feet long in one or more cultivation areas on private property, or knowingly allows such cultivation on private property that the person owns, occupies, or controls, commits a drug petty offense, and upon conviction, is subject to a fine of not more than $1,000.[130] In addition, it is a drug felony for a person who is not licensed under the law to knowingly manufacture natural medicine product using an inherently hazardous substance or for a person who owns, manages, operates, or otherwise controls the use of a property to allow a person to do so.[131]

As of July 2023, Colorado's regulatory framework is currently under development and expected to begin accepting healing center applications by the end of calendar year 2024. Although Colorado has generally taken steps to legalize and decriminalize psilocybin, the federal Controlled Substances Act provides federal sanctions for the possession, manufacture, distribution, and dispensing of Schedule I controlled substances, including psilocybin, except in limited circumstances.[132] Figure 8 provides an overview of the legislative and administrative components involved in the state's legalization of psilocybin.

---

[128] Colo. Rev. Stat. § 18-18-434(1).

[129] Colo. Rev. Stat. § 18-18-434(2).

[130] Colo. Rev. Stat. § 18-18-434(3)(a).

[131] Colo. Rev. Stat. § 18-18-434(4).

[132] 21 U.S.C. §§ 841, 844.

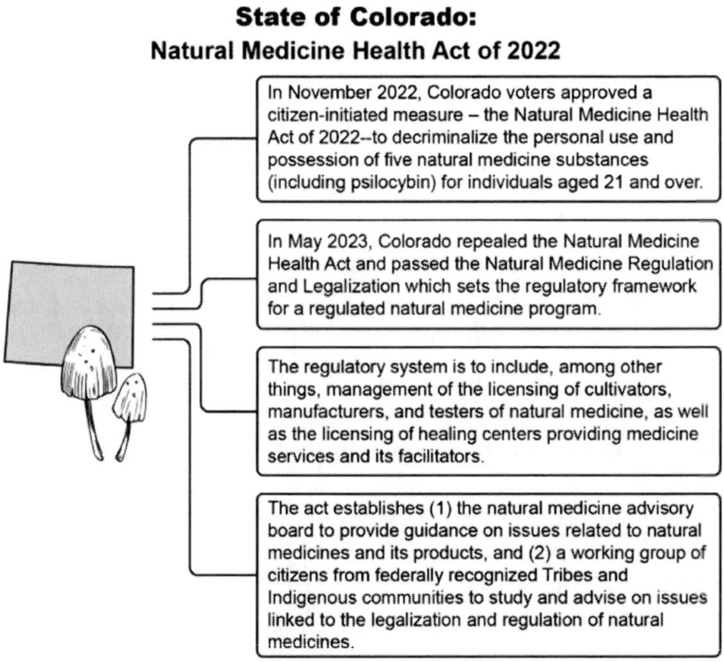

Source: GAO analyis of the State of Colorado Natural Nedicine health Act of 2022. | GAO-24-106630.

Figure 8. Overview of State of Colorado's Legislative and Administrative Components Involved Legalizing Psilocybin.

Appendix III: Selected States with Initiatives Focusing on Psilocybin

Some states have passed state laws establishing state-level pilot or research programs. For example, in Connecticut, the Department of Mental Health and Addiction Services was required to establish, within available appropriations, a psychedelic-assisted therapy pilot program, to be administered by a medical school in Connecticut, no later than January 1, 2023.[133] In addition, Maryland established the Post-Traumatic Stress Disorder and Traumatic Brain Injury Alternative Therapies Fund for the purpose of supporting the Maryland Department of Health in studying the effectiveness of and improving access to alternative therapies for post-traumatic stress disorder and traumatic brain

133 Conn. Gen Stat. § 17a-484g.

injuries in veterans.[134] Table 4 provides a description of selected states with state laws related to pilot programs for psilocybin services or studies of psilocybin for therapeutic use.[135]

Table 4. Descriptions of the selected states initiatives focusing on psilocybin related therapies and treatments

Selected States	Characteristics of Selected States Psilocybin-Based Initiatives
Arizona	In Arizona, the Director of the Arizona Department of Health Services is required to provide from monies appropriated, competitive research grants for whole mushroom psilocybin phase one, two, and three clinical trials that are capable of approval by the U.S. Food and Drug Administration (FDA) to evaluate the effects of whole mushroom psilocybin on treating conditions such as post-traumatic stress disorder, symptoms associated with long COVID-19, symptoms associated with end-of-life distress, depression, substance use disorder and addiction disorders, chronic pain, and eating disorders.[a]
Connecticut	In Connecticut, the Department of Mental Health and Addiction Services was required to establish, within available appropriations, a psychedelic-assisted therapy pilot program, to be administered by a medical school in Connecticut, no later than January 1, 2023. The pilot program is required to provide qualified patients with 3,4-methylenedioxymethamphetamine (MDMA)-assisted or psilocybin-assisted therapy as part of a research program approved by FDA.[b]
Maryland	Maryland established the Post-Traumatic Stress Disorder and Traumatic Brain Injury Alternative Therapies Fund for the purpose of supporting the Maryland Department of Health in studying the effectiveness of and improving access to alternative therapies for post-traumatic stress disorder and traumatic brain injuries in veterans. "Alternative therapies"

[134] Md. Code Ann., Health-Gen. § 24-2102.

[135] We reviewed the controlled substances laws of the 50 States and Washington, D.C., related to psilocybin to provide information related to the criminalization, deprioritization, decriminalization, or legalization of the use, possession, manufacture, and/or sale of psilocybin. During our research, we identified states that have passed state laws establishing state-level pilot research programs or studies of the therapeutic use of psilocybin. We randomly selected several of these programs to provide an overview of some of the characteristics of these programs.

Table 4. (Continued)

Selected States	Characteristics of Selected States Psilocybin-Based Initiatives
	includes hyperbaric oxygen therapy and psychedelics including 3,4-Methylenedioxymethamphetamine (MDMA), psilocybin, and ketamine.[c] Generally, the Fund may be used only for studying the use of alternative therapies for veterans with post-traumatic stress disorder and traumatic brain injuries; providing cost-free access to alternative therapies for veterans with post-traumatic stress disorder and traumatic brain injuries; administrative expenses of the Maryland Department of Health; and the Department's periodic consultation with certain entities, such as the Department of Veterans Affairs, The Johns Hopkins University, the University of Maryland, and Walter Reed National Military Medical Center.[d]
Washington	In Washington, subject to amounts appropriated, a psilocybin therapy services pilot program is established within, and administered by, the University of Washington's Department of Psychiatry and Behavioral Sciences. No later than January 1, 2025, the University of Washington's Department of Psychiatry and Behavioral Sciences must implement a psilocybin therapy pilot program that generally, must offer psilocybin therapy services through pathways approved by FDA, to populations including first responders and veterans who are: 21 years of age or older; and experiencing post-traumatic stress disorder, mood disorders, or substance use disorders. Generally, the pilot program must offer psilocybin therapy services facilitated by a licensed advanced social worker, independent clinical social worker, or mental health counselor; a licensed physician; or a licensed psychiatric advanced registered nurse practitioner. In addition, the pilot program must ensure psilocybin therapy services are safe, accessible, and affordable.[e]

Source: GAO's analysis of the some of the characteristics of selected states with legislation establishing a pilot program or study of psilocybin for therapeutic use. | GAO-24-106630.

[a] 2023 Ariz. Legis. Serv. Ch. 139, § 6 (Ariz. Rev. Stat. 36-132 note).

[b] Conn. Gen Stat. § 17a-484g.

[c] Md. Code Ann., Health-Gen. § 24-2101.

[d] Md. Code Ann., Health-Gen. § 24-2102.

[e] Wash. Rev. Code § 19.410.010.

Appendix IV: Key Federal Agencies Involved in Combating the Illegal Use, Manufacture, Distribution, and Transport of Controlled Substances, Including Psilocybin

As previously noted, the Drug Enforcement Administration (DEA) investigates and enforces potential violations of the Controlled Substances Act. The Federal Bureau of Investigation (FBI) also investigates cases related to violations of the Controlled Substances Act.[136] DEA coordinates and collaborates with state and local law enforcement agencies to implement or enforce the Act by sharing information and partnering in investigations and enforcement actions. DEA also manages and reviews petitions seeking religious exemptions from the Controlled Substances Act under the Religious Freedom Restoration Act to permit the use of controlled substances, including psilocybin. Within DEA, the Diversion Control Division's Diversion Regulatory Section and the Import/Export Section are the two main components that carry out this process. In addition to DEA and FBI, several other federal departments and agencies are involved in efforts to address controlled substances, including psilocybin, in the United States. Table 5 provides some examples of the key federal agencies involved in these efforts.

Table 5. Examples of key federal agencies involved in combating the illegal use, manufacture, distribution, and transport of controlled substances, including Psilocybin

Federal Agency	Tasks
Department of Justice	
Drug Enforcement Administration (DEA)	Enforces the controlled substances laws and regulations of the United States. Coordinates with the Food and Drug Administration to review DEA registration applications requesting authorization to conduct research with a Schedule I controlled substance. Completes on-site inspections of the research facilities associated with DEA registration applicants.

[136] Under 28 C.F.R. § 0.85, the FBI has the authority to investigate violations of the laws, including the criminal drug laws, of the United States and collect evidence in cases in which the United States is or may be a party in interest, except in cases in which such responsibility is by statute or otherwise exclusively assigned to another investigative agency.

Table 5. (Continued)

Federal Agency	Tasks
	Develops guidance, policies, procedures, and other documentation that outlines DEA's process for reviewing religious exemption petitions from the Controlled Substances Act under the Religious Freedom Restoration Act. Accepts and reviews petitions seeking exemptions under the Religious Freedom Restoration Act to permit the use of controlled substances, including psilocybin.
Executive Office for United States Attorneys (EOUSA)	Provides executive and administrative support for the U.S. Attorney's offices across the United States.
U.S. Attorneys' Offices	Enforce federal laws throughout the country, including drug trafficking and production offenses. U.S. Attorneys serve as the nation's principal litigators and conduct most of the trial work in which the United States is a party, including prosecuting drug cases. There are 93 U.S. Attorneys located in districts throughout the United States and its territories.
Executive Office of The President	
Office of National Drug Control Policy (ONDCP)	Leads and coordinates the federal government's drug policy. ONDCP's primary functions include: (1) developing and overseeing the implementation of the National Drug Control Strategy, (2) developing and overseeing the implementation of the National Drug Control Budget, and (3) administering programs to address overdoses, disrupt drug trafficking, and support community-led efforts to reduce youth substance use disorder.
Health and Human Services	
Food and Drug Administration (FDA)	Coordinates with DEA to review DEA registration applications requesting authorization to conduct research with a Schedule I controlled substance. Protects public health by ensuring the safety, efficacy, and security of human and veterinary drugs, biological products, and medical devices.

Federal Agency	Tasks
	Coordinates with DEA on scheduling drugs under the Controlled Substances Act. May authorize the use of experimental drugs in emergency situations that do not allow time for prior submission of an Investigational New Drug application if done in accordance with 21 C.F.R. pt. 312, subpt. I. Collaborates with the U.S. Customs and Border Protection (CBP) and Immigration and Customs Enforcement's Homeland Security Investigations to prevent the importation of unapproved drugs and investigates their distribution. Inspects registered facilities that manufacture drugs approved for marketing in the United States.
Department of Homeland Security	
U.S. Customs and Border Protection (CBP)	Responsible for securing the United States borders—protecting against terrorist threats and to prevent the illegal entry of inadmissible persons and contraband, while also facilitating lawful travel, trade, and immigration.
U.S. Immigration and Customs Enforcement	Enforces federal laws governing border control, customs, trade, and immigration. Homeland Security Investigations investigates the illegal movement of goods into and out of the United States, including narcotics. Collaborates with FDA and CBP to prevent the importation of unapproved drugs and investigates their distribution.
Department of the Interior	
Bureau of Indian Affairs (BIA)	Responsible for controlling the use of psilocybin on Tribal Nation lands. Tribal Nations are subject to federal law, but as sovereign entities, they operate under their own constitutions, enact their own laws, and provide services to their citizens. At the time of this review, the Bureau of Indian Affairs officials stated that no federally recognized Indian tribes have legalized the use of psilocybin for religious or spiritual practices.[a]

Table 5. (Continued)

Federal Agency	Tasks
U.S. Postal Inspection Service (USPIS)	Protects against and prevents criminal attacks to postal employees, customers, infrastructure, and the U.S. Mail. Enforces laws that defend the nation's mail system from illegal or dangerous use. As the federal law enforcement arm of the U.S. Postal Service, investigates cases and prepares them for court along with U.S. Attorneys, other law enforcement, and local prosecutors.

Source: GAO analysis of agency documents. | GAO-24-106630.

[a] In August 2023, we attempted to meet with officials representing selected Tribal Nations throughout the United States to obtain their perspectives on the legalization of psilocybin for religious or spiritual purposes. A majority of the Tribal Nations were not responsive; however, we spoke with a representative from one Tribal Nation and the representative stated that the Tribe has no history of psilocybin use for religious, Indigenous, spiritual or any other practices.

Appendix V: Additional Perspectives Related to Challenges and Barriers Obtaining Exemptions

Along with the stakeholders' perspectives mentioned earlier in the report, we obtained additional perspectives related to the challenges and barriers that exist in the legal access and use of psilocybin for religious practices under the Religious Freedom and Restoration Act. As stated earlier, we interviewed a non-generalizable sample of nine individuals from law firms and advocacy organizations selected to represent a range of perspectives on the barriers, if any, that exist in the legal access to and use of psilocybin for religious, Indigenous, or spiritual practices under the Religious Freedom Restoration Act. In addition, we attempted to meet with officials representing various Tribal Nations to obtain their perspectives on the petitioning for the use of psilocybin for religious or spiritual purposes. A representative from one of the eleven Tribal Nations we contacted responded to our request and stated the Tribe has no history of psilocybin use for religious, Indigenous, spiritual or any other practices. We also interviewed DEA officials to identify their perspectives on the agency's process to review petitions for a religious exemption.

Table 6 provides an overview of the additional perspectives we obtained related to the challenges and barriers that exist in the legal access and use of psilocybin for religious practices under the Religious Freedom and Restoration Act.

Table 6. Additional perspectives related to challenges and barriers obtaining exemptions

Category	Perspectives of Challenges and Barriers Obtaining Exemptions
Fear of Drug Enforcement Administration (DEA) prosecution	According to four of nine selected stakeholders, some citizens of Tribal Nations fear that DEA will investigate and prosecute them for having used psilocybin for spiritual practices such as coming of age ceremonies and introducing religious chiefs prior to submitting their Religious Freedom Restoration Act petition. This fear stems from preexisting emotional and mental trauma from racial persecution, according to select stakeholders. Additionally, other selected stakeholders shared that members of religious communities also had concerns regarding prosecution by acknowledging any previous unlawful or illegal conduct with psilocybin. DEA's guidance indicates that "[t]he petition must be signed by the petitioner, who must declare under penalty of perjury that the information provided therein is true and correct See 28 U.S.C. § 1746."[a] DEA officials noted that entities and individuals submitting a petition under the Religious Freedom Restoration Act remain subject to the Controlled Substances Act and its regulations. DEA described the collection of information as an important component of its investigation to understand a petitioner's ability to properly handle a controlled substance. DEA stated that it does not use information about a petitioner's use of a controlled substance in granting or denying a petition, and that it does not use this information to threaten civil or criminal sanctions against a petitioner during the review process, however this information is not included in the public guidance.
Legal costs of the Religious Freedom	According to two of nine selected stakeholders, petitioners incur legal costs from attorneys who assist the petitioner to navigate the complex DEA process. Individuals or

Table 6. (Continued)

Category	Perspectives of Challenges and Barriers Obtaining Exemptions
Restoration Act exemption process	organizations may not be able to afford these costs. Facing the prospect of retaining an attorney for a process that may take years, we were told by stakeholders that this could discourage petitioners from applying for religious exemption. According to DEA officials, each petition is unique and calls for a case-specific review and agency decision as to whether, and under what conditions, a religious exemption under the Religious Freedom Restoration Act should be granted.
Prohibition of ceremonial use of psilocybin during petition process	DEA's guidance requires petitioners to abstain from sacramental ceremonies involving controlled substances as petitions undergo review by the DEA. According to four of nine selected stakeholders, this requirement is burdensome to petitioners and becomes amplified by the absence of a clear processing timeframe.[b] DEA officials stated that as a Schedule I controlled substance, unless a substance has specifically been exempted under federal law, any person engaging in activities with any controlled substance must acquire a DEA registration. Pursuant to 21 U.S.C. § 823(a), the Attorney General generally is required to register an applicant to manufacture controlled substances in Schedule I if the Attorney General determines that such registration is consistent with the public interest and with United States obligations. In determining the public interest, one of the factors to be considered is the maintenance of effective controls against diversion of particular controlled substances and any controlled substance in schedule I compounded therefrom into other than legitimate medical, scientific, research, or industrial channels, by limiting the importation and bulk manufacture of such controlled substances to a number of establishments which can produce an adequate and uninterrupted supply of these substances under adequately competitive conditions for legitimate medical, scientific, research, and industrial purposes. Similarly, pursuant to 21 U.S.C. § 823(b), the Attorney General generally is required to register an

Category	Perspectives of Challenges and Barriers Obtaining Exemptions
	applicant to distribute a controlled substance in Schedule I unless the Attorney General determines that the issuance of such registration is inconsistent with the public interest. In determining the public interest, one of the factors to be considered is the maintenance of effective control against diversion of particular controlled substances into other than legitimate medical, scientific, and industrial channels. Under 21 U.S.C. § 822(d), the Attorney General may, by regulation, waive the requirement for registration of certain manufacturers, distributors, or dispensers if the Attorney General finds it consistent with the public health and safety. While DEA initiated the drafting of a notice of proposed rulemaking related to DEA's process for petitioning for religious exemptions to the Controlled Substances Act under the Religious Freedom Restoration Act in 2019 and it is under review, DEA has no estimated timeline for issuing the notice of proposed rulemaking due to the multi-step interagency review process, according to DEA officials.

Source: GAO analysis of perspectives provided by selected attorney and advocacy organization stakeholders. | GAO-24-106630.

[a] Pursuant to 18 U.S.C. § 1621(2), whoever in any declaration, certificate, verification, or statement under penalty of perjury as permitted under 28 U.S.C. § 1746, willfully subscribes as true any material matter which he does not believe to be true; is guilty of perjury and shall, except as otherwise expressly provided by law, be fined under this title or imprisoned not more than five years, or both. This section is applicable whether the statement or subscription is made within or without the United States.

[b] As described in a decision by the Court of Appeals for the Eleventh Circuit, in 2017, a church requested a religious exemption from the Controlled Substances Act permitting them to import, possess, and distribute plants containing DMT to make ayahuasca. The DEA initially did not respond to Soul Quest's petition. After three years with no response from the DEA, Soul Quest filed a complaint against the DEA in federal district court and an accompanying motion seeking declaratory and injunctive relief. Soul Quest claimed that through the DEA's failure to respond to its petition, the agency violated its right to the free exercise of religion and its rights under the Religious Freedom Restoration Act. Soul Quest also filed a motion for a preliminary injunction, seeking an order prohibiting the DEA from arresting, prosecuting, or threatening Soul Quest or its members for importing, distributing, or ingesting the sacramental tea. According to the decision, this action apparently got the DEA's attention because, soon after, the DEA responded

to Soul Quest with an undated letter confirming receipt of the petition. DEA denied that request on April 16, 2021, advising petitioners that the decision constituted a final determination of petitioners' exemption request under 21 U.S.C. § 877. Soul Quest Church of Mother Earth, Inc. v. Attorney General, No. 22-110722, 2023 WL 8714320 (11th Cir. 2023).

Appendix VI: GAO Contact and Staff Acknowledgments

GAO Contact:

Triana McNeil, (202) 512-8777 or McNeilT@gao.gov.

Staff Acknowledgments

In addition to the contact named above, Frederick T. Lyles, Jr. (Assistant Director), Katrina Taylor (Analyst in Charge), Janet Temko-Blinder, Caroline Christopher, Billy Commons, Benjamin Crossley, Michele Fejfar, Geovana Mendoza, Kevin Reeves, and Candace Strickland made key contributions to the report. Also contributing to the report were Tyler Autry, Wendy Dye, Susan Hsu, and Gabriel Jimenez.

Related Products

High-Risk Series: Efforts Made to Achieve Progress Need to be Maintained and Expanded to Fully Address All Areas, GAO-23-106203. Washington, D.C.: April 20, 2023.

Drug Control: Office of National Drug Control Policy Met Some Strategy Requirements but Needs a Performance Evaluation Plan, GAO-23-105508. Washington, D.C.: December 19, 2022.

Drug Policy: Preliminary Observations on the 2022 National Drug Control Strategy, GAO-22-106087, Washington, D.C.: June 15, 2022.

Drug Control Grants: ONDCP Should Document Its Process for Identifying Duplication, Overlap, and Fragmentation, GAO-22-104666, Washington, D.C.: December 8, 2021.

Synthetic Opioids: Considerations for the Class-Wide Scheduling of Fentanyl-Related Substances, GAO-21-499. Washington, D.C.: April 12, 2021.

High-Risk Series: Dedicated Leadership Needed to Address Limited Progress in Most High-Risk Areas, GAO-21-119SP. Washington, D.C.: March 2, 2021.

Substance Use Disorder: Reliable Data Needed for Substance Abuse Prevention and Treatment Block Grant Program, GAO-21-58. Washington, D.C.: December 14, 2020.

Drug Misuse: Agencies Have Not Fully Identified How Grants That Can Support Drug Prevention Education Programs Contribute to National Goals, GAO-21-96. Washington, D.C.: November 18, 2020.

Prescription Drug Monitoring Programs: Views on Usefulness and Challenges of Programs, GAO-21-22. Washington, D.C.: October 1, 2020.

Bureau of Prisons: Improved Planning Would Help BOP Evaluate and Manage Its Portfolio of Drug Education and Treatment Programs, GAO-20-423, Washington, D.C.: May 26, 2020.

Workforce Innovation and Opportunity Act: Additional DOL Actions Needed to Help States and Employers Address Substance Use Disorder, GAO-20-337, Washington, D.C.: May 21, 2020.

Drug Misuse: Sustained National Efforts Are Necessary for Prevention, Response, and Recovery, GAO-20-474. Washington, D.C.: March 26, 2020.

Drug Control: Actions Needed to Ensure Usefulness of Data on Suspicious Opioid Orders, GAO-20-118. Washington, D.C.: January 29, 2020.

Opioid Use Disorder: Barriers to Medicaid Beneficiaries' Access to Treatment Medications, GAO-20-233. Washington, D.C.: January 24, 2020.

Drug Control: The Office of National Drug Control Policy Should Develop Key Planning Elements to Meet Statutory Requirements, GAO-20-124. Washington, D.C.: December 18, 2019.

Veterans Health Care: Services for Substance Use Disorders, and Efforts to Address Access Issues in Rural Areas, GAO-20-35. Washington, D.C.: December 2, 2019.

Drug Policy: Preliminary Observations on the 2019 National Drug Control Strategy, GAO-19-370T. Washington, D.C.: March 7, 2019.

Drug Control: DOD Should Improve Its Oversight of the National Guard Counterdrug Program, GAO-19-27. Washington, D.C.: January 17, 2019.

Colombia: U.S. Counternarcotics Assistance Achieved Some Positive Results, but State Needs to Review the Overall U.S. Approach, GAO-19-106. Washington, D.C.: December 12, 2018.

Illegal Marijuana: Opportunities Exist to Improve Oversight of State and Local Eradication Efforts, GAO-19-9. Washington, D.C.: November 14, 2018.

Opioid Crisis: Status of Public Health Emergency Authorities, GAO-18-685R. Washington, D.C.: September 26, 2018.

Prescription Opioids: Medicare Needs Better Information to Reduce the Risk of Harm to Beneficiaries, GAO-18-585T. Washington, D.C.: May 29, 2018.

VA Health Care: Progress Made Towards Improving Opioid Safety, but Further Efforts to Assess Progress and Reduce Risk Are Needed, GAO-18-380. Washington, D.C.: May 29, 2018.

Illicit Opioids: Office of National Drug Control Policy and Other Agencies Need to Better Assess Strategic Efforts, GAO-18-569T. Washington, D.C.: May 17, 2018.

Illicit Opioids: While Greater Attention Given to Combating Synthetic Opioids, Agencies Need to Better Assess their Efforts, GAO-18-205. Washington, D.C.: March 29, 2018.

Substance Use Disorder: Information on Recovery Housing Prevalence, Selected States' Oversight, and Funding, GAO-18-315. Washington, D.C.: March 22, 2018.

Opioid Use Disorders: HHS Needs Measures to Assess the Effectiveness of Efforts to Expand Access to Medication-Assisted Treatment, GAO-18-44. Washington, D.C.: October 31, 2017.

Counternarcotics: Overview of U.S. Efforts in the Western Hemisphere, GAO-18-10. Washington, D.C.: October 13, 2017.

Preventing Drug Abuse: Low Participation by Pharmacies and Other Entities as Voluntary Collectors of Unused Prescription Drugs, GAO-18-25. Washington, D.C.: October 12, 2017.

Prescription Opioids: Medicare Needs to Expand Oversight Efforts to Reduce the Risk of Harm, GAO-18-15. Washington, D.C.: October 6, 2017.

Drug Control Policy: Information on Status of Federal Efforts and Key Issues for Preventing Illicit Drug Use, GAO-17-766T. Washington, D.C.: July 26, 2017.

Drug-Free Communities Support Program: Agencies Have Strengthened Collaboration but Could Enhance Grantee Compliance and Performance Monitoring, GAO-17-120. Washington, D.C.: February 7, 2017.

State Marijuana Legalization: DOJ Should Document Its Approach to Monitoring the Effects of Legalization, GAO-16-1. Washington, D.C.: December 30, 2015.

Office of National Drug Control Policy: Office Could Better Identify Opportunities to Increase Program Coordination, GAO-13-333. Washington, D.C.: March 26, 2013.

ONDCP Media Campaign: Contractor's National Evaluation Did Not Find That the Youth Anti-Drug Media Campaign Was Effective in Reducing Youth Drug Use, GAO-06-818. Washington, D.C.: August 25, 2006.

Marijuana: Early Experiences with Four States' Laws That Allow Use for Medical Purposes, GAO-03-189. Washington, D.C.: November 1, 2002.

GAO's Mission

The Government Accountability Office, the audit, evaluation, and investigative arm of Congress, exists to support Congress in meeting its constitutional responsibilities and to help improve the performance and accountability of the federal government for the American people. GAO examines the use of public funds; evaluates federal programs and policies; and provides analyses, recommendations, and other assistance to help Congress make informed oversight, policy, and funding decisions. GAO's commitment to good government is reflected in its core values of accountability, integrity, and reliability.

Connect with GAO

Connect with GAO on Facebook, Flickr, Twitter, and YouTube. Subscribe to our RSS Feeds or Email Updates. Listen to our Podcasts. Visit GAO on the web at https://www.gao.gov.

To Report Fraud, Waste, and Abuse in Federal Programs

Contact FraudNet:

Website: https://www.gao.gov/about/what-gao-does/fraudnet Automated answering system: (800) 424-5454 or (202) 512-7700.

Congressional Relations

A. Nicole Clowers, Managing Director, ClowersA@gao.gov, (202) 512-4400, U.S. Government Accountability Office, 441 G Street NW, Room 7125, Washington, DC 20548.

Public Affairs

Chuck Young, Managing Director, youngc1@gao.gov, (202) 512-4800.

U.S. Government Accountability Office, 441 G Street NW, Room 7149 Washington, DC 20548.

Strategic Planning and External Liaison

Stephen J. Sanford, Managing Director, spel@gao.gov, (202) 512-4707.

U.S. Government Accountability Office, 441 G Street NW, Room 7814, Washington, DC 20548.

Index

A

B

C

S

T

U

V

W